Hand and Wrist Therapy

Grégory Mesplié

Editor

Hand and Wrist Therapy

Clinical Examination and Advanced Rehabilitation Tools

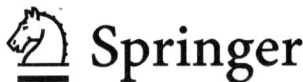 Springer

Editor
Grégory Mesplié
ISAMMS
BIARRITZ, France

ISBN 978-3-030-94941-9   ISBN 978-3-030-94942-6   (eBook)
https://doi.org/10.1007/978-3-030-94942-6

To my mother, the illustrator, for her incredible work and kindness.

To my family and closed ones for their support, this book is also yours.

Foreword

Hand and Wrist Therapy is a fusion of science and skilled perception (more commonly called clinical reasoning). Therapists can learn the science from many sources, but clinical reasoning is a personal skill developed only when we apply what we see during a patient examination with what we know from our science learning. In this book, Grégory Mesplié helps you connect the science to your clinical examination, which is the basis of all treatment decisions.

Not all examinations provide relevant information. It is important to know both what to examine and how to examine. This is required so the information gleaned is focused, relevant, and helpful. This volume emphasizes what to examine as well as how to examine and then discusses the examination findings considering the science and options for treatment. For therapists who are learning to be a skilled hand and wrist therapist, such a resource is valuable!

This book should be your springboard to a rich and exciting career in hand and wrist therapy where each patient encounter more sharply hones your skills at combining the science with clinical reasoning.

Enjoy learning!!

Judy C. Colditz
Occupational Therapist, Hand Therapist, President of the International
Federation of Societies of Hand Therapists
and the American Society of Hand Therapists

Contents

Contributors

Baptiste Arrate Institut Sud Aquitain de la Main et du Membre Supérieur, Biarritz, France

Rémy Dehez Institut Sud Aquitain de la Main et du Membre Supérieur, Biarritz, France

Cap Kiné, Capbreton, France

François Delaquaize Hôpitaux Universitaires de Genève, Genève, Switzerland

Chantal Donapetry Institut Sud Aquitain de la Main et du Membre Supérieur, Biarritz, France

Xabi Ezpeleta Institut Sud Aquitain de la Main et du Membre Supérieur, Biarritz, France

Coline Geoffroy Institut Sud Aquitain de la Main et du Membre Supérieur, Biarritz, France

Grégory Mesplié Institut Sud Aquitain de la Main et du Membre Supérieur, Biarritz, France

Doriane Parmentier Institut Sud Aquitain de la Main et du Membre Supérieur, Biarritz, France

Romain Prolonge Institut Sud Aquitain de la Main et du Membre Supérieur, Biarritz, France

Marie Schwebel Hôpitaux Universitaires de Strasbourg, Strasbourg, France

Part I

Clinical Examination and Clinical Reasoning

Clinical Examination of the Wrist and Hand

Grégory Mesplié and Marie Schwebel

1.1 Notion of Multidisciplinary Team and Position in the Care Protocol

In physiotherapy, the assessment is a clinical examination allowing to establish a treatment plan and to communicate with the rest of the healthcare team. It must be simple, repeatable, and compared to the healthy side (or to the standard). It must also be dated to assess the patient's evolution.

1.1.1 The Notion of "Team"

The notion of healthcare team is essential in the hand rehabilitation, as well as the communication between its members. Paraclinical exams, surgical reports, and letters between caregivers must be conducted regularly, and easily accessible to all members of the team. Therefore, the medium of communication must be secured and accessible only to the healthcare team members.

The lack of these elements can lead to approximations that can have disastrous consequences, especially in case of injuries causing an important tissue weakness.

G. Mesplié (✉)
Institut Sud Aquitain de la Main et du Membre Supérieur, Biarritz, France

M. Schwebel
Hôpitaux Universitaires de Strasbourg, Strasbourg, France

Stanley's observation summarizes well this crucial interaction, as well as the importance of rehabilitation in hand pathologies:

"Good surgeon + good physical therapist = good results
Good surgeon + bad physical therapist = mediocre results
Bad surgeon + good physical therapist = acceptable results
Bad surgeon + bad physical therapist = disastrous results"

The dressings also play an important part in this multidisciplinary care, as they allow early mobilizations, which guarantee an optimal functional recovery. How is the healing going? What areas must not suffer from temperature variations? Hot and cold temperatures are often used in physiotherapy, so the rehabilitation must be adapted in case of a controlled wound healing, a transplant, or a bolster dressing. How to realize a dressing that does not interfere with the mobilization and rehabilitation.

The dressing is an occluding and sterile device allowing to:

- protect the wound against friction, irritation, and infection, thus reducing pain
- keep the wound's "moist environment" for better healing
- stop the bleeding by compressing the small blood vessels, especially during the first days after surgery
- absorb an exudate that would slow the healing down because of maceration
- deal with the wound better, as the hand washing and showering are allowed, thanks to waterproof or silicon dressings, convenience, and "aesthetic covering" of the wound

Changing a dressing requires strict compliance to specific hygiene rules. Moreover, regarding the hand and/or fingers, the dressing should also meet the following criteria:

- The dressing must be as small as possible: the commissures of the fingers should be free, as well as the joints. The fingertips should not be "blinded," and the palm should not be covered to maintain the main functions of the hand: touching and grabbing (Fig. 1.1).
- The dressing must be adapted to the injury, if it is too big it might block several proximal joints or prevent the orthosis from fitting correctly.
- The dressing must not prevent an early mobilization; therefore, it must be as light as possible. Cotton bandages should not be used anymore, except as a temporary compression device in case of important bleeding (Fig. 1.2).
- The dressing must stay clean: it is usually changed every 2 days, but this can be adapted to the wound and the patient's activities.
- The removal should be painless.

The nurse must act gently:

- Removing the dressing under a continuous stream of room-temperature tap water. The tap water combines the mechanical action of the water flowing, and the humidification, which helps in case of a dry dressing (that often happens for the first dressing). The patient should then wash his hands, as it helps removing the scab. It

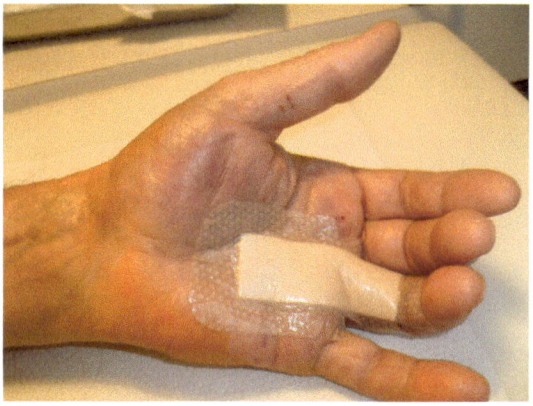

Fig. 1.1 The rule of a dressing as small as possible is essential to allow a precise early mobilization

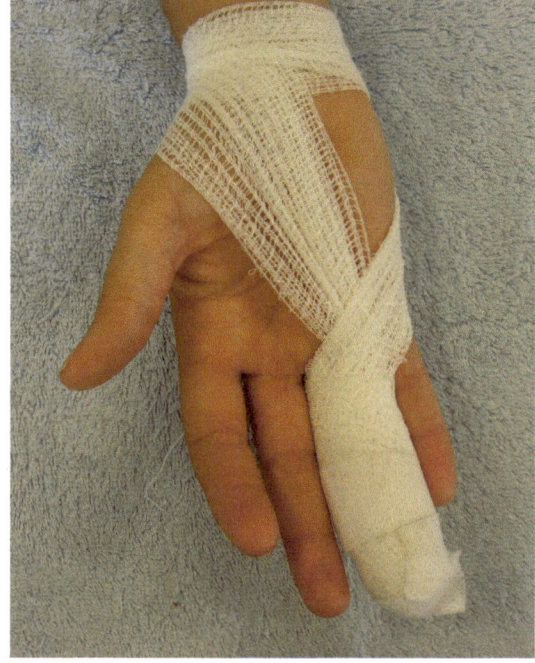

Fig. 1.2 The dressings are too thick for mobilizing

is also a first step towards re-including his hand and familiarizing with the wounded hand.
- Using non-adhesive dressings or protecting the wound.
- Applying tension in a tangential direction from the wound: distorting the meshes of the compress or the "tulle gras" to remove it without tugging on the wound.
- Making sure the patient takes his analgesics and adjusting the time when he does if needed

so that it is most efficient during the dressing replacement. Most of the time, it should be taken at least 30 min before.

If there is the slightest doubt when removing the dressing (aspect, redness, smell), the nurse will advise the patient to see his doctor or surgeon, as a wound can evolve towards an infection, a local inflammation, or a torpid wound, even with the best care. The wound could be trimmed, or even surgically revised, an antibiotic treatment or a different protocol can be implemented.

The nurse can spot signs of complications like allergies, infection, hematoma, necrosis, skin separation, protrusion of the surgical material, complex regional pain syndrome, or pathological scaring. The nurse will also have an important monitoring role in finger re-implantations, grafts, and skin flaps. Finally, the nurse gives the patient advice, so that he can adapt his daily life to deal with his wound better (fight against edema and pain, positions to take, or mobilizations to do).

For a good healing, some rules must be followed:

- Never wet the dressing (call the nurse if it is the case).
- Do not smoke.
- Avoid getting the dressing dirty.
- Do not take the dressing off alone, as nothing and no one should be in direct contact with the wound.
- Have a healthy diet, rich in proteins.
- Stay hydrated.
- Control the body temperature.
- Respect the surgeon's prescription for drugs.

The wound healing usually takes approximately 15 days. This time frame can vary depending on natural parameters such as the type of the wound (traumatic, surgical, burn, necrosis), as well as individual parameters as certain pathologies or risk factors (tobacco, alcohol, diabetes, unhealthy diet) can increase the healing time.

When the wound is healed, the scar must be left out in the open air, even with absorbable suture material—which can be taken off too. It is important to regain rapidly both the motricity and function of the hand.

The scar will change during the following 6 months, so it will be important to:

- Watch for a retraction or a hypertrophic or keloid scar.
- Apply a hydrating cream daily.
- Avoid sun exposure on the scar without sunscreen (50-index or higher), during a year.

1.1.2   The Clinical Assessment in the Care Protocol

The patient coming to a physical therapist's office already has a medical diagnosis. Based on this diagnosis, the initial physiotherapy examination must allow us to identify priorities (edema, pain, stiffness), thus leading to an appropriate care depending on our primary goals.

It is also a way to check the patient's administrative information, as well as other specific elements (job, hobbies, medical history) that can modify the primary goals of the treatment.

The following assessments will evaluate the efficiency of rehabilitation and lead to possible adjustments if the priorities have changed.

1.2   Tools Needed

The tools we use must allow us to realize an assessment as complete as possible, while respecting the requirements of reproducibility and simplicity. Touch pads can be an interesting solution to realize and securely store the assessments: a model can be made in advance, allowing the realization of a complete assessment in a coherent period of time.

1.2.1   Visual Analog Scale (VAS)

It evaluates pain intensity. It is a subjective self-evaluation, but it allows to understand how the patient perceives the nociceptive message.

The visual analog scale is a ruler with two sides: one with a graduation from 1 to 10 corresponding to the pain intensity, the other with a chart on which the patient locates his pain level (Fig. 1.3).

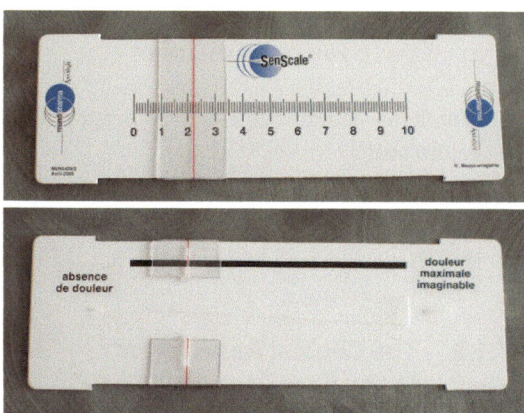

Fig. 1.3 Example of a visual analog scale

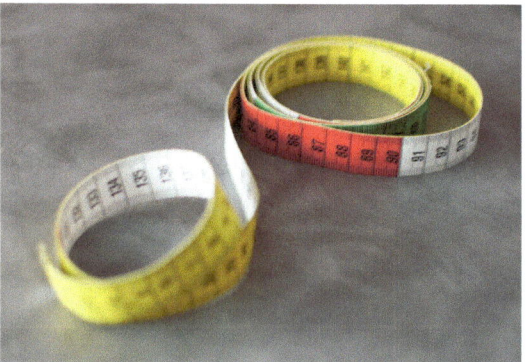

Fig. 1.4 Measuring tape for measuring edemas and muscular atrophies

1.2.2 Measuring Tape

It is used to measure the perimeters of the concerned areas and to compare them to the healthy side. It helps to objectively evaluate edema and amyotrophy after a traumatism and/or immobilization (Fig. 1.4).

1.2.3 Laser Thermometer

It is used to evaluate the variations of cutaneous temperature and must be compared to the healthy side as it can vary from 28 to 36 °C depending on the individual (Fig. 1.5).

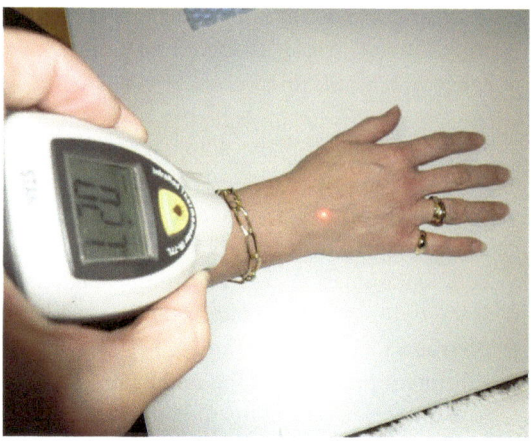

Fig. 1.5 Laser thermometer for skin temperature

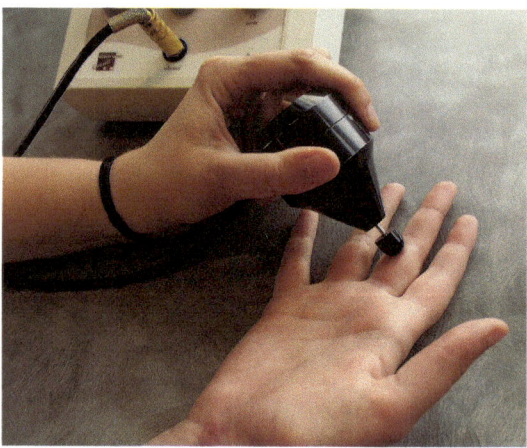

Fig. 1.6 The Vibralgic can be used to assess the vibratory perception threshold (VPT)

1.2.4 Transcutaneous Vibratory Stimulating Device

With a frequency of 100 Hz, we increase the vibration intensity to determine the vibratory perception threshold (Fig. 1.6).

1.2.5 Semmes-Weinstein Monofilaments

They are calibrated monofilaments used to know the pressure applied on the concerned cutaneous zone. They allow to evaluate the pressure perception threshold and participate in the quantitative and qualitative evaluation of allodynia.

1.2.6 Goniometers

These tools measure the angle and are used to objectively assess active and passive joint amplitudes. The results are compared to the healthy side or to the standard, depending on the case.

There are several types of goniometers in terms of size and type of studied mobility.

1.2.6.1 Cochin Goniometer
The stationary arm is placed along the segment adjacent to the mobilized segment. The point of rotation is placed at the level of the center of the joint. The moveable arm is placed along the mobilized segment (Fig. 1.7).

1.2.6.2 Rippstein Goniometer
The reference is the vertical or the horizontal. We use it to measure pronosupination, with the elbow at 90° of flexion (the reference being the vertical) (Fig. 1.8).

1.2.7 Dynamometers

We use them to evaluate the patient's strength and compare it to the healthy side.

They also allow to determine the muscle balance, which must be readjusted if the ratio between the agonist and antagonist muscles is modified.

These muscle imbalances are essential, must be looked for, and rebalanced if needed as they can cause compensations and important joint disorders.

There are several types of dynamometers.

1.2.7.1 Dynamometer Measuring Grasp (Jamar)
It is used to measure the clamping force of the hand. There are several notches that can change the spacing between the two resistances (Fig. 1.9).

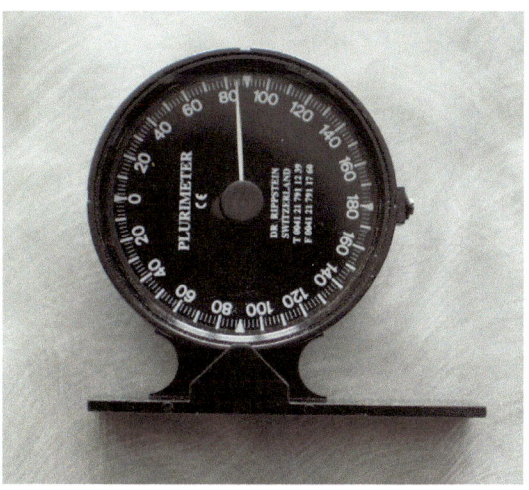

Fig. 1.8 Rippstein goniometer

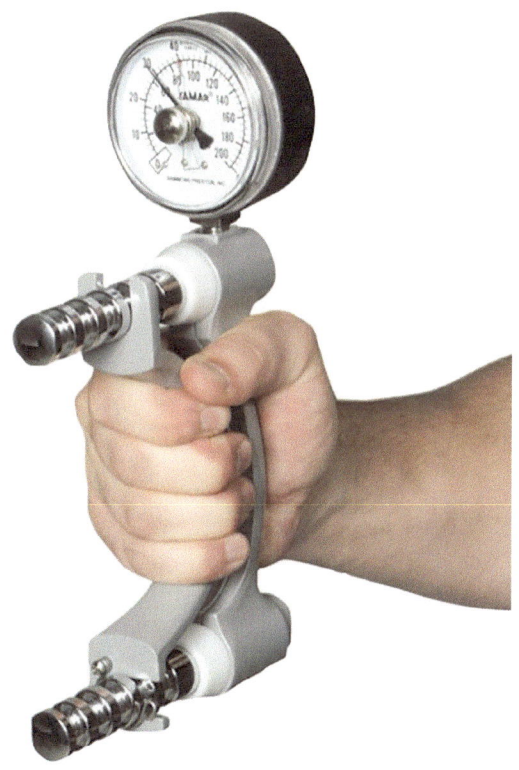

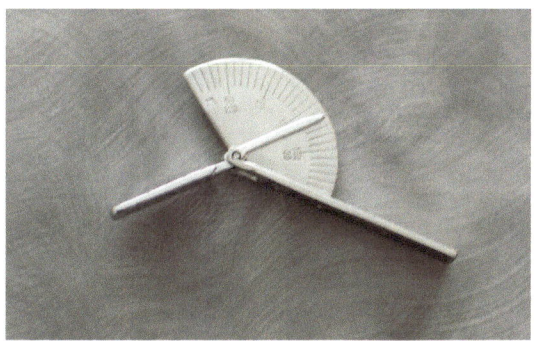

Fig. 1.7 Cochin goniometer

Fig. 1.9 Jamar© dynamometer for grasp

1.2.7.2 Vigorimeter Measuring Grip (Martin)

It is used to assess the patient's global gripping strength, with the intrinsic and extrinsic muscles working in synergy (Fig. 1.10).

1.2.7.3 Dynamometer Measuring the Pinch

It is used to assess the strength between the thumb and the fingers, especially the key pinch and the pinch (Fig. 1.11).

1.2.7.4 Measuring the Clamp

We evaluate the intrinsic strength specifically as clamping is achieved by the interosseous and thenar muscles.

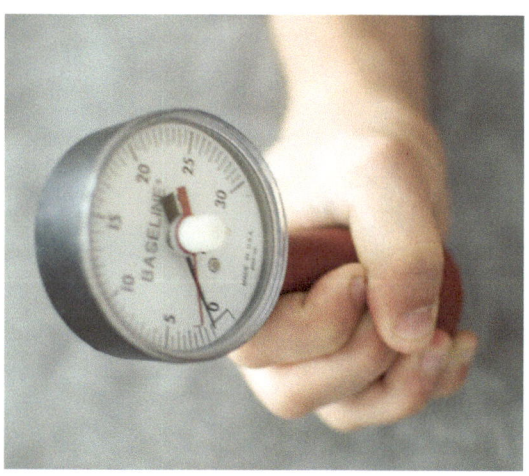

Fig. 1.10 Martin vigorimeter for grip

1.2.7.5 Dynamometer Measuring the Wrist Strength in Flexion and Extension, and Ulnar and Radial Inclinations

It is used to assess the strength of the flexor and extensor muscles of the wrist, as well as the radial and ulnar stabilizers (Fig. 1.12).

1.2.7.6 Dynamometer Measuring the Strength in Pronosupination

It allows us to assess the strength of the patient's pronator and supinator muscles, with the elbow in a 90° flexion to avoid the participation of shoulder rotators.

1.2.8 Ruler

It is used to measure the straight distance between two points. We use it to measure the span of the hand (Fig. 1.13).

1.2.9 Camera

Compact cameras are used to keep a picture of the hand at a given time, regarding a vicious attitude, an edema, or any visual element.

They also allow to realize videos that complete the assessment regarding the qualitative and quantitative aspect of the global hand or wrist mobility.

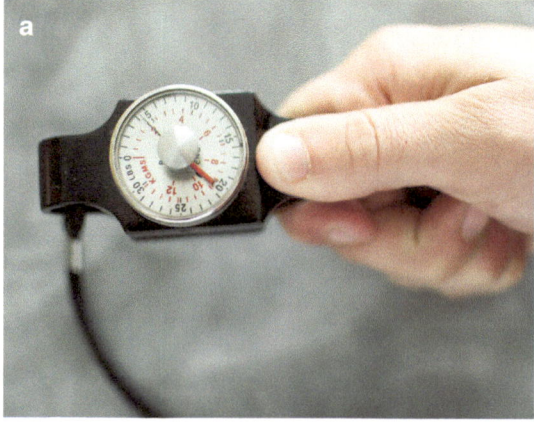
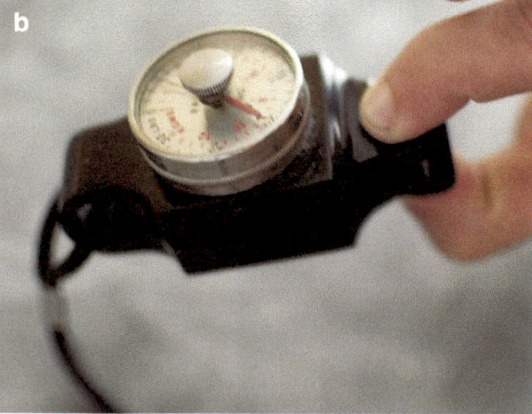

Fig. 1.11 (**a**) Key pinch (**b**) Pinch

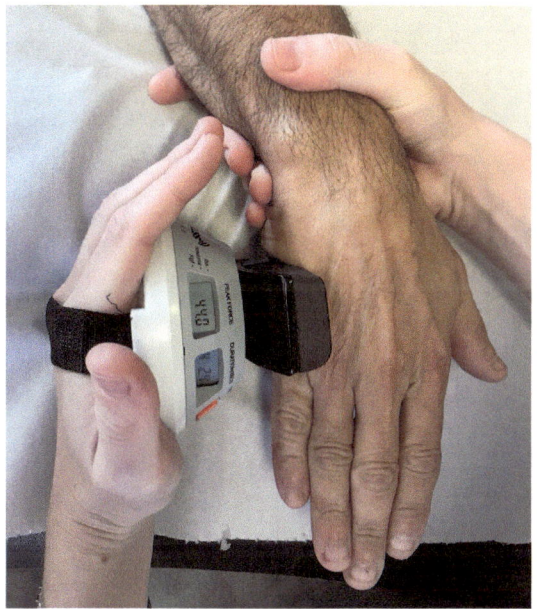

Fig. 1.12 Dynamometer for thrust force

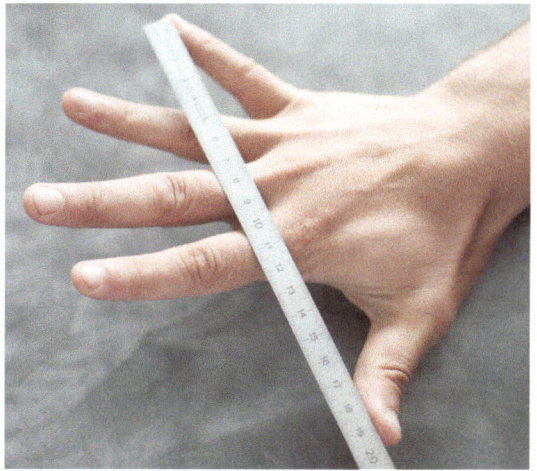

Fig. 1.13 Using a ruler to measure the span

These videos and pictures can have a positive effect on the patients' morale, especially when they are undergoing a long-term rehabilitation: this way, they can visualize the advances they have made, even when they are not spectacular from day to day (Fig. 1.14).

1.2.10 Echograph

Echography, based on the use of ultrasounds, is an operator-dependent technique that requires a good initial formation and a frequent use. It offers several advantages [1]:

- Noninvasive technique with no radiation.
- There is no risk and no counterindication.
- The exam itself is cheap (the expensive part is buying the device).
- Real-time and dynamic imagery technique with a real interest for movement specialists.
- More precise and sensitive than X-ray, it is the perfect examination for exploring tendons and detecting tenosynovitis.

In the hand and wrist, the probes must have a high frequency (>15 MHz) to get a good quality image.

1.3 General Organization of the Assessments

1.3.1 Anamnesis

1.3.1.1 Environment
To be thorough, the therapist must analyze the patient's environment in a multifactorial manner by taking into consideration their personal characteristics (age, gender, history, former treatments, or surgeries), their social and professional environments, eventual sports played, as well as their motivations and goals.

1.3.1.2 Observation
By simple observation of the patient's hand and gesture, different elements can be identified such as:

- Functional exclusion of injured parts of the hand.
- Finger deformity (essentially boutonnière and swan-neck deformities) or global deformities (ulnar claw, wrist drop, or ape hand in particular).

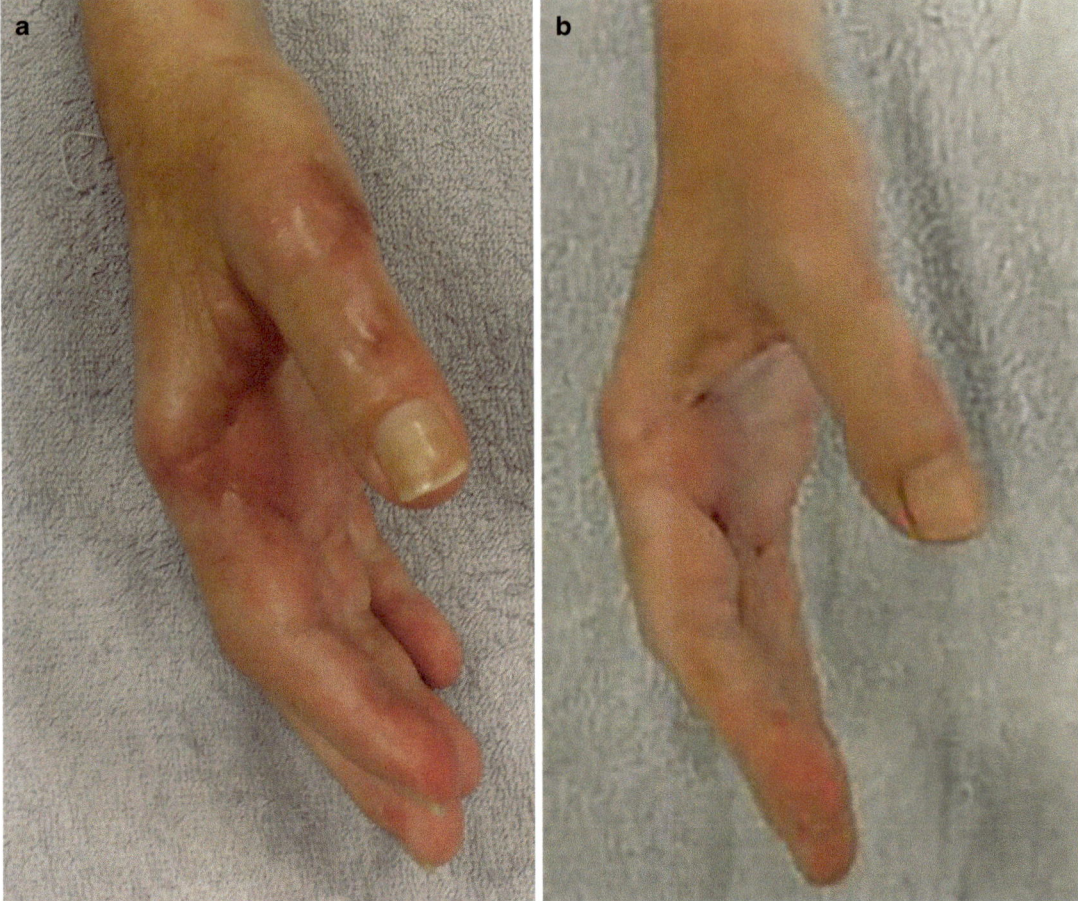

Fig. 1.14 (**a** and **b**) Using a photo and/or video camera can help the patient and the therapist to assess the improvement, especially if it is slow

- Obvious presence of edema that can be associated with a modification of the appearance of the skin or not (glossy or blotched skin, etc.)
- Appearance of skin appendages (thickness and structure of the fingernails, dorsal pilosity) compared to the healthy side (if present).
- Dermatoglyphic patterns (that will tend to fade with functional exclusion).
- Muscle atrophy that can show nerve damage.

Taking photographs or videos of the patient's hand and wrist can complete the therapist's global analysis.

1.3.1.3 Etiology
The situation in which the symptoms appeared must be investigated. It could be a single trauma, several repeated micro-traumas or the symptoms

could have appeared without any known trauma at all. This information, along with the idea of quick or slower onset of symptoms, will help the therapist guide their approach towards severe tissue damage in the first case, or towards more degenerative and/or positional damage in the second case.

1.3.1.4 Functional Signs
Functional signs reflect the different issues that the patient experiences. These signs do not meet any objective criteria; however, they help the therapist focus his clinical examination on the dominant complaint. Verbal exchanges with the patient will inform the therapist in terms of pain, loss of strength, diminished hand mobility, cracking or jumping during gripping, as well as the

presence of "strange feelings," which often correlate with cutaneous sensory disorders.

Pain

The International Association for the Study of Pain (IASP) defines pain as "an unpleasant sensory and emotional experience associated with, or resembling that associated with, actual or potential tissue damage."

This definition helps understand the multifactorial [2] side of pain (Fig. 1.15) and the fact that its level is not necessarily correlated with the severity of the tissue damage.

This paragraph concerns peripheral pain and not central pain, which is often treated in specialized facilities, but it is important to know how to identify this type of pain to address the patients to an establishment offering the adapted global treatment (Table 1.1).

Nociceptive Pain

Nociceptive pain means severe pain related to tissue damage.

The lesion responsible for the pain signal must be the therapist's main concern during treatment and the therapeutic approach will depend on the other elements of the clinical examination.

The idea is to define the patient's experience as precisely as possible regarding the type of pain, its rate, localization, intensity, and the calming and exacerbating factors. It is important to specify if the patient is on pain medication during the evaluation or not, to not bias comparison with future evaluations.

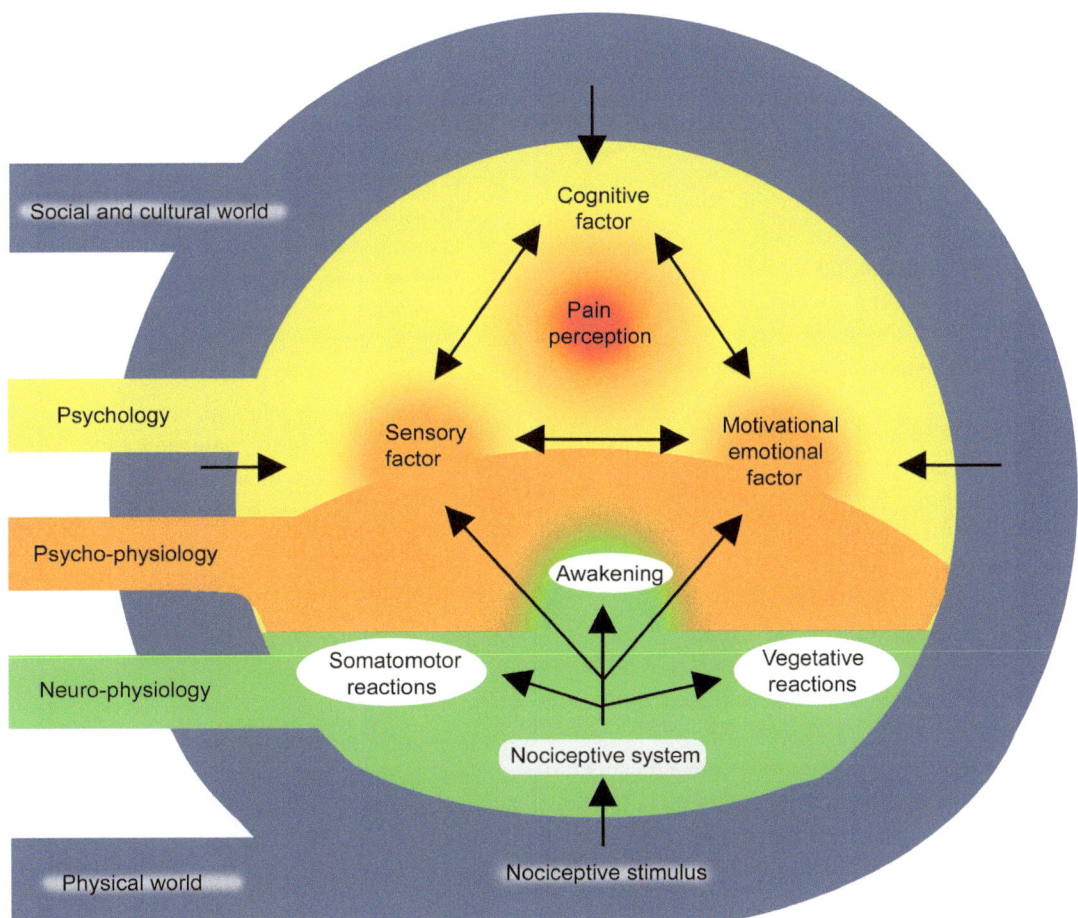

Fig. 1.15 Multifactorial aspect of pain (according to Le Bars and Plaghki [2])

Table 1.1 Factors participating in differentiating neuropathic pain and central sensitization

Neuropathic pain	Non-neuropathic central sensitization
The patient's history and the related medical diagnoses (stroke, diabetes, cancer, herpes zoster, etc.) suggest an injury or a disease affecting the somatosensory system	The patient's history and the related medical diagnoses don't suggest a pathology affecting the somatosensory system
There is evidence (clinical/laboratory/imagery) confirming an injury or a disease affecting the somatosensory system	There is no evidence confirming an injury or a disease affecting the somatosensory system
Pain is logical, from a neuro-anatomical point of view	The location of the pain does not match a peripheral nerve territory or the body schema in the central nervous system
The pain is typically described as burning, throbbing, and tingling	The pain is mostly described as dull and diffuse
Sensory dysfunctions (hypoesthesia, allodynia) are found in the symptomatic area	Sensory dysfunctions are found outside and far away from the symptomatic area

Table 1.2 Proposal for a standardized questionnaire for painful patients

Questionnaire for painful patient
Location of the pain
Where does it hurt? (The patient must point to the painful area)
Is your pain deep or superficial? (Aside from joint pain)
Nature of the pain
Is your pain constant or sporadic?
If constant, does its intensity change?
If sporadic, when does it hurt?
How long does your pain last?
What is its frequency? (often, on occasions)
How long have you been in pain?
Are you hurting now?
Expression of the pain
Describe your pain (pulsating, widespread, cutting, dull)
Does the pain move towards other areas?
Does the pain increase when you move?
Does the pain increase in certain postures?
Can you show the movement and/or postures that increase your pain?
Do you feel some stiffness linked with your pain?
Do you feel pain when you are at rest?
Do you feel pain during the night or in the morning?
Does the pain wake you up?
Do you feel pain during the activity?
Do you feel pain after the activity?
What increases your pain?
What helps decrease your pain?
What do you do to relieve yourself from pain?

The pattern can be mechanic (due to effort) or inflammatory (nocturnal with morning stiffness). Pain can be sudden, throbbing, burn-like, with a compressing feeling, electric, etc.

The therapist must precisely determine what triggers the pain, if it can be identified, to define the cause.

The idea is to test the different structures of the painful area using technical palpation and tissue constraint. For example, pain caused by active mobilization that disappears during passive mobilization most likely has a musculotendinous origin.

The localization can be diffuse or precise. Using a drawing on the assessment sheet can help communication with the rest of the rehabilitation team.

The intensity of the pain is evaluated using the VAS (Visual Analog Scale), described in the previous paragraph), and must include pain during the assessment, as well as the maximal and minimal pain experienced during the last 15 days.

Knowing the calming factors can be very useful to identify the cause of pain and especially to guide the therapist in their treatment choices.

Using a questionnaire for painful patients is extremely helpful and improves inter- and intra-therapist reproducibility (Table 1.2).

Neuropathic Pain (No Allodynia)

This type of pain signifies chronic pain where tissue is no longer the source of the problem. Tissue nociception, if it still exists, is no longer part of the clinical picture: tempting to reduce it will often have very little positive impact on the patient [3].

The NP4 (Table 1.3) can be interesting to reveal the presence of neuropathic pain (sensitivity 80% and specificity 92%) [4] and may be

Table 1.3 NP4 participating in the diagnoses of neuropathic pain if the patient checks at least four items

NP4 assessment

Neuropathic pain
5/12/2020

To evaluate the probability of neuropathic pain,
Tick the boxes corresponding to your sensations.

Does your pain have one or several of theses caracterics ?	
Burn	▨
Painful cold sensation	✓
Electric shock	▨

Is your pain associated with one or several symptoms in the same area ?	
Tingling	✓
Stinging	▨
Numbness	✓
Itching	✓

PN 4 scoring (out of 7)	4

A «yes» is worth 1 point and a «no» is worth 0 point.
If the score is 4 or higher, the pain is probably neuropathic (sensitivity 80% - specificity 92%)

completed by other criteria that help differentiate neuropathic pain and non-neuropathic central sensitization (Table 1.1).

Other tests such as the NPSI (Neuropathic Pain Symptom Inventory) can help identify neuropathic pain that can be associated with mechanical allodynia.

In the case of chronic pain, and considering the multifactorial aspect of pain, the McGill Pain Questionnaire can be very useful because it combines investigation of the sensory and the emotional aspects of pain (and does not limit itself to assessing pain intensity), with good validity [5].

Allodynia
Allodynia is pain triggered by a stimulus that typically does not cause pain (definition of the International Association for the Study of Pain).

There are two forms of allodynia: mechanical allodynia (pain triggered by a static stimulus such as pressure) and dynamic allodynia (pain triggered by a mobile stimulus such as water running over the skin, air blowing against the skin or something brushing against the skin).

The therapist can realize two types of assessment:

- **Quantitative assessment**: establishing the allodynic zone (allodynography).

  Materials: to identify the allodynic zone, two permanent factors are used: pressure (15 g esthesiometer) and pain intensity (VAS scale).

  Preamble to the test: allodynia is present in a tested territory if the patient experiences no pain without a stimulus and when pain with a score of 3 (VAS scale) is caused by the pressure of the 15 g esthesiometer, or if the score of the pain already present is increased by two points.

Localization of the stimulus: during the assessment, the patient is asked to localize the most painful zone which will help the therapist identify the nerve branch that is likely damaged of which the cutaneous distribution territory matches the zone described by the patient (the atlas of cutaneous territories of the human body [6] can be very helpful).

Characteristics of the stimulus: exactly like an aesthesiography, the applied pressure corresponds to the minimal pressure needed to bend the monofilament.

Duration of the stimulus: the application time is about 2 s, with a 10 s delay in between each stimulation.

Test protocol: the assessments aim to identify the most precise territory possible in comparison with a permanent reference such as a crease in the skin and a scar. The first mark is placed along the longitudinal axis of the damaged nerve branch going in a distal to proximal direction, centimeter by centimeter, towards the painful zone. The patient is asked to give the therapist a sign such as saying "it's starting" when discomfort appears and thus, when the therapist approaches the allodynic zone. From then on, the therapist shall continue millimeter by millimeter until the patient says "stop," when their pain can be evaluated at 3 points on the VAS (for patients with no pain at the beginning of the assessment) or increased by two points (for patients that already experienced pain before starting the assessment). The same protocol is applied to find the second mark on the longitudinal axis proximally, and then the two marks along the transversal axis. The allodynography identifies the range of the allodynic zone but not its intensity which is objectified by using the rainbow pain scale.

Qualitative assessment: measuring the intensity of the allodynia (rainbow pain scale).

Preamble to the test: it is preferable to evaluate the intensity of the allodynia using the rainbow pain scale during the session that follows the allodynography to shorten assessment time and reduce pain experience for the patient.

Materials: after the allodynography is complete, the therapist shall define the severity of the allodynia by identifying the lowest esthesiometer that triggers pain evaluated at 3 points on the VAS in the most painful zone located by the patient among 6 established esthesiometers: 0.03 g (red), 0.2 g (orange), 0.7 g (yellow), 1.5 g (green), 3.6 g (blue), 8.7 g (indigo), and 15 g (purple), starting with the lowest monofilament.

Characteristics of the stimulus: the same method is used during the allodynography; the applied pressure must be just enough to bend the monofilament.

Duration of the stimulus: Each stimulation lasts 2 s, with a 10 s delay in between each stimulation.

Test protocol: the defined esthesiometer can then be used to circumscribe the rainbow zone with the same color as the esthesiometer (red if the esthesiometer is 0.03 g, for example). The identified territory is smaller than the zone on the allodynography since the tested zone and the "reference" pain (VAS = 3) are the same, but the esthesiometer is lower (Fig. 1.16).

Three rainbow pain scales are completed after the first allodynography, then a second allodynography is drawn, followed by three new rainbow pain scales, and so on.

Mobility

The patient can describe an alteration of wrist and hand mobility, whether it be towards mobility deficiency or increased mobility.

Loss of Strength

The patient can describe loss of strength secondary to genuine muscle weakness or due to diminished elements that guarantee passive stability

Fig. 1.16 Pain rainbow

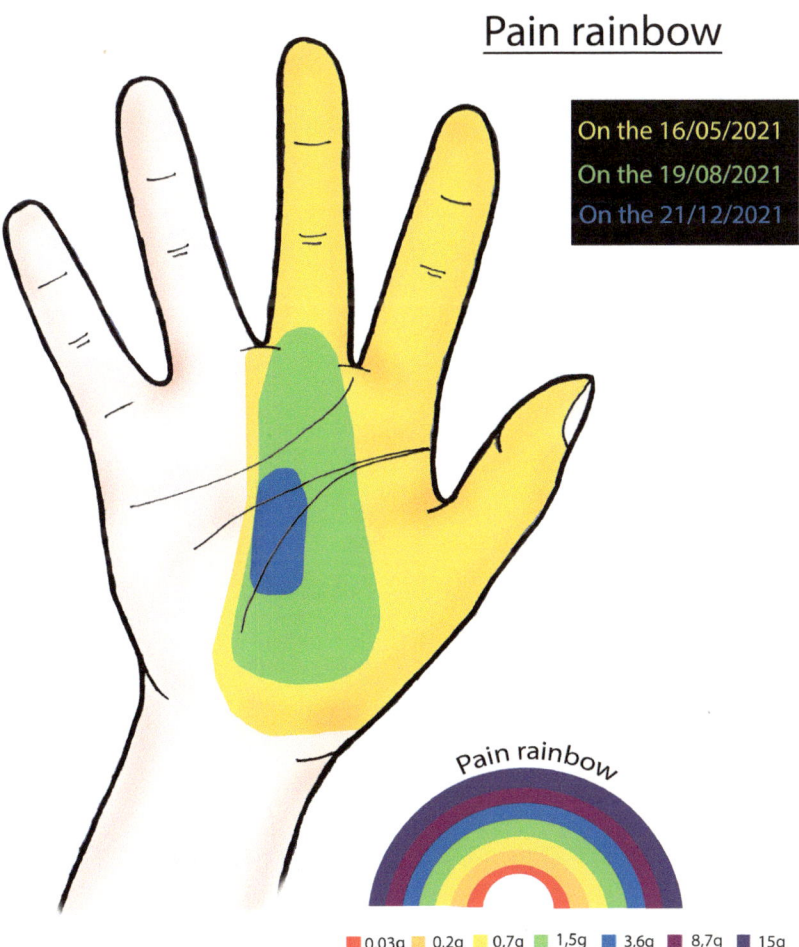

Pain rainbow

On the 16/05/2021
On the 19/08/2021
On the 21/12/2021

Pain rainbow

0,03g 0,2g 0,7g 1,5g 3,6g 8,7g 15g

(ligament injury, loss of skeletal congruence) that lead to functional insufficiency of the active elements.

"Jumps" and Cracking

The patient can experience cracking and jumping sensations during strength or mobilization activities, due to a disruption of joint dynamics, often related to an alteration of the ligaments or bones of the responsible joint.

1.3.2   Clinical Signs

1.3.2.1 Palpation (Fig. 1.17)

This step is crucial to identify the location of the injury which is often painful during palpation and tensioning.

Correct palpation requires solid morpho-palpatory knowledge of the hand and wrist. The potentially sensitive zones are countless, and the assessment must be completed a few days after trauma (after eliminating injuries that could call for medical or surgical treatment) to avoid false-positive results that are frequent during the acute phase.

1.3.2.2 Trophic Examination

This assessment concerns all problems related to the injured zone's trophicity, meaning the expression of tissue nutrition by the vascular mechanisms.

- **Regarding the integument**, the therapist shall observe pilosity, color (hyperemia, white or blotched skin), and the secretions that can inform them on the alteration of

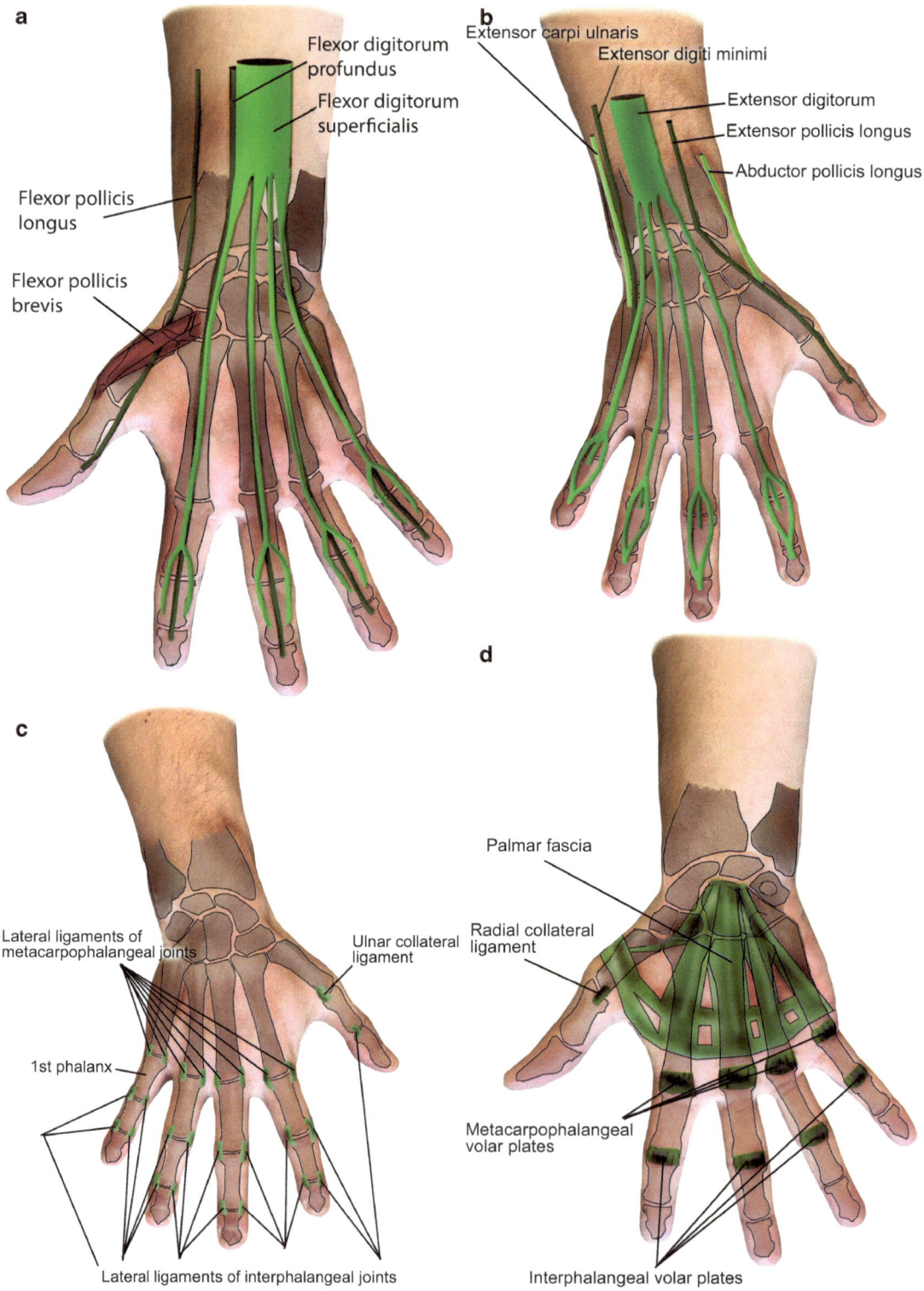

Fig. 1.17 Cutaneous elements that can be palpated. Hand: (**a**) Palmar tendons, (**b**) Dorsal tendons, (**c**) Lateral ligaments, (**d**) Volar plates. Wrist: (**a**) Palmar tendons, (**b**) Dorsal tendons, (**c**) Ulnar tendons, (**d**) Radial tendons, (**e**) Bones (frontal plane), (**f**) Ulnar bones, (**g**) Radial bones, (**h**) Nerves on the anterior side, (**i**) Nerves on the ulnar side, (**j**) Nerves on the radial side

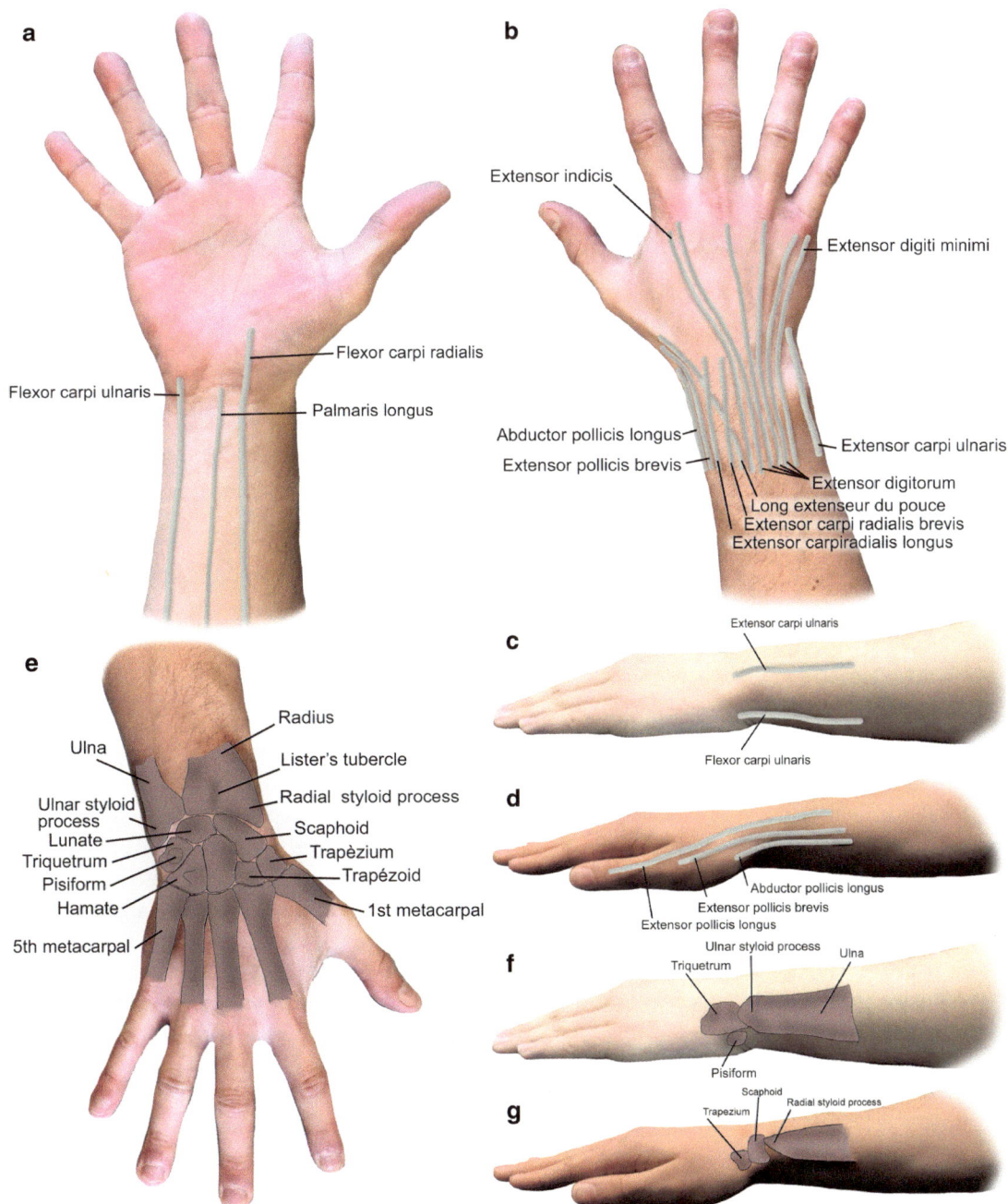

Fig. 1.17 (continued)

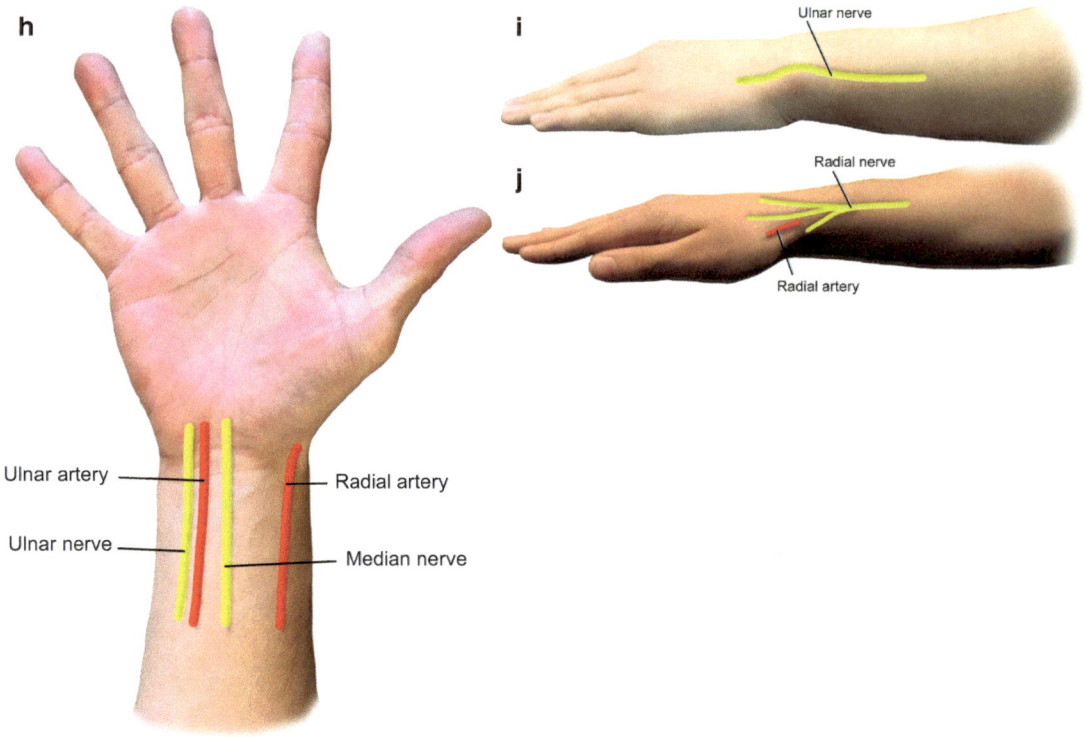

Fig. 1.17 (continued)

local vascular mechanisms. Palpation must help the therapist evaluate the mechanical integumentary properties (extensibility, elasticity, consistency, and mobility compared to adjacent tissue). The skin's temperature is measured using a laser thermometer and compared to the healthy side or to the norm (28–36°C).

- **Regarding skin appendages**, they can be brittle, hypertrophic, or dry, which are signs of trophic alteration.
- **Regarding post-traumatic edema**, which can cause fibrosis and adhesion, which can jeopardize the functional prognosis. To assess it quantitatively, circumferential measuring is appropriate for finger and wrist edema, but the "8 method" is most suitable when the edema in the hand is global [7] (Fig. 1.18). Volumetric measuring, in addition to being complicated to set up in an office, is less reliable than the "8 measuring method" for global edema in the hand, especially because the

measurements can change due to the temperature of the water [7]. A qualitative assessment is associated with the measurements, paying particular attention to skin temperature and consistency of the edema.

- **Regarding the muscles**, the therapist shall observe their mechanical properties (excitability, contractility, extensibility, and elasticity). In practice, the therapist shall evaluate the basic tone using perpendicular than longitudinal pressure and kneading on the muscle fibers. These palpation methods inform the therapist on the muscle tone by detecting indurated or painful spots and the muscle's mobility compared to the adjacent tissues. The evaluation of muscle extensibility is mainly used for polyarticular muscles by comparing them to the healthy side. Presence of muscle atrophy can be observed visually and objectified by comparative perimeter measuring. The perimeter of an intrinsic atrophy is measured across the metacarpal diaph-

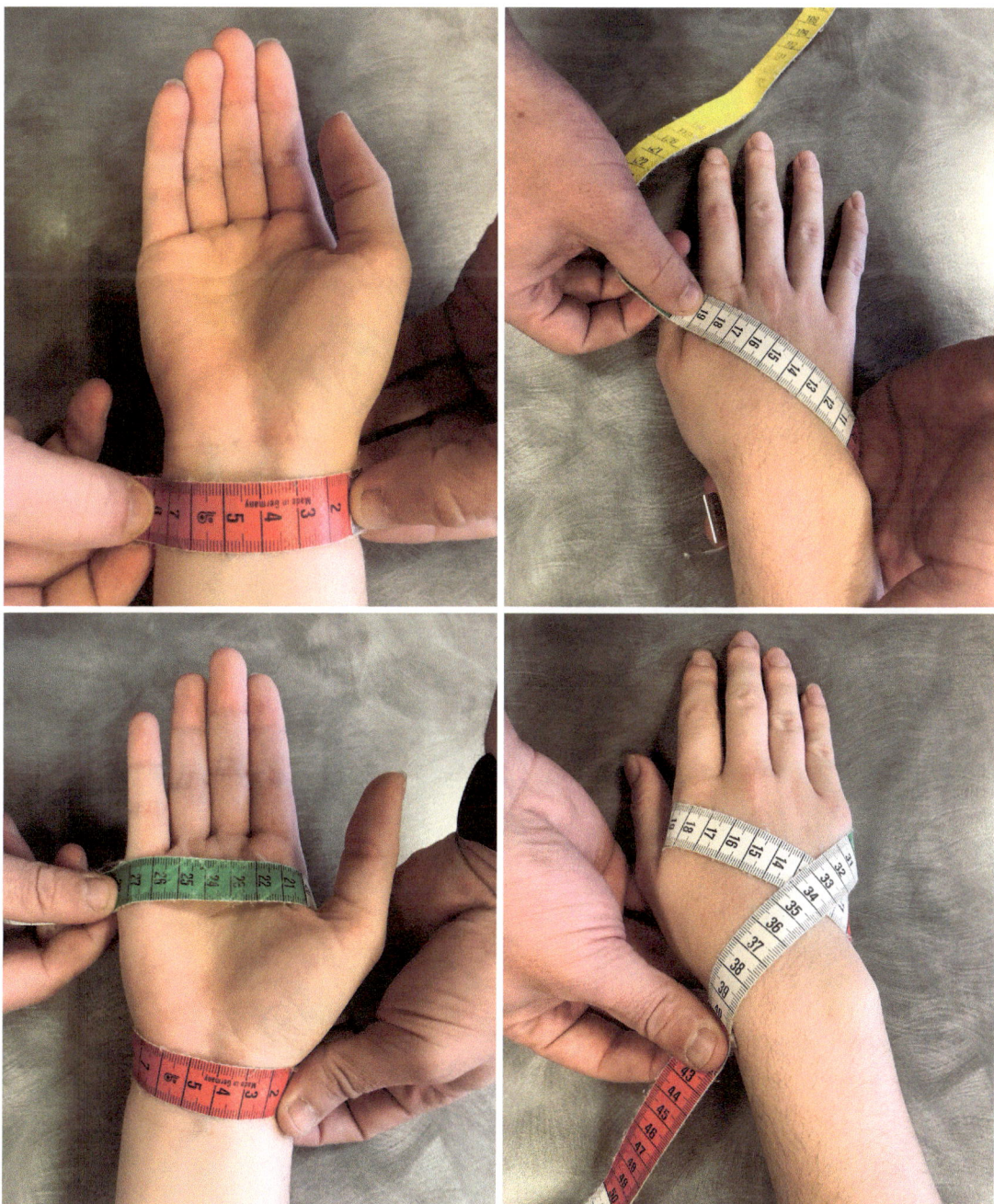

Fig. 1.18 Height measurement for assessing a global hand edema

ysis and around the upper third of the forearm for the extrinsic muscles (Fig. 1.19). Taking pictures is useful for thenar and hypothenar atrophies that are more difficult to quantify with measurements.

1.3.2.3 Scar Examination

To examine a scar, therapists rarely have access to specific objective assessment tools like a Cutometer to measure the skin's elasticity, a derma-spectrometer to evaluate the pigmentation

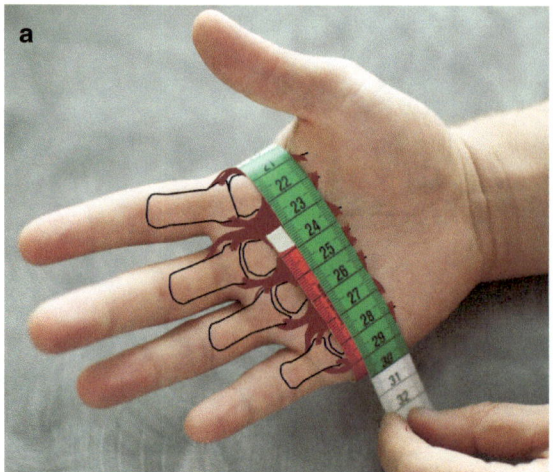
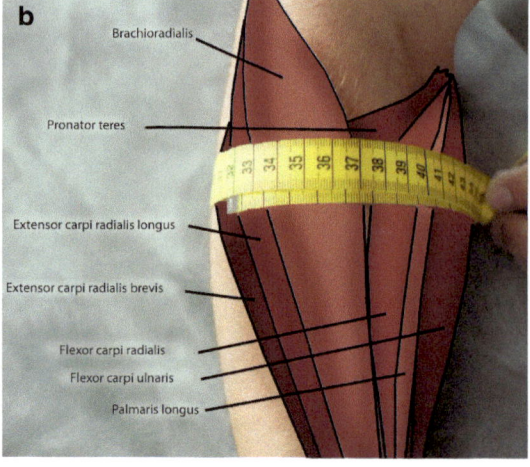

Fig. 1.19 (**a**) Measuring the amyotrophy of interosseous muscles at the level of the metacarpal diaphyses (where their muscle bodies are located) (**b**) measuring the amyot-rophy of extrinsic muscles at the level of the superior one-third of the forearm

and the redness of the skin, or 3D photography for volume measurement. However, therapists can make some simple measurements with common equipment.

There are also several subjective assessment tools to evaluate scars, for example, pain and pruritus. These characteristics can be observed by the therapist, or directly by the patient.

In this paragraph, two hybrid tools shall be presented that are both objective and subjective: the Vancouver Scar Scale (VSS) and the POSAS scale. Other tools exist [8]: Seattle scar scale (1997), Hamilton (1998), Manchester (1998), Stony Brooks scar evaluation (2007), and more.

Objective Assessment Tools

Wound Size
The size of the lesion (length, width, thickness) can be easily measured with a graduated ruler or a caliper.

A scar that develops beyond the limits of the initial injury is one of the characteristics of keloid scarring (relatively rare in the hand), whereas a thick scar can be a sign of an evolution towards hypertrophic scarring [9].

The differences between a linear scar and a keloid or hypertrophic scar, which are two types of pathological scars, must be identified by the therapist because their treatments are different (see Chap. 4) (Fig. 1.20) [9].

Wound Location
The direction and the localization of the scar also have an impact on its development. In fact, there can be strain in some skin lines related to the direction of the collagen fibers, called Langer lines, which are parallel to the flexion creases of the hand. To avoid scar contractures, surgical incisions tempt to comply with these lines, using Z-plasties for example. However, when the scar is caused by a burn or an injury and its direction is perpendicular to the flexion creases, there is more risk to develop scar contractures. Let us not forget that scar retraction is a normal process [10], but its intensity is variable. Shall be distinguished simple or flat retractile scars and raised retractile scars or scar contractures (Fig. 1.21).

Diascopy (Skin Recoloring)
This test uses a chronometer to measure the amount of time the scar needs to recolor after applying vertical pressure with a slightly convex transparent blade or lens. Pressure is applied until the skin is evenly white, then the therapist removes the tool and measures the

SCAR TYPE	AT THE BEGINNING	AFTER 3 MONTHS	AFTER 6 MONTHS	AFTER 12 MONTHS

Linear scar (post-surgery or traumatic)	- Avoid sun exposure.
	 - Preventive treatment :
	  - hydratation
	  - taping
	  - silicon
	  - compression ?
	 - Always reevaluate the scar after 6 weeks.
		- Normal maturation of the scar : stop the treatment at 3 months.
		 - Beginning of hypertrophy :
		  - continue or intensify the treatment as long as needed
		  - pressotherapy
			- Late maturation of the scar : continue with the silicon as long as needed.
			 - Hypertrophy :
			  - continue the previous treatment
			  - send to a specialist for corticosteroid injections
			  - consider surgery.
				Differential diagnosis between permanent hypertrophic scar or not.
				 - Send to a specialized surgeon
				 - Continue the preventive treatment (pressotherapy, silicon …)

Hypertrophic extensive scar (after prolonged healing)	- Avoid sun exposure
	 - Preventive treatment :
	  - silicon + compression
	  - hydratation
	 - Always reevaluate the scar after 6 weeks
		- Normal maturation of the scar (rare) : stop the treatment at 3 months.
		 - Beginning of hypertrophy :
		  - custom-fit compressive clothing
		  - corticosteroid injections with a specialist
		  - surgery if needed.
			- On hypertrophy : continue or intensify the treatment :
			  - custom-fit compressive clothing + silicon
			  - send to a specialist for corticosteroid injections
			  - surgery if needed
				- Permanent hypertrophic scar :
				  - send to a specialized surgeon
				  - continue the preventive treatment (pressotherapy, silicon …)

Keloid scar	- Avoid sun exposure.
	 - Starting keloid :
	  - silicon + compression
	  - hydratation
		- Evolving keloid :
		  - silicon + compression
		  - send to the specialist for corticosteroid injections
				- If no improvement : send to a specialized surgeon (scar excision)

Fig. 1.20 Main differences between linear, hypertrophic, and keloid scars

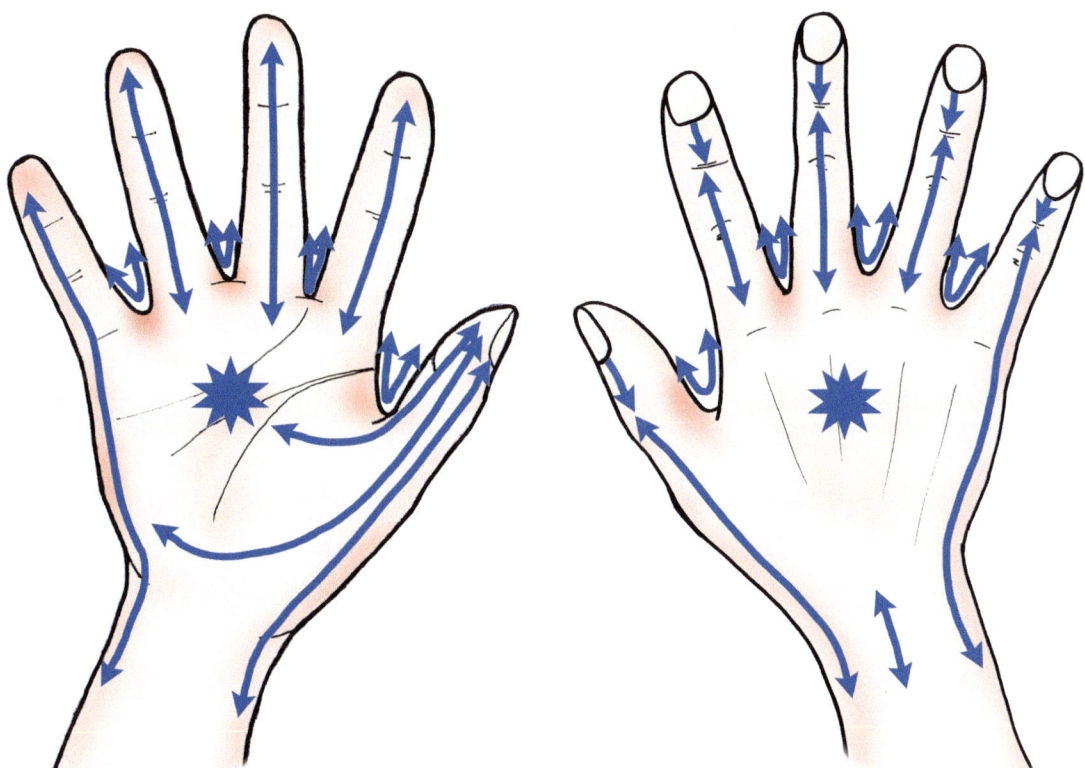

Fig. 1.21 Predictable bands locations

amount of time the depressed zone needs to regain its original color.

The greater the inflammation is, the faster the whitening of the skin will disappear since all inflammatory skin mechanisms lead to an increase in peripheral capillary flow.

Recoloring of healthy skin will take over 3 s. Under 3 s, the scar can thus be considered inflammatory. Some authors, specialized in burn injuries [11], recommend massaging the lesion starting at a result of 2 s of recoloring time with the test.

If recoloring time is under 3 s, there is inflammatory activity in the scar, whereas if it is over 3 s, the result is normal (Fig. 1.22).

Skin Stretching and Pulling Tests

Adhesion is defined by restricted mobility of scar tissue compared to subjacent tissue. Two tests help evaluate adhesion and shall be completed by a joint range assessment.

For the skin stretching test, the therapist holds a graduated ruler or a tape measure at one extremity of the scar, while the other hand creates horizontal traction of the skin to measure its elongation.

> It should be noted that there is also a specific measuring tool for this test called an Adherometer, developed by Ferriero et al. [12] That can easily be printed on a transparent plastic sheet (Fig. 1.23).

The skin pulling test consists of pulling the skin outwards between the thumb and index finger and evaluating the scar adhesion with a scale that goes from 1 to 5 (Fig. 1.24).
Hybrid Assessment Tools (Objective and Subjective)

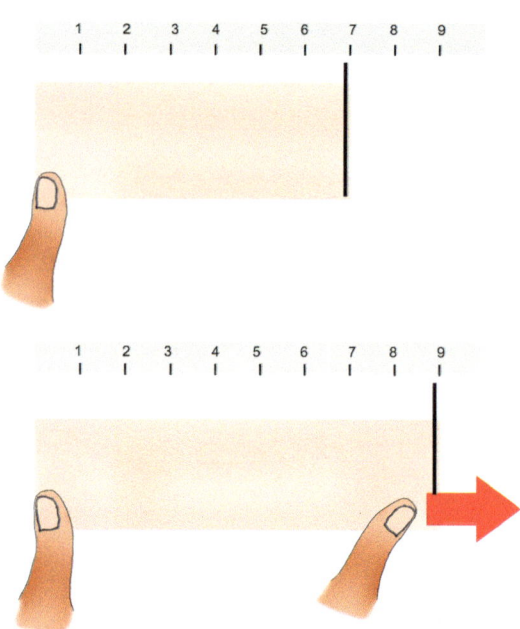

Fig. 1.23 Skin stretching test. One of the assessor's hands holds a graduated ruler or a measuring tape at the extremity of the wound, while the other hand applies a horizontal traction on the skin to assess how much it can lengthen

Vancouver Scar Scale

The Vancouver Scar Scale (VSS) was introduced in 1990 by Sullivan and al. and was modified multiple times. The most commonly used version is that of Baryza and Barysa revised in 1995 [13]. This version includes inflammation, color, thickness, and skin pliability using a skin wrinkling test (Fig. 1.25).

POSAS

The Patient and Observer Scar Assessment Scale (POSAS) was developed by Draaijers et al. in 2004 [14]. Both the patient and the therapist fill out a sheet that each has seven items, rated from 1 to 10. The lower the score is, the more the scar is considered close to normal skin and accepted by the patient. The patient evaluates pain, itching (pruritis), color, pliability, thickness, and the irregularities compared to healthy skin. The therapist evaluates vascularity (using the diascopy test), pigmentation, thickness, relief, pliability, and surface area. Both scales also include an item regarding the evaluator's general opinion on the scar (Fig. 1.26).

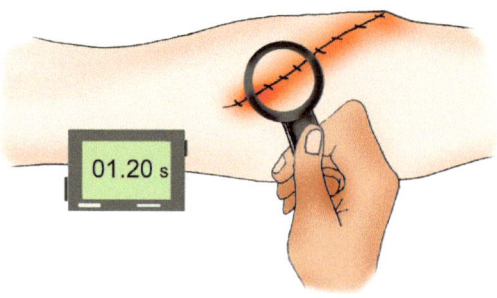

Fig. 1.22 Diascopy test. If it takes the skin more than 3 s to get back to its normal color, the scar is inflammatory. If it takes less than 3 s, the test is normal

Fig. 1.24 Skin pulling test. By pulling the skin between the thumb and the index fingers (**a**), we assess the scar adhesion with a scale from 1 to 5 (**b**)

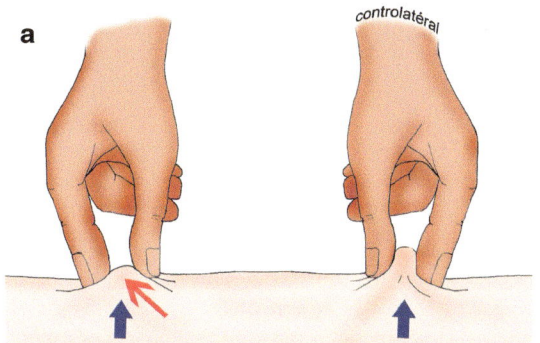

b

Scale for skin pulling test	
1	It is possible to roll a skin fold.
2	The skin is supple with a little tension
3	The skin is firm, not very extensible, and resists to manual tension
4	Bands with the skin getting white when stretched
5	The skin cannot be pulled

VANCOUVER SCAR SCALE		
INFLAMMATION	0 1 2 3	Normal Hypopigmentation Mixed pigmentation Hyperpigmentation
COLOR	0 1 2 3	Normal Pink Red Purple
THICKNESS	0 1 2 3	Normal < à 2mm < à 5mm > à 5mm
PLIABILITY	0 1 2 3 4 5	Normal skin Supple skin, flexible with minimal resistance Supple skin but beginning of tension Firm skin : not very extensible or mobile, resists to manual tension Banding with the skin getting white when stretching the scar Permanent shortening of the scar, producing deformity

Fig. 1.25 Vancouver scar scale

| 1= Normal skin ⟶ worst scar imaginable = 10 | | | | | | | | | | | |
Parameter	①	②	③	④	⑤	⑥	⑦	⑧	⑨	⑩	Catégory
Vascularity	○	○	○	○	○	○	○	○	○	○	Pale/pink/red/purple/mix
Pigmentation	○	○	○	○	○	○	○	○	○	○	Hypo/Hyper/Mix
Thickness	○	○	○	○	○	○	○	○	○	○	Thicker/thinner
Relief	○	○	○	○	○	○	○	○	○	○	More/less/mix
Pliability	○	○	○	○	○	○	○	○	○	○	Supple/stiff/mix
Surface area	○	○	○	○	○	○	○	○	○	○	Expansion/contraction/mix
Overall opinion	○	○	○	○	○	○	○	○	○	○	

Explanation:

The Patient and Observer Scar Assessment Scale has 6 items: vascularity, pigmentation, thickness, relief, pliability, and surface area. Each item is scored on a scale from 1 (normal skin) to 10 (the worse imaginable scar). The addition of the 6 items gives the total score for the assessor's POSAS. Each item has been associated with a qualitative category that must be evaluated circling the right information. Moreover, a general opinion about the scar is given by a scale from 1 to 10. All these parameters should be compared to an anatomically similar and healthy zone.

Explanatory notes about each item:

Vascularity: presence of blood vessels in the scar tissue evaluated by the redness due to the blood return after pressing a plexiglass on the scar (until it whitens).

Pigmentation: brownish color of the scar due to melanin pigments. Apply a plexiglass on the skin with a moderate pressure to rule out vascularity issues.

Thickness: average distance between the subcutaneous edges of the dermis and the epidermic surface of the scar.

Relief: area on which the irregularities are present (compared with the adjacent healthy tissue).

Pliability: assessed by folding the skin between the thumb and index finger.

Surface area: area occupied by the scar, in relation with the surface area of the initial wound.

	1 = No, not at all ⟶ Yes, very much = 10									
	①	②	③	④	⑤	⑥	⑦	⑧	⑨	⑩
Has the scar been painful the past few weeks ?	○	○	○	○	○	○	○	○	○	○
Has the scar been itching the past few weeks ?	○	○	○	○	○	○	○	○	○	○
	1 = No, as normal skin ⟶ Yes, very different = 10									
Is the scar color different from the color of your normal skin at present ?	○	○	○	○	○	○	○	○	○	○
Is the stiffness of the scar different from your normal skin at present ?	○	○	○	○	○	○	○	○	○	○
Is the thickness of the scar different from your normal skin at present ?	○	○	○	○	○	○	○	○	○	○
Is the scar more irregular than your normal skin at present ?	○	○	○	○	○	○	○	○	○	○
	1 = As normal skin ⟶ very different = 10									
What is your overall opinion of the scar compared to normal skin ?	○	○	○	○	○	○	○	○	○	○

Fig. 1.26 Patient and Observer Scar Assessment Scale (POSAS)

1.3.2.4 Sensory Examination

Spatial and Temporal Conditions

Time

A sensory evaluation should never exceed 20 min because over that amount of time, the patient's attention abilities are not optimal [15, 16]. It is also important to respect the delay between each stimulation to avoid causing receptor overload.

Environment

A sensory evaluation must be completed without any possible visual control from the patient. The patient can be blindfolded, or their hand can be hidden behind a folding screen on a comfortable cushion. The patient's hand must remain still; otherwise, the test could be biased by stimulating the kinesthetic receptors (Fig. 1.27).

It must be remembered that a sensory examination is subjective and is based on the patient's interpretation of applied stimuli. Therefore, it is very important that the patient fully understands the instructions before starting. The patient must be able to verbalize their sensations. This assessment must be completed by a neuropathic pain evaluation (NP4, NPSI, McGill Pain Questionnaire) and a motor evaluation (see Chap. 7) given that most nerves are sensory and motor.

Nomenclature

Before tackling sensory examination, it is essential to clarify the different terms used to characterize it. These definitions are outlined by the IASP (International Association for the Study of Pain) and are classified in alphabetical order:

- **Allodynia**: pain triggered by a stimulus that typically does not cause pain.
- **Painful anesthesia**: pain in an area or region that is anesthetized.
- **Burn**: baking sensation or a firing pain (as if fire were burning the surface of the skin).
- **Nociceptive pain**: pain caused by potential or real non-neural tissue damage that is due to the activation of nociceptors.
- **Neuropathic pain**: pain caused by damage to or an illness of the somatosensory nervous system.
- **Dysesthesia**: abnormal or unpleasant sensation that can be spontaneous or induced.
- **Hyperalgesia**: increased response to a stimulus that is typically painful.
- **Hyperesthesia**: increased sensitivity to a stimulation whether it be painful or not (this term includes allodynia and hyperalgesia).
- **Hypoalgesia**: reduced response to a stimulus that is typically painful.
- **Hypoesthesia**: reduced sensitivity to a stimulation, excluding particular senses.
- **Paresthesia**: abnormal but not unpleasant sensation that can be spontaneous or induced.

Quebec's Disability Creation Process Model described by Fougeyrollas [17] speaks of "abilities related to the senses and perception" of which are distinguished interoceptive, proprioceptive, and exteroceptive functions, which the "sense of touch" is part of. The definitions below that seem

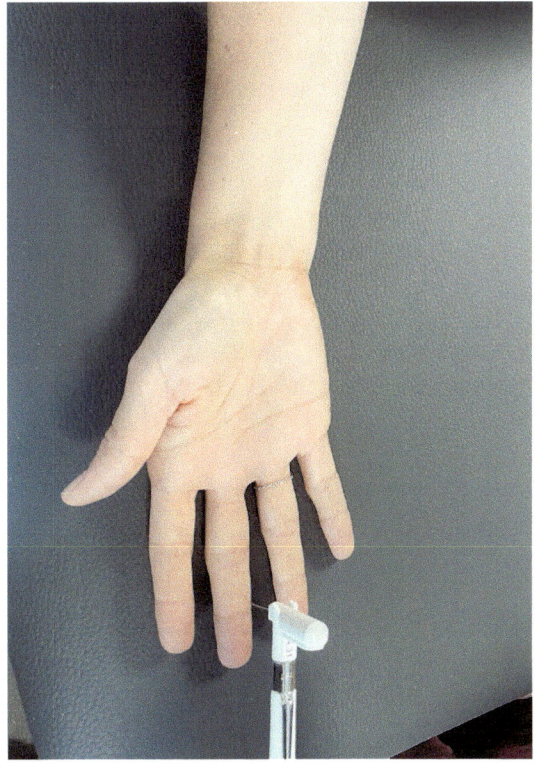

Fig. 1.27 Installing the patient for the sensory examination

relevant for rehabilitation purposes have the additional advantage of offering a vocabulary to therapists to help them evaluate their patients.

- **Topoaesthesia**: the ability to locate a stimulus on the skin.
- **Pallaesthesia**: the ability to feel vibrations.
- **Morphognosia**: the ability to distinguish shapes by touch.
- **Hylognosia**: the ability to recognize and identify textures.
- **Baresthaesia**: the ability to distinguish weight.
- **Stereognosis**: the ability to identify objects by touch from their shape and texture.
- **Graphesthesia**: the ability to identify a figure or symbol drawn on the skin.

However, it must be remembered that this classification is very theoretical. In practice, the abilities stated are rarely used in an isolated manner. It is more suitable to speak of the haptic sense that includes motor and sensory functions.

"What matters is not really the quantity of receptors that recover after nerve damage, but more the use that is made of them." (Winn-Parry).

Stages of Cutaneous Sensorial Recovery [18–20]

Before using any assessment, it is important to keep in mind sensory recovery chronology after peripheral nerve damage.

On a peripheral level, new sensory receptors do not regenerate after suffering from damage. However, the denervated sensory receptors can reconnect by the regenerating axons of the damaged nerve and the axons of the healthy adjacent nerves ("collateral sprouting" phenomenon).

Free nerve endings (nociceptors and thermoreceptors) in charge of thermal and pain information recover first. This is because during the first months of regeneration, there is an imbalance between myelinated fibers and non-myelinated fibers: the non-myelinated fibers that are connected to free nerve endings proportionately outnumber the myelinated fibers that are connected to the mechanoreceptors [19].

Mechanoreceptors do not all react in the same way after peripheral nerve damage. Merkel mechanoreceptors degenerate faster than Meissner corpuscles after peripheral nerve damage [21]. Pacini corpuscles seem to remain rather stable after denervation, even if their shape is altered. There is little knowledge regarding the evolution of Ruffini corpuscles.

Thus, the ability to detect a stimulus that moves across the skin (that Meissner corpuscles are responsible for) generally recovers before the ability to identify a static stimulus (that Merkel discs are responsible for). This explains why the moving two-point discrimination test can often be completed before the static two-point discrimination test.

Lastly, low frequency vibration perception recovers before that of high frequency vibration [19].

There are several classifications of the stages of dermal sensory recovery. The simplified classification of Spicher is a good reference since it synthesizes the different preexisting classifications (Zachary in 1946 and Dellon in 1988) [22] (Fig. 1.28).

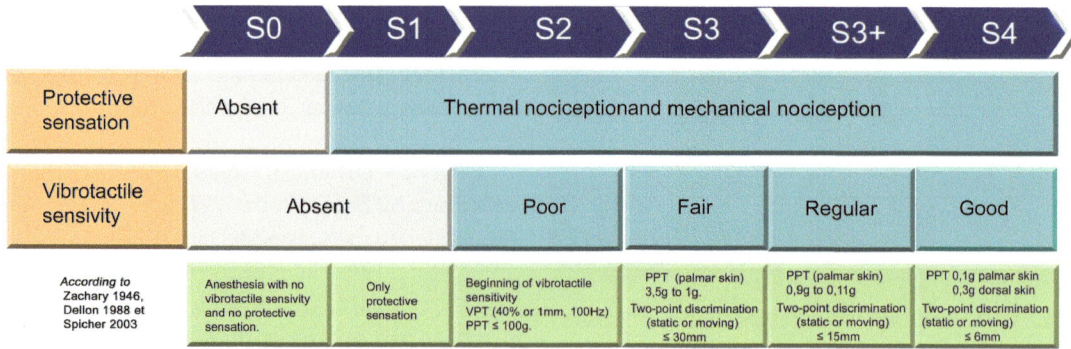

Fig. 1.28 Classification of stages of cutaneous sensorial recovery (according to Zachary and Dellon)

The assessment of dermal sensitivity shall be related to the recovery stage (Fig. 1.29).

Quantitative Test: Aesthesiography

The first assessment to complete when confronted with partial nerve damage is an aesthesiography that helps identify the hypoesthetic zone.

- **Reference values**: On average, the pressure perception threshold (PPT) of the hand is 0.1 g for palmar skin, 0.3 g for dorsal skin, and 0.6 g for the rest of the body.
- **Materials**: Depending on the zones to evaluate, the 0.2, 0.4, and 0.7 g esthesiometers (Semmes-Weinstein monofilaments) are used.
- **Test protocol**: The patient is asked to close their eyes or place their hand behind a folding screen and respond "yes" when they feel the contact of a monofilament.
- **Duration and characteristics of the stimulus**: During the stimulus, the monofilament must bend under the pressure applied by the

therapist and the contact must last about 2 s. The delay time between each stimulus is 10 s.

- **Localization of the stimulus**: The evaluations are completed to identify the most precise territory possible in comparison with a permanent reference such as a crease in the skin and a scar.

The first mark is placed along the longitudinal axis of the damaged nerve branch going in a distal to proximal direction, centimeter by centimeter until the patient does not detect the stimulus. Then the therapist continues millimeter by millimeter in the opposite direction until the patient detects a stimulus. The therapist then continues in a distal to proximal direction one last time, millimeter by millimeter, until the patient does not detect the stimulus. This mark is drawn on the graph paper used for the evaluation.

The same protocol is applied to find the proximal spot where the patient does not detect the stimulus, and then the two spots along the transversal axis of the zone (Fig. 1.30).

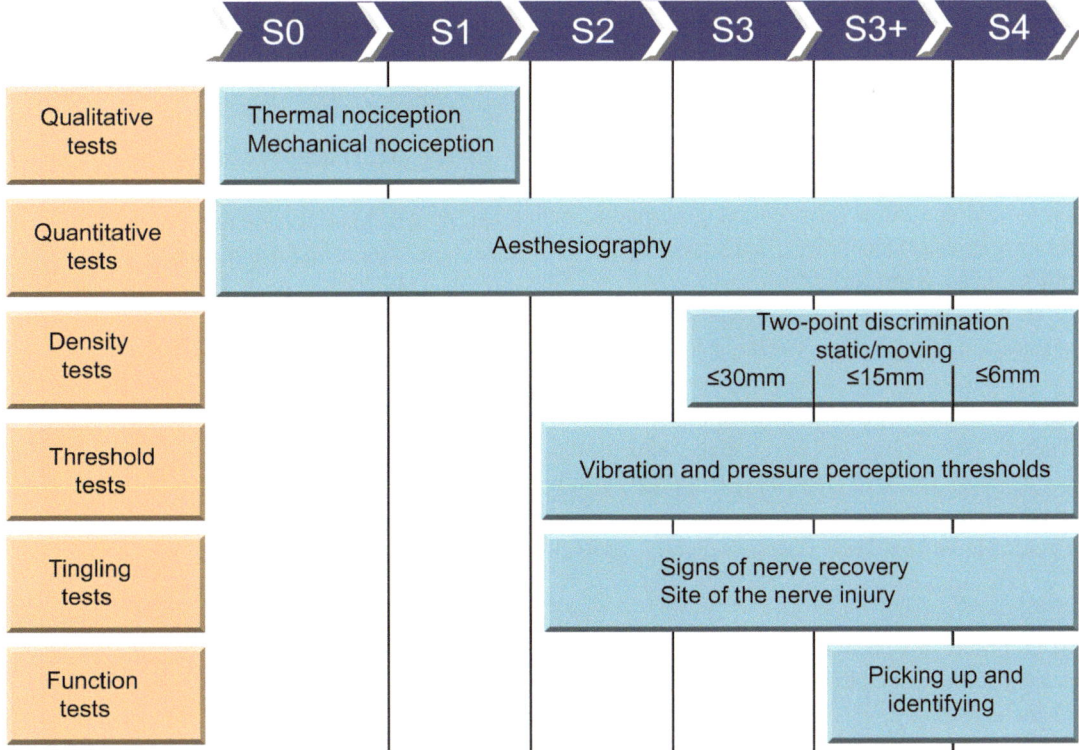

Fig. 1.29 Assessment techniques for cutaneous sensitivity depending on the stage of recovery

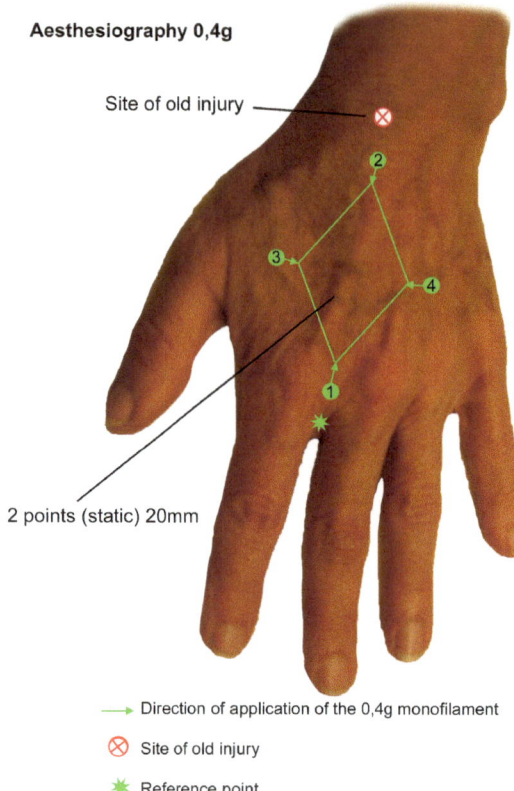

Aesthesiography 0,4g

Site of old injury

2 points (static) 20mm

→ Direction of application of the 0,4g monofilament

⊗ Site of old injury

✳ Reference point

Fig. 1.30 Aesthesiography (example)

Qualitative Tests

Thermal Nociception and Mechanical Nociception

Protective sensation (also called protopathic or thermo-algesic sensibility) helps avoid injuries due to invasive agents.

It includes mechano-nociception, protective sensation against intense mechanical stimuli such as a prick, and thermo-nociception, protection against intense thermal stimuli (over 45°C). Thermo-nociceptors are also called multi-modal nociceptors because they also react to certain chemical stimulations.

Preamble to the Test: Chronologically, protective sensation is the first to recover after peripheral nerve damage. Therefore, it is not necessary to complete this test and pointlessly prick the patient if they have already recovered their vibrotactile sensitivity.

Materials: For thermo-nociception, the applied stimulus is a glass receptacle (test tube) with hot water (maximal temperature obtainable from the faucet, over 45 °C). For mechano-nociception, the stimulus is a prick with a single-use needle applied on previously disinfected skin.

Duration of the Stimulus: In both cases, the patient must respond maximum 2 s after application of the stimulus to be accepted.

Test Result: Sunderland [23] proposed a specific classification for the results of these tests (Fig. 1.31).

> It should be noted that the "prick-touch" test is neither specific nor valid to evaluate protective sensitivity [24] because it also assesses vibrotactile sensitivity. Its use is not recommended.

Sympathetic Nervous System

If the patient cannot detect a skin prick, nor heat, or if they are unable to understand the instructions, it is possible to assess the sympathetic innervation of the hand, considering sensitive and sympathetic fibers are damaged simultaneously.

To test the sympathetic fibers, perspiration can be evaluated by the "corn flour and Betadine®" test [15]. The hand is coated with Betadine®, then a mixture of paraffin oil and corn flower is applied onto the skin. The spots that blacken show recovering perspiration.

The O'Ryan test [15] observes the reaction of the hand when submerged in hot water. In fact, when under hot water for an extended amount of time, the nerves will cause decreasing in the diameter of the blood vessels at the fingertips, which will reduce in volume. Since the skin will maintain the same surface, this will result in the appearance of creases in the skin.

These tests can only confirm complete anesthesia and are not often used in common practice.

a

Thermal nociception	
T°0	Anesthésia
T°1	Simple perception of an undefined change of state
T°2	Distinction between stinging and touching with painful, radiating, and non-localized paresthesia
T°3	Radiating stinging or tingling, poor localized
T°4	Painful sensation, with little or no radiation

b

Mecanical nociception	
P0	Anesthesia
P1	Simple perception of an undefined change of state
P2	Distinction between stinging and touching with painful, radiating and non-localized paresthesia
P3	Radiating stinging or tingling, poor localized
P4	Painful sensation, with little or no radiation
P5	Normal perception

Fig. 1.31 Specific classification for thermal nociception (**a**) and mechanical nociception (**b**)

It should be noted that the ninhydrin test described by Moberg [25] is not recommended anymore due to the toxicity of ninhydrin.

Threshold Tests

They are qualitative assessments that aim to evaluate two aspects of mechanoreceptor activity: their perception threshold in response to a stimulus (the quantity of stimulus that needs to be provided) and its density (enabling discriminative abilities).

- **Pressure Perception Threshold (PPT):**
  Preamble to the test: The PPT test is completed on a rotating basis with density tests because passing the two tests during the same session requires a lot of concentration from the patient.

  Materials: A kit of 20 esthesiometers (Semmes-Weinstein monofilaments). It should be noted that for each monofilament, the values used correlate with the logarithm of its pressure force, in grams per square centimeter multiplied by 10^{-4}. To begin, therapists can equip themselves with a kit of 5 monofilaments also called WEST (Weinstein Enhanced

Sensory Test) [26, 27] but the test's sensitivity to change will obviously decrease [28].

It should be noted that an esthesiometer to evaluate the cornea exists. It is called the Cochet-bonnet esthesiometer, and it has been compared to the Semmes-Weinstein monofilaments in a study [29]. However, the digital Von Frey esthesiometer, sometimes used in research on animals, is not sensitive enough to evaluate the hand.

Characteristics of the stimulus: During the stimulus, the monofilament must bend under the pressure applied by the therapist. It must be applied perpendicularly to the surface of the tested skin.

Duration of the stimulus: The contact should last about 2 s. The delay in between each application is 10 s.

Localization of the stimulus: The stimulus is applied in the zone identified by the aesthesiography during the first session.

Test protocol [27, 30–33]: It is interesting to start by passing the test on the healthy side with the patient's visual control to make sure that they understand the instructions. The therapist then applies genuine and fake stimuli while asking the patient "and now?" The patient, whose eyes are closed, answers "yes" when they feel the contact of the monofilament and "no" in the opposite case. For this description, we have decided to not present the protocol using six passages (3 ascendant/3 descendant following the pattern ADADAD) described by Malenfant et al. [33] and used again by Spicher. We prefer Bell-Krotoski's protocol [31], used again by Novak [30] who propose one ascendant series. The monofilaments are applied from the thinnest to the largest, until the patient feels the stimulus. This monofilament shall be the reference. It is recommended to apply the reference monofilament at least three times (according to Krotoski and Novak) to ensure the test's reliability, and optimally five times (according to Weinstein [27]).

Test result: The pressure perception threshold correlates with the last monofilament that the patient feels during the ascending series (with at least two correct responses over 3, or 4 correct responses over 5). For this description, we choose not to retain the color code proposed by Bell-Krotoski because it does not have good sensitivity to change [28].

Reference values [22]: Less than 0.1 g on the palmar side of the fingers (monofilament 2.83) and less than 0.2 g (monofilament 3.22) on the dorsal side. Factors like age, lifestyle habits, and the dominant hand can make the normal perception threshold vary (Fig. 1.32).

- **Vibration Perception Threshold (VPT):** This test evaluates the ability to detect the

Fig. 1.32 Reference values for Pressure Perception Threshold (PPT)

Palmar face of the fingers	Other cutaneous territories	Stage
100g to 3,6g	100g to 5,1g	S2
3,5g to 1g		S3
0,99g to 0,11g		S3+
< 0,1g	< 0,4-0,2g	S4

Table 1.4 Perceived frequency and maximal sensitivity of the hand cutaneous receptors

	Narrow receptive field		Wide receptive field	
	Merkel	Meissner	Pacini	Ruffini
Frequency range	0–100 Hz	1–300 Hz	5–1000 Hz	0–? Hz
Maximal sensitivity at	5 Hz	50 Hz	200 Hz	0.5 Hz

lowest vibration possible in one specific spot, using a TVS (Transcutaneous Vibratory Stimulation) device.

Materials: TVS (Transcutaneous Vibratory Stimulation) device such as Vibralgic® or Vibradol®.

Duration of the stimulus: The stimuli last around 2 s interrupted by 10 s pauses in between each of them.

Characteristics of the stimulus: The frequency is set at 100 Hz and the vibration amplitude at 8% (Vibralgic 5®) or 0.2 mm. If the intensity of the stimulus is not felt by the patient as "vibrated," the therapist can set the vibration amplitude at 40% (or 1 mm) which corresponds to the strongest vibratory perception of stage S2.

Test protocol: The therapist conducts an ascendant series by blocks of 1% (or 0.025 mm).

Test result: The VPT is the lowest vibration felt by the patient as "vibrated."

Reference values [34]: According to Roll, "With regard to skin, almost all of the mechanoreceptors are extremely sensitive to low frequency mechanical vibrations between 1 and 300 Hz. The slowly adapting receptors, which are constantly activated during stimulation of their receptive field (Merkel discs and Ruffini endings), respond linearly up to vibration frequencies around 200 Hz, and thereafter, they respond to subharmonic frequencies of order two. The rapidly-adapting receptors (Meissner, Pacini and Golgi-Mazzoni corpuscles), on the other hand, which are only activated at the beginning and at the end of a stimulation, respond to vibration frequencies up to 200–300 Hz and stop responding abruptly when the frequency increases." The exact frequencies

felt remain controversial and the recent data proposed by Purves and al. does not completely match that of Roll (Table 1.4) [35].

Density Tests (Fig. 1.33): Static Two-Point Discrimination Test (Weber Test)

This test is the first discrimination test to be described, in 1885 by Weber [24, 36]. According to Dellon et al., it is the best "predictor" of hand function. It is used to evaluate the smallest distance at which the patient can distinguish the perception of one static point from two static points applied by the blunted tips of a compass. It tests the density of the slowly adapting receptors. To be precise, this test is valid to measure the neurological system's identification abilities (which include detection of a stimulus and its sensory integration) but is not valid to measure detection of the somatosensory neurological system [37].

- **Materials**: This test requires a compass with two blunted tips, called a "Weber compass," an esthesiometer with two blunted tips or a "Touch Test ©" disc or "Diskriminator ©," with blunted tips 1–25 mm apart (Fig. 1.34). The use of a paper clip, sometimes described, is not recommended because it is not sufficiently accurate [38].
- **Preamble to the test**: Before starting, the test can be completed on the healthy hand by applying one and then two points under the patient's visual control and asking them what they felt to make sure they understand the instructions. For the real test on the injured hand, the patient will be asked to respond "one" or "two" with their eyes closed.
- **Localization of the stimulus**: The test is done within the hypoesthetic territory. The compass is aligned in parallel with the longitudinal axis

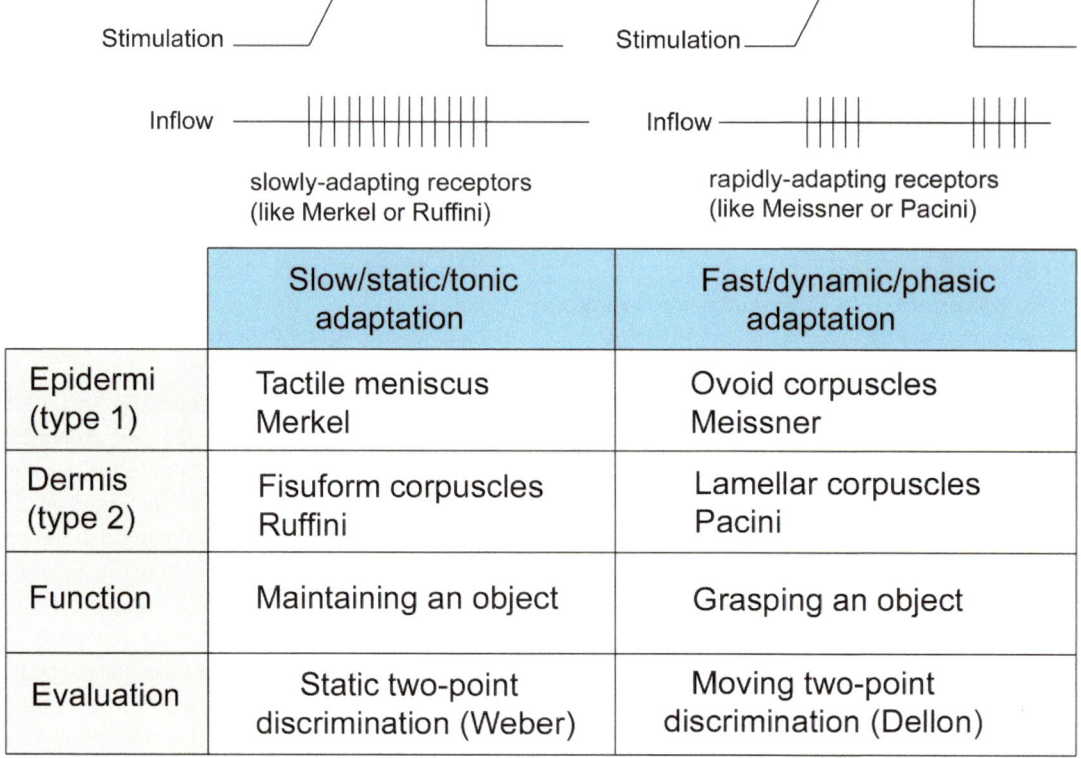

Fig. 1.33 Characteristics of cutaneous mechanoreceptors

of the damaged nerve (to limit the possible substitution of the adjacent territories) except for the fingertips, for distances equal or inferior to 8 mm, the axis of the compass will be perpendicular to the tested finger.

- **Duration of the stimulus**: The duration of the stimulus is 2 s and the delay between two stimuli is 10 s [30].
- **Characteristics of the stimulus**: The pressure must be below the limit of skin whitening to not stimulate other distant mechanoreceptors. To choose the distance to start with, the therapist applies two points in a descendant series until the patient hesitates in their response or commits an error: 25 mm > 20 mm > 15 mm > 12 mm > 10 mm > 8 mm > 7 mm > 6 mm > 4 mm. The distances over 25 mm have been voluntarily removed to reduce assessment time in the case of the hand, but it could be useful to use larger distances for evaluations of the forearm and the wrist.

- **Test protocol**: Next, 10 stimuli of one or two points (at the reference distance set by the descendant series) are successively applied in random order: five one-point stimuli and five two-point stimuli. If the patient gives 7 correct responses over 10, the test can be pursued with a smaller distance. If the patient fails, the therapist will write down the minimal distance for which they correctly identified 7 over 10 one- or two-point stimuli. If the evaluation is done in the case of hypoesthesia subjacent to mechanical allodynia, the static two-point discrimination test is shortened (5 stimuli instead of the 10 normally required) in order to avoid causing pain.
- **Test result**: The result is the minimal distance for which the patient correctly identified 7 over 10 one- or two-point stimuli.
- **Reference values**: The normal perception threshold is 2–6 mm for the fingertips, 7–10 mm for the palmar side of the hand and fingers,

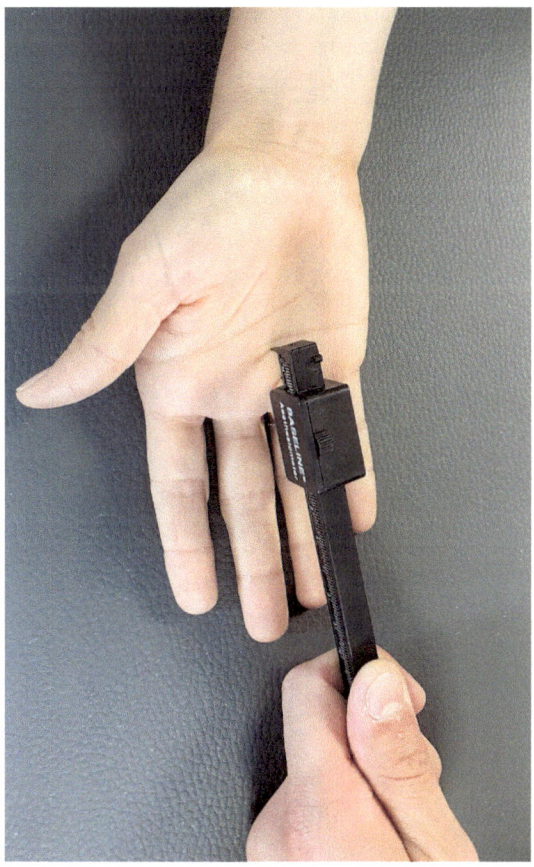

Fig. 1.34 Installation and tool adapted to the static two-point discrimination test (Weber)

7–12 mm for their dorsal side, and about 20 mm for the wrist and the forearm [23].

Density Tests: Moving Two-Point Discrimination Test (Dellon Test)

This test is based on the same principles as the Weber test, but it evaluates the density of the rapidly adapting receptors [15].

The tips of the compass are moved across the surface of the skin making sure to apply the same pressure on each side. The average discriminative values are similar to that of the Weber test.

According to the recovery chronology, these receptors recover before the slowly adapting receptors.

Density Tests: Tingling Test (Table 1.5)

The aim is to distinguish the different types of tingling signs. A tingling sign is "a sensation trig-

gered by a mechanical stimulation of the nerve at the distal portion of a damaged nerve or at the site of an axonal injury […] This tingling feeling can be compared to a low electric current." [39]. The sign of nerve regeneration and the nerve injury location are distinguished.

- **Materials**: The evaluation of tingling signs is completed using a device that generates vibrations, but the test can also be done using hand percussion along the presumed damaged nerve's trajectory [15].
- **Looking for peripheral tingling or nerve regeneration sign (Tinel sign or Dellon advancing tingling sign)**: The sign is a tingling sensation triggered by stimulation of the extremities of the nerve fibers that are regenerating. The investigation is done in a distal to proximal direction using small hand-percussions along the trajectory of the damaged nerve (or with a large zig-zag motion with the Vibralgic or Vibradol sensor). The tingling sensation should radiate towards the periphery, feel uncomfortable but not painful and should not persist in time. Once the distal regeneration sign is identified, the spot shall be marked on the aesthesiography to follow its progress, and therefore the nerve's regeneration, by repeating the test periodically. It is difficult to precisely evaluate nerve regeneration speed, but according to some authors it can be considered 8.5 mm/day for the arm, 2 mm/day for the wrist and 0.5 mm/day for the fingers, and not 1 mm/day in a homogeneous manner as often heard [40]. According to other authors, regrowth progresses 1 mm/day for the hand, but can reach 3 mm/day for more proximal injuries [41]. The site of the nerve regeneration sign should not be and cannot be desensitized.
- **Looking for tingling at the site of nerve damage**: The investigation is done in a proximal to distal direction along the trajectory of the nerve. First, the therapist identifies the spot from which the radiation sensation migrates towards the periphery. This spot is localized (less than 3 mm² according to Spicher), if the spot is wider, the diagnostic of mechanical allodynia should be considered. Unlike the nerve regeneration sign, this

Table 1.5 Situations met when doing a tingling test. A—After a nerve section, there is a Wallerian degeneration of the distal part of the injured nerve. B—The research for the axonal injury site is done from proximal to distal along the injured nerve, until we trigger an electric sensation. C—A severed nerve that hasn't been repaired always results in a neuroma. D—The research for a sign of recovery is done from distal to proximal until we trigger an electric sensation to the periphery. E—A repaired nerve can result in a neuroma. F—Neuroma on amputation stump

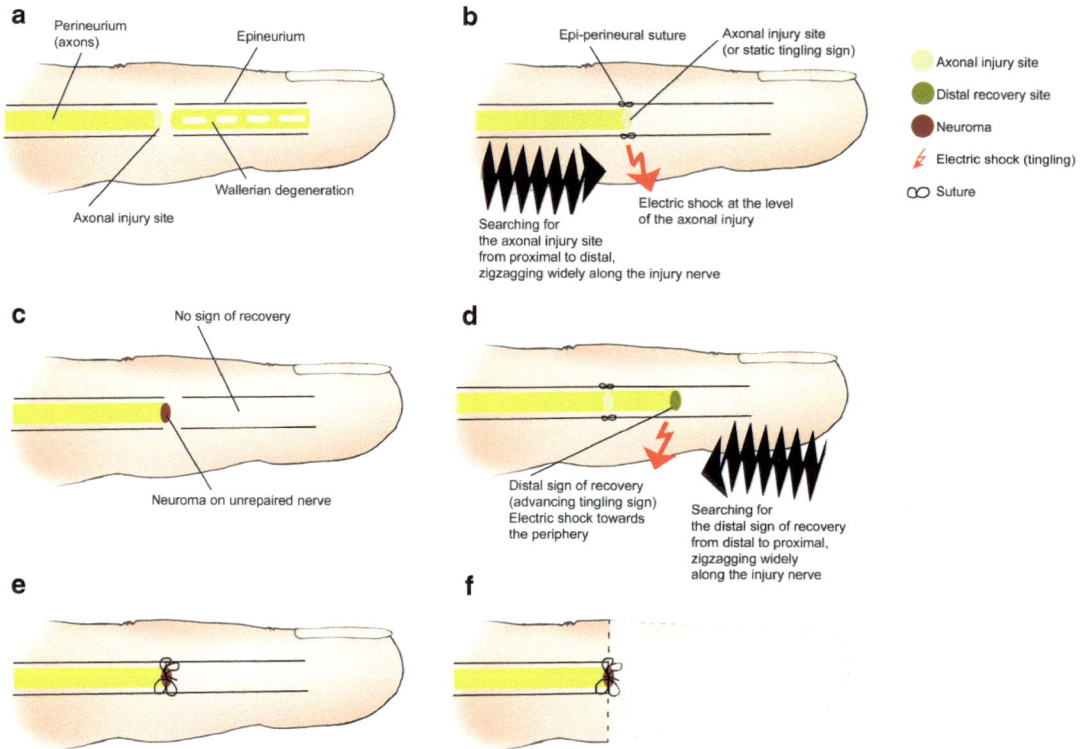

spot is stationary [22]. If there is a neuroma is a tumor-like lesion that occurs in peripheral nerves that is generally related to a traumatic cause. Sunderland and then Herndon differentiate several types of neuromas: continuous neuromas, neuromas on completely severed nerves and neuromas on amputation stumps. Continuous neuromas can be pseudo-neuromas also called continuous neuromas with intact perineurium. They can occur due to repeated local trauma such as the case of damage to the ulnar digital nerve of the thumb in bowlers or damage to the posterior interosseous nerve also called the arcade of Fröhse. A severed nerve that is not repaired will inevitably result in a neuroma at the axonal lesion. However, a repaired severed nerve can also result in a neuroma. A neuroma can also appear after amputation because nerve regrowth is impossible.

> It should be noted that a painful stump is not necessarily a sign of neuroma. Post-amputation pain can also be caused by ungual tissue residue, a bone splinter or phantom pain, for example.

Various criteria help objectify the diagnosis of a neuroma [42]:

- Presence of neuropathic pain (burning, electric discharge, tingling, intolerance to cold).
- Pain that radiates in a zone that correlates with the cutaneous distribution territory of

a nerve branch. Pain is triggered by the stimulation of one specific spot (trigger point) and not a whole zone (differential diagnosis between type 2 CRPS and mechanical allodynia) [43].

- Pain that can be at least partially relieved by local anesthetic infiltration.
- Presence of the Tinel sign (regeneration sign), but that remains static and does not move towards the periphery during healing.

Therefore, it is important to distinguish the two different tingling signs because the rehabilitation protocol can be different. In sensitivity rehabilitation, one of the most common methods is "desensitization," that is based on the gate-control theory which consists in tolerating progressively strong tactile stimuli, to obtain maximal occupation of the conduction path and suppress the pain signal. This method is recommended in neuroma treatment, but the distal regeneration sign should not be and cannot be desensitized. On the contrary, the nerve must be given the time to heal naturally for sensitivity to recover [40].

Functional Tests

According to Tubiana [44], "Tactile sense is passive, touch is voluntary." Touch is a functional tactilo-proprio-kinesthetic system that covers more than just the sensation of contact and includes finger movement. The nomenclature described earlier differentiates stereognosis which is the ability to identify objects (tactile symbolism), hylognosia (ability to identify substances and materials), and morphognosia (the ability to identify shapes), but to obtain this information, the fingers have to move.

Hence, the importance of the concept of haptic perception, term introduced in psychology by Reversz in 1934, that comes from "hapto" in Greek meaning "touch," and "haptiko" meaning "capable of touching." The haptic system can be defined as tactilo-proprio-kesthetic perception.

Haptic perception is active, and it is the result of active exploration movements of the hand as it meets objects. These exploration movements induce mechanical deformities of the skin and the muscles, giving proprioceptive and motor information in addition to sensory information. Debrégeas et al. [45] emphasizes the importance of dermatoglyphs for texture perception. In fact, the ridges and creases in the fingertips enhance vibrations and enable us to feel fine textures.

Access to characteristics such as shape, size, and orientation requires exploratory procedures. To compensate for the limited tactile perception field, the patient uses "exploratory procedures," meaning specific groups of movements that are characterized by the amount of information they can provide and therefore the range of properties to which they are adapted. Lederman and Klatzky [46] observed an exploration strategy in two phases: first, non-specialized procedures are used involving the whole hand and providing global information on several properties, which gives general knowledge on perception, and then specific procedures are implemented. For example, for shape, adults start with Envelopment, then pursue with Contour Following. Some procedures are specifically specialized, and others are more general. For example, Lateral Friction is only appropriate for texture, Lifting for weight, and Pressure for material toughness. Static Contact mainly informs on temperature and, more approximately, on shape, size, texture, and toughness. Envelopment also gives global information on these properties, whereas Contour Following gives precise knowledge on shape and size, and a vaguer idea about texture and toughness. These different procedures are either necessary (essential for a given property), sufficient, or optimal, meaning that they have the maximal efficiency for a given property. Therefore, Lateral Friction is optimal for texture, whereas Lifting is necessary and optimal for weight.

Functional Tests: Stereognosis and Morphognosia Assessment

The modified Moberg test: in 1989, Dellon developed a modified version (modified Moberg test or Dellon pick-up test) that consists of using 12 similar standard metal objects [47, 48] and asking the patient to identify them without visual control.

- **Materials**: A chronometer and 12 metal objects (screw, key, nail, wingnut, big square bolt, hexagonal bolt, small square bolt, 1€ coin, 50 cent coin, washer, safety pin, paper clip).
- **Test protocol**:

  Pick up: This part of the test is timed. The patient picks up each object and places it in a box, first with their healthy hand and then with their injured hand. The patient is timed for each hand. If the ulnar nerve is not damaged, the last two fingers should be bent.

  Identification: This part of the test is timed, and the patient has their eyes closed. The therapist places each object in the patient's hand, and they must identify it in less than 30 s.

  Both parts of this test strongly rely on the hand's motor function. It is true that if hand function is diminished, it will be difficult to differentiate failure due to motor deficit and that due to sensory deficit. If the motor deficit is considered too severe, the test can be done authorizing the patient's visual control [31].

  The protocols and scores vary according to authors and are rarely described in detail [36, 49]. However, Berthe and Orset propose a functional interpretation scale of Dellon's pick up and identification test, based on their personal experience [23] (Fig. 1.35).

  Various other tests have been proposed to assess function, among which:

- **The "Shape Texture Identification" test (STI)** developed by Rosén and Lundborg in 1998 [50]. It is a codified test that evaluates shape and texture recognition. It is available for sale and has a standardized protocol, but it will not be selected for this publication because the material is very costly. The pick-up identification test seems more suitable for practical and fast assessment.
- **The Seddon coin-test** that consists in recognizing different coins of different values.
- **The Riddoch test** where the patient is asked to differentiate coins that have flat or crenellated edges.
- **The Porter test** where the patient is asked to recognize different small letters of the alphabet (H, O, V, Y) in less than 30 s. If the patient takes more time, the test is considered negative.

Functional Tests: Hylognosia Assessment

GDR TACT and evaluation of stimulated sensitivity: A CNRS multidisciplinary research group, the GDR Tact (Touch: Analysis Knowledge Simulation—https://gdr.tact.uha.fr/), aims to combine skills (tribology of materials, electrical engineering, cognitive psychology, biology, and neuroscience) to unite academic, hospital, and industrial counterparts that share issues related to touch. The objective is to create a standardized

Picking up	Identifying (total time /12)	Functional value
< 15 seconds	< 3 seconds	Excellent
15 to 20 seconds	3 à 8 seconds	Good
20 to 25 seconds	8 à 15 seconds	Medium
25 to 30 seconds	15 à 30 seconds	Poor
> 30 seconds	> 30 seconds	Null

Fig. 1.35 Interpretation of the results of the modified Moberg test or Dellon test, according to Berthe and Orset [22]

assessment of hylognosia, meaning texture recognition, which requires both motor and sensory abilities. The goal is to transpose this evaluation on a sort of touch pad that would simulate textures by varying the vibrations sent to the fingertips.

1.3.2.5 Mobility Assessment

Quantitative Aspects

Goniometric measures are realized with the following reference positions:

- **For pronosupination**: 90° of elbow flexion, thumb spread and directed upwards (Fig. 1.36).
- **For wrist flexion/extension and radial/ulnar inclinations**: The longitudinal axes of the forearm and the third finger are aligned (Fig. 1.37).
- **For fingers flexion/extension**: The metacarpal bones and the phalanges are aligned.
- **For the thumb**: The most used position is the thumb's resting position (electromyographic silence) for the trapezio-metacarpal joint (25°

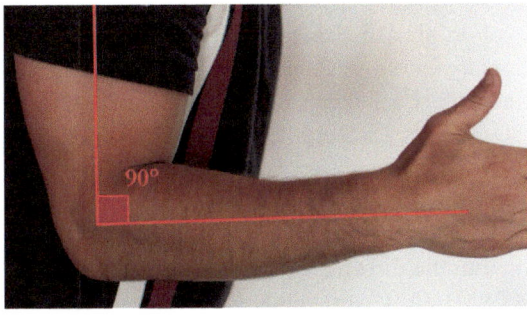

Fig. 1.36 Measuring pronosupination with a 90° flexion of the elbow to avoid the participation of shoulder rotators

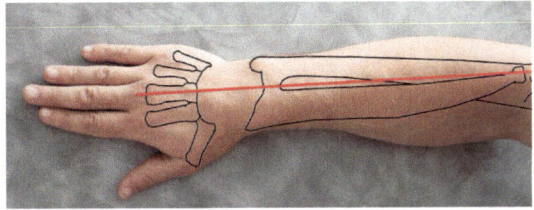

Fig. 1.37 Measuring flexion/extension and radial/ulnar inclinations of the wrist, making sure that the third metacarpal and the forearm axis are aligned

of flexion and 25° of abduction) [51]. For the metacarpophalangeal joint, it corresponds to the alignment of the first metacarpal bone and the first phalanx. For the interphalangeal joint, it corresponds to the alignment of the first and second phalanges.

The quantitative assessment is realized for active and passive mobilities and compared to the healthy side or to the standard.

This assessment is realized after having placed the concerned polyarticular muscles in a shortened position, so that the range of motion's limit is not due to a muscle hypo-extensibility.

Wrist

The radiocarpal and mediocarpal joints are jointly involved in the wrist's global mobility that is usually: 45° of ulnar inclination, 15° of radial inclination, and 90° of flexion/extension. These values vary a lot from one individual to the other [52].

These amplitudes are measured with a Cochin goniometer, with the proximal arm aligned with the forearm axis and the distal arm aligned with the third metacarpal bone. The center of rotation is placed at the level of the capitate's proximal pole (articular center of the wrist).

To assess wrist flexion and extension, placing the goniometer at a dorsal level and at a palmar level seem to be the most precise and reproducible technique [53].

Pronosupination is measured with a Rippstein goniometer placed at the level of the distal radio-ulnar joint. With the elbow flexed at 90°, the standard pronation amplitude is between 60° and 80° and the standard supination amplitude is between 80° and 95° [54].

Hand

The mobilities are assessed with a small Cochin goniometer for more precision in small fingers amplitudes.

Even if the range of motion varies widely from one patient to another, the metacarpophalangeal joint's flexion is usually 90° for the index finger, with a growing evolution towards the fifth finger. The usual passive extension is between 30° and 40°, and they allow varus/valgus movements in extension when the collateral ligaments are relaxed. It should also be noted that there is an automatic axial rotation movement in the four fingers during flexion, which favors the opposition with the thumb.

The interphalangeal joint of the index has a flexion of 90°. As for the metacarpophalangeal joints, this amplitude has a growing evolution from the index finger to the fifth finger. The proximal interphalangeal joint has no extension, while the distal interphalangeal joint usually allows a few degrees of passive extension [52].

In the thumb, the trapezio-metacarpal joint is essential in oppositions: it is shaped like a "scoliotic horse saddle" [52] to allow the automatic rotation in pronation during the flexion, for a good opposition between the thumb and the fingers. The international standard defines the mobilities in flexion/extension and abduction/adduction (Fig. 1.38).

The thumb's metacarpophalangeal joint usually allows a flexion between 60° and 70° and no extension. The interphalangeal joint allows a flexion between 75° and 80° and an extension around 10° [55].

This goniometric assessment is combined with the realization of the Kapandji score that rates the mobility of the thumb in opposition from 0 to 10 (Fig. 1.39).

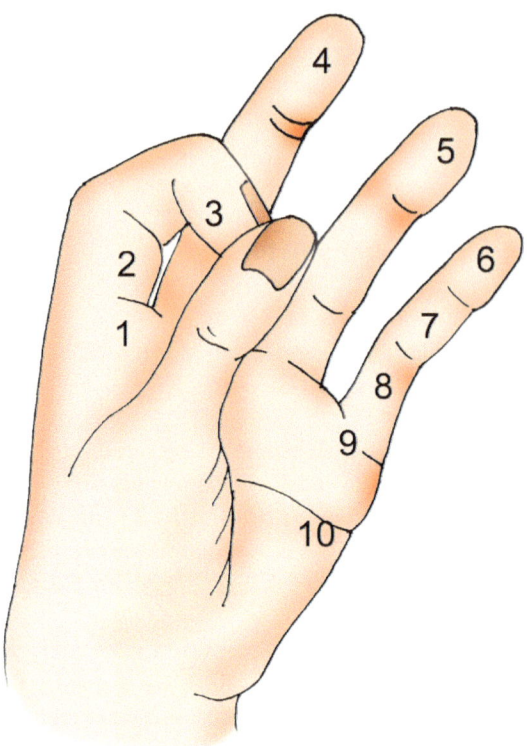

Fig. 1.39 Kapandji score

For all these measures, passive and active range of motions should be assessed, as the differences between them can help to guide the diagnosis towards a musculotendinous limitation.

In passive measurements, the therapist can use a dynamometer to quantify the strength applied to realize the mobilization to avoid biases [56].

For the fingers, using the Total Active Motion (TAM) [57] can be interesting, especially in cases with tendon damages or with several joints involved. It is the sum of the amplitudes measured at the level of the metacarpophalangeal joints, and the proximal and distal interphalangeal joints. The result can be compared to one of the contralateral hands or to the standard (even if it is widely variable depending on the individuals). The TAM (percentage) corresponds to the division of the damaged hand's TAM by the contralateral one or the standard (260°) [58].

The Total Passive Motion (TPM) follows the same principles but concerns the passive mobility

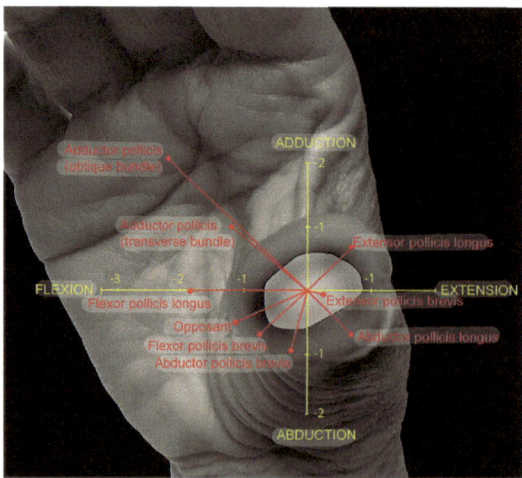

Fig. 1.38 International standard defining the movements of the trapezio-metacarpal joint in flexion/extension and abduction/adduction

of the metacarpophalangeal joints, and the proximal and distal interphalangeal joints.

Qualitative Aspects

Type of "Stop" and Range of Motion Limitation Depending on the Adjacent Joints

This analysis is operator-dependent, so it is not very reproducible. However, the kind of "stop" felt by the therapist can guide the diagnosis towards the limitation's tissular origin.

A hard "stop" that does not change with mobilizations is compatible with an osseous or osteophytic origin, whereas a hard "stop" that changes with mobilizations is compatible with a ligamentous or capsular origin.

A hard or soft "stop" that depends on the adjacent joints' positions guides us towards a muscular origin such as hypo-extensibility or peritendinous adhesion of the antagonist muscles.

Significant Difference Between Active Range of Motion and Passive Range of Motion

A significant difference between passive and active mobilities (compared with the healthy side) should guide the therapist towards a potential tendon injury, a disorder of the motor nerve responsible for the requested movement, or an injury of an element stabilizing the tendon responsible for the requested movement.

Joint Glidings

Intra-articular glidings must be studied in the joint's unlocked position to avoid any tension on the ligaments, capsules, or muscles. The therapist realizes glidings, axial rotations, coaptations, and decoaptations. These elements are assessed comparing them to the healthy side.

1.3.2.6 Neuromotor Assessment

The motor assessment can concern three elements: reflex, automatic, and voluntary motricities.

Reflex Motricity

It corresponds to a reproducible motor reaction triggered by a well-identified sensorial stimulus and executed through predetermined nervous circuits. Its evaluation is determined by osteotendinous reflexes.

To assess them, the patient must be relaxed, and the tested muscle should be placed in medium race. The therapist realizes a quick percussion on the tested muscle's tendon and evaluated the intensity of the observed response:

- **Grade 0**: No response.
- **Grade 1**: A little reduced compared to the healthy side (if present).
- **Grade 2**: Normal (compared to the healthy side).
- **Grade 3**: More intense than the healthy side (or than standard).
- **Grade 4**: Very intense.

In peripheral nerve injuries, we observe grades 0, 1, and 2. Grades 3 and 4 are mostly related to pyramidal syndromes, which we will not describe here.

Automatic Motricity

It corresponds to stereotypical and reproducible movements generated by innate neuronal networks (breathing, swallowing, etc.) or built by learning (driving, sports, etc.). Its evaluation in the hand is difficult to quantify but its alteration has an impact on the hand's dexterity.

Voluntary Motricity

Muscular Testing

It corresponds to intentional movements triggered by and external stimulus or an "internal instruction." This motricity is the most complex, and there is a wide range of intentional movements differentiated by the number of mobilized segments, their repetition, their speed, or their spatiotemporal precision. Assessing this mobility is complex and must consider the elements of the motor control with a precise neurologic evaluation. In case of peripheral nerve injury, we will use the following grading based on Daniels and Worthingham's testing:

- **Grades 5 or "normal" and 4 or "good"**: We can differentiate them if the contralateral muscles are normal. The resistance is applied in the whole amplitude until the breaking point. We ask the patient to "hold" a position, and the therapist applies a resistance as opposed as possible to the muscle traction. This test must not produce pain.

- **Grade 3 or "acceptable"**: It corresponds to the ability to mobilize the concerned segment in all its range of motion and against gravity.
- **Grade 2 or "mediocre"**: It corresponds to the ability to mobilize the concerned segment in all its range of motion without gravity, or in part of its range of motion against gravity.
- **Grade 1 or "trace" and 0**: It requires a careful inspection and a precise palpation as it is about determining whether there is a contraction of the requested muscle or not. This can be done for superficial muscles but is unreliable (unrealistic?) for deep muscles.

For the wrist:

- **The flexor carpi radialis** is innervated by the median nerve (C6) and flexes the wrist.
- **The flexor carpi ulnaris** is innervated by the ulnar nerve (C8-T1) and realizes a flexion/ulnar inclination of the wrist.
- **The extensor carpi radialis longus** is innervated by the radial nerve (C6-C7) and realizes and extension/radial inclination of the wrist.
- **The extensor carpi radialis brevis** is innervated by the radial nerve (C6-C7) and extends the wrist with a minor component of radial inclination.
- **The extensor carpi ulnaris** is innervated by the radial nerve (C7) and realizes and extension and ulnar inclination of the wrist, especially in forearm supination when its angle of attack is most favorable to this movement.

For the fingers:

- **The flexor digitorum superficialis** is innervated by the median nerve (C7-C8-T1) and flexes the proximal interphalangeal joint. We test it by asking for a flexion of the second phalanx towards the first phalanx, with the other fingers maintained extended (Fig. 1.40).

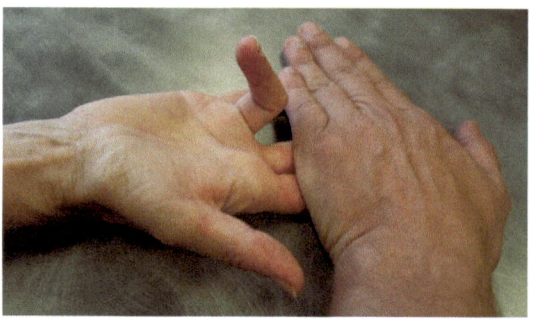

Fig. 1.40 Assessment of voluntary motor control in the flexor digitorum superficialis of the fourth finger

- **The flexor digitorum profundus** is innervated by the median nerve (C8-T1) for the index and third fingers, and by the ulnar nerve (C8-T1) for the fourth and fifth fingers. It is tested by asking for a flexion of the third phalanx towards the second phalanx, with the two proximal phalanges maintained in extension.
- **The extensor digitorum** is innervated by the radial nerve (C7) and extends the metacarpophalangeal joints. It is tested by asking for an extension of this joint at the level of the third and fourth fingers as the index and fifth fingers both have their own extensor muscles that can disturb the movement analysis.
- **The extensor indicis** is innervated by the radial nerve (C7) and extends the index finger's metacarpophalangeal joint. It is tested by asking for this movement, with the third and fourth fingers' metacarpophalangeal joints flexed to remove the action of the extensor digitorum.
- **The extensor digiti minimi** (Fig. 1.41) is innervated by the radial nerve (C7) and extends the fifth finger's metacarpophalangeal joint. It is tested by asking for an extension of the fifth finger's first phalanx, with the third and fourth fingers' metacarpophalangeal joints flexed.
- **The interossei muscles** are innervated by the ulnar nerve (C8) and all flex the metacarpophalangeal joints and extend the interphalangeal joints. The dorsal interossei muscles abduct the fingers while the palmar interossei muscles adduct the fingers. Their common actions can be tested by asking for a flexion of the first phalanx and extension of the interpha-

langeal joints. Their specific actions can be tested by asking the patient to spread his fingers with the metacarpophalangeal joints extended (dorsal interossei) or to bring his fingers together (palmar interossei).

- **The abductor digiti minimi** is innervated by the ulnar nerve (C8) and moves the fifth finger away from the fourth finger. It also participates in the flexion of the fifth finger's metacarpophalangeal joint, along with the flexor digiti minimi brevis and the fourth palmar interosseous muscle.
- **The opponens digiti minimi** is innervated by the ulnar nerve (C8) and flexes the fifth metacarpal bone.
- **The flexor digiti minimi brevis** is anatomically very close to the abductor digiti minimi, but its main action is the flexion of the fifth finger's metacarpophalangeal joint. It cannot be analytically tested.

For the thumb:

- **The flexor pollicis longus** is innervated by the median nerve (C8-T1) and flexes the interphalangeal joint.
- **The extensor pollicis longus** is innervated by the radial nerve (C7) and extends the interphalangeal joint while participating in the extension of the metacarpophalangeal joint. It also participates in the retro-position, the adduction and supination, and the adduction of the trapezio-metacarpal joint. It is tested by asking for an extension of the interphalangeal joint or an adduction of the thumb column.
- **The extensor pollicis brevis** is innervated by the radial nerve (C7) and extends the metacarpophalangeal joint. It is tested by asking for this movement, with the interphalangeal joint slightly flexed.
- **The abductor pollicis longus** is innervated by the radial nerve (C7) and extends and abducts the first metacarpal bone. It is tested by asking the patient to move his thumb away from the palm of his hand.
- **The abductor pollicis brevis** is innervated by the median nerve (C6-C7). It realizes and

abduction of the first metacarpal bone in a plane perpendicular to the palm of the hand and a pronation/abduction of the first phalanx.

- **The opponens pollicis** is innervated by the median nerve (D6-D7) and abducts the first metacarpal bone.
- **The flexor pollicis brevis** is innervated by the median nerve (C6-C7) for its superficial bundle and by the ulnar nerve (C6) for its deep bundle. It realizes a flexion/adduction of the first metacarpal bone and a flexion/pronation of the metacarpophalangeal joint. It is difficult to test it analytically as it can be compensated by the adductor pollicis for adduction, and by the abductor pollicis brevis (or even the inconstant first palmar interosseous muscle) for the flexion of the metacarpophalangeal joint.
- **The adductor pollicis** is innervated by the ulnar nerve and brings the first metacarpal bone closer to the second metacarpal bone with a flexion/adduction. It is also responsible for the flexion of the metacarpophalangeal joint.

Dynamometric Measurements

Aside from peripheral and central motor damages that require a specific assessment, the neuromuscular evaluation is mainly realized with dynamometers [59] to assess:

- **Grasp**: It allows to assess the grasping force and must be realized with a calibrated dynamometer. The patient is placed with his elbow close to his body, and with 90° of flexion (ideally placed on an armrest), a neutral pronosupination, and a neutral wrist position (Fig. 1.42). The contraction lasts 3 s with a 15 s recovery time between the three measurements. The result is the average of the three contractions. The patient must not exceed the pain threshold [60].
- **Clamp (thumb/index finger)**: The modalities are the same as the grasp measurement, but the goal is to assess the clamping force between the thumb and the index finger. The

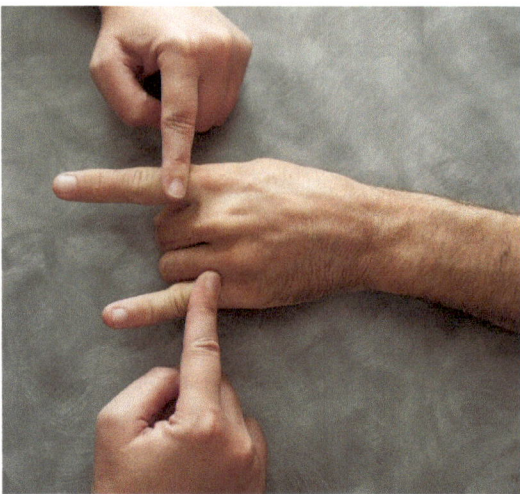

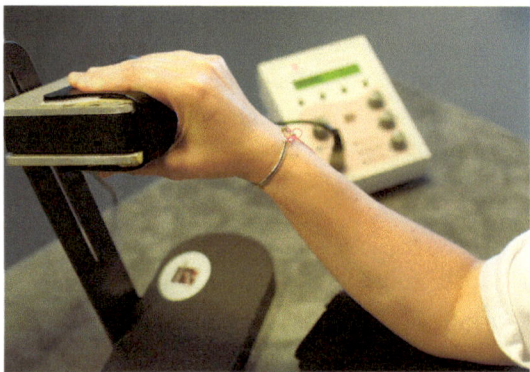

Fig. 1.43 Specific dynamometer to evaluate clamping (intrinsic muscles)

Fig. 1.41 Assessment of voluntary motor control in the extensor indicis and extensor digiti minimi

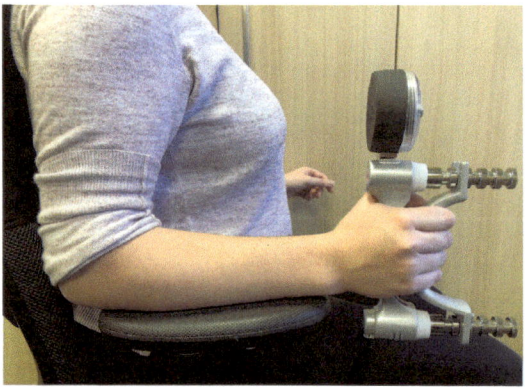

Fig. 1.42 Installation of a patient to measure grasp

most used measures are the key pinch, the pinch, and the pinch between three fingers.

- **Clamp (hand)**: It allows to selectively assess the intrinsic strength as the general clamping movement is realized by the interossei and thenar muscles (Fig. 1.43).

Other dynamometers can be used to assess and analyze the agonist/antagonist muscles ratios and therefore show the muscular imbalances (Fig. 1.44).

1.3.2.7 Clinical Tests
There are many clinical tests we can use to improve our assessment, but their specificity and

sensitivity are highly variable. They are "easy" tools, but they can also mislead us.

We will describe here the most used tests in hand and wrist rehabilitation. More specific tests will be described in the second and third volumes with the corresponding pathologies.

Mobility

Finochietto Test
The patient can flex his interphalangeal joints if the metacarpophalangeal joint is flexed but not if it is extended.

This test shows a retraction of the interossei muscles if the limitation appears in passive and active movements, or a retraction of the lumbrical muscles if the limitation appears only in active movements.

Kilgore Test
It is the opposite of the Finochietto test. The patient can flex his interphalangeal joints if the metacarpophalangeal joint is extended but not if it is flexed.

This test shows adhesions in the extensor system at the level of the back of the metacarpal bones (Fig. 1.45).

Haines Test
The distal interphalangeal joint can be flexed if the proximal interphalangeal joint is flexed but not if it is extended.

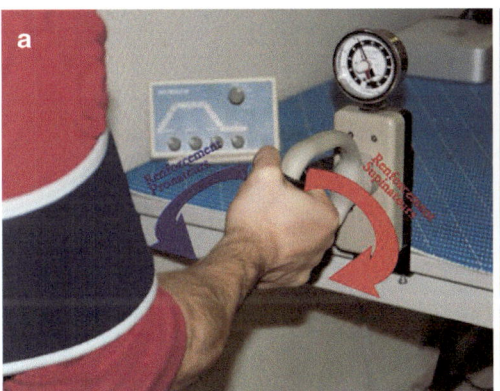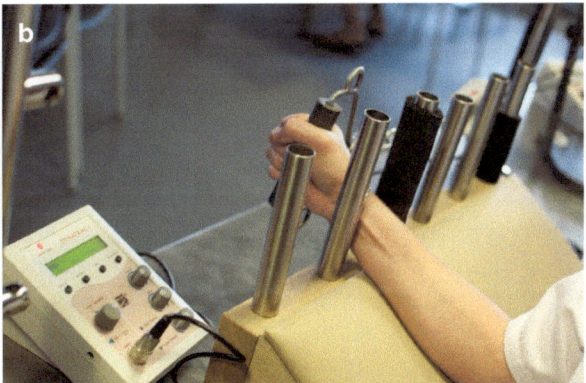

Fig. 1.44 Specific dynamometer to evaluate strength in wrist pronation/supination (**a**) and wrist flexion/extension (**b**)

This test shows a retraction of the oblique retinacular ligament that is tensed in this position.

Blocked Finger After Active fFexion

When the patient flexes his finger, it gets stuck after a certain position, and can be unlocked with a passive extension—we can sometimes hear a typical "clunk" sound.

It is the clinical sign of a trigger finger, due to the presence of a nodule on the flexor system. This nodule conflicts with the beginning of the tendon sheath when the tendon glides during the finger flexion.

Instability

In the Hand: Joint Laxity Tests

They allow to assess a joint's level of instability. The idea is to put the injured ligament under tension and to assess the pain, the stop, and the range of motion, comparing them with the healthy side.

If there is pain but no laxity at the end of the movement, the ligament is slightly injured. If there is a laxity with a firm stop, more fibers are injured. If there is an important laxity (sometimes with no pain), the ligament can be completely broken, which must be confirmed with paraclinical exams.

In the fingers, the volar plate can be tested by placing the joint in maximal extension and trying to bring it towards hyperextension. The collateral ligaments of the metacarpophalangeal joints are tested with 70° of flexion to evaluate all the bundles, and with 90° of flexion to evaluate the posterior bundles. The collateral ligaments of the

interphalangeal joints are tested in extension to evaluate all the bundles, and in 45° of flexion to evaluate the main dorsal bundle.

In the thumb, the longitudinal palmar ligaments of the metacarpophalangeal joint are tested by placing the joint in maximal extension and bringing it towards hyperextension. The collateral ligaments are tested in extension to evaluate both bundles, and in 30° of flexion to evaluate the main bundle (Fig. 1.46).

In the Wrist

- **Radioulnar ballottement test**: It is based on the specific mobilization of the distal radioulnar joint (see Chap. 5). The test is positive if the patient feels pain when mobilizing (compared to the healthy side). It shows joint suffering. It is realized in pronation, neutral position, and supination, for a complete assessment of the distal radioulnar ligaments.
- **Compression test for the triangular fibrocartilage complex (TFCC) (sensitivity 66%, specificity 64%)**: The patient is placed with his elbow in 90° of flexion and maximal ulnar inclination. The therapist applies a longitudinal compression and a complete passive forearm pronation. The test is positive when it recreates the patient's pain. It shows injuries of the TFCC's meniscus homolog.
- **Scaphoid's bell sign**: This test consists in evaluating the scaphoid's dynamics. The therapist places his thumb on the scaphoid tubercle, at the level of the proximal pole. In wrist

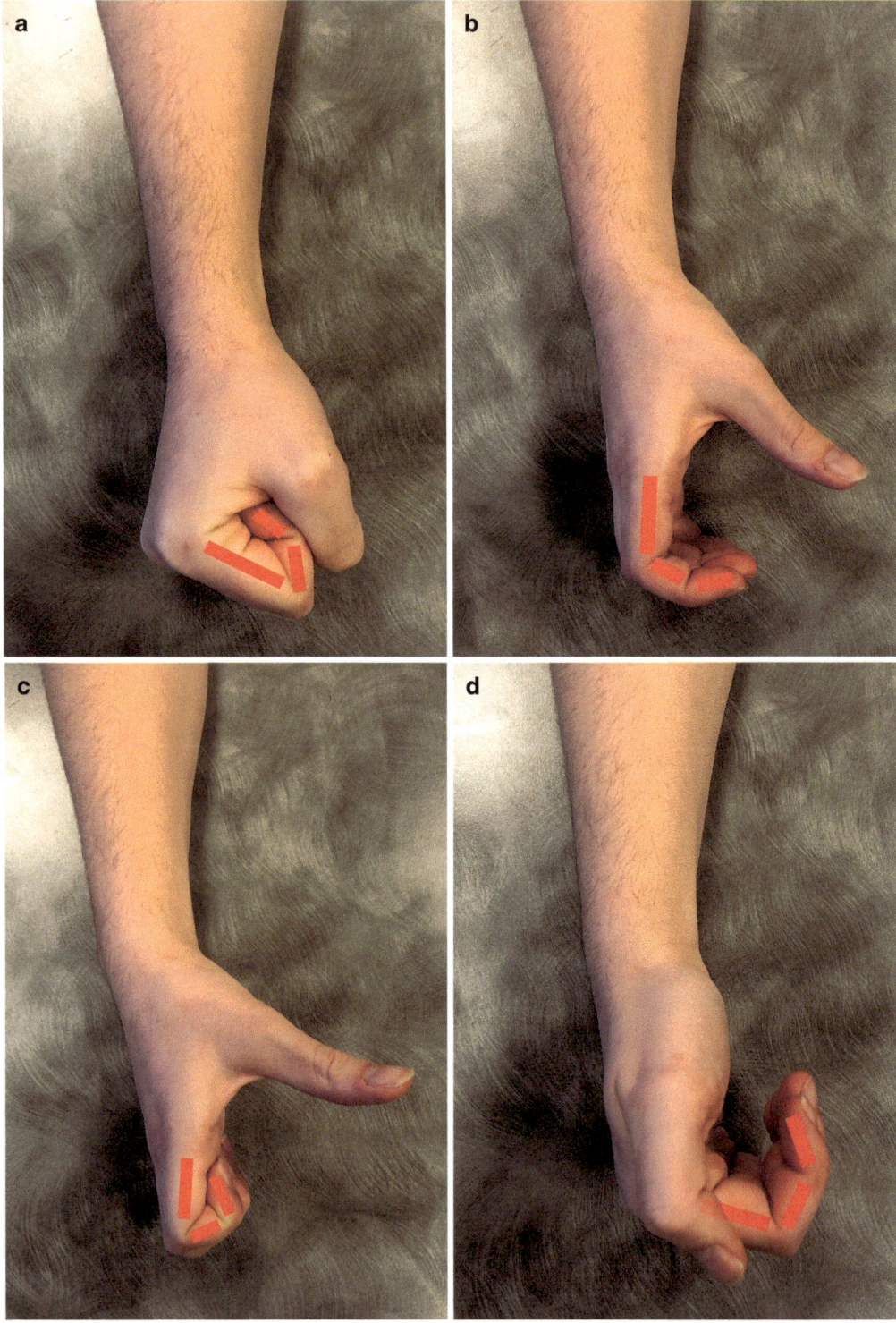

Fig. 1.45 Finochietto (**a** and **b**) and Kilgore (**c** and **d**) tests are very useful in loss of motion, for a differential diagnosis between a hypo-extensibility in intrinsic muscles allowing interphalangeal flexion if the metacarpophalangeal joint is flexed (**a**) but not if it is extended (**b**), or an adhesion between the extensors and the back of the metacarpals allowing interphalangeal flexion if the metacarpophalangeal joint is extended (**c**) but not if it is flexed (**d**)

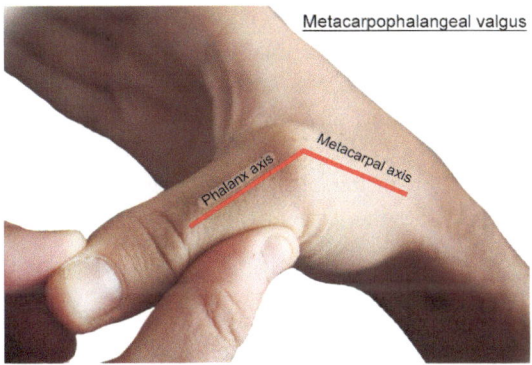

Fig. 1.46 Tensioning and palpating the main bundle of the ulnar collateral ligament of the thumb is realized with 30° of flexion in the metacarpophalangeal joint to relax the accessory bundle

radial inclination, the scaphoid goes in flexion ("lies down") because the distance between the radius and the trapezium and trapezoid bones decreases. This causes the tubercle to push the therapist's thumb and creates a depression under his index finger. In wrist ulnar inclination, the scaphoid goes in extension ("straightens up") which causes its proximal pole to push the therapist's index finger and causes a depression under his thumb. If these movements do not occur, there can be a ligamentous injury (scapholunate ligament or scapho-trapezio-trapezoid ligaments) as the movements of the scaphoid are abnormal.

- **Pisiform test**: The patient's forearm is in a vertical position. With one hand, the therapist places the wrist in slight flexion to relax the pisiform's stabilizing muscles. With the thumb and index finger of his other hand, he glides the pisiform against the underlying triquetrum. Any pain during this test should trigger a specific X-ray to confirm the hypothesis of joint suffering. A wide translation of the pisiform compared to the other side suggests a laxity of the pisohamate ligaments.
- **Watson's test (sensitivity 48%, specificity 67%)**: The therapist faces the patient in an "arm wrestling" position. The scaphoid is held in place between the therapist's thumb and index finger. The therapist applies a firm pressure on the tubercle while he places the wrist in ulnar inclination (scaphoid in extension). He then brings the wrist in radial inclination

while keeping the pressure on the scaphoid's tubercle, blocking the scaphoid flexion. If the scapholunate ligament is injured, the proximal pole of the scaphoid will cause pain as it will move dorsally—the therapist can even feel a "jump" under his index finger. This test must be realized on both sides as it can be positive in people with laxity without pathology [9].

- **Scapholunate ballottement (sensitivity 69%, specificity 66%)**: As for the radioulnar ballottement, if pain appears when mobilizing the scaphoid in relation to the lunate, it means that there is intra-articular suffering in the scapholunate joint.
- **Reagan's test or lunotriquetral ballottement (sensitivity 64%, specificity 44%)**: The test is positive if it is painful to mobilize the triquetrum in relation to the lunate.
- **Mediocarpal "jump" when moving from radial inclination to ulnar inclination**: This shows a palmar mediocarpal instability that gets less important in ulnar inclination as the first carpal row moves towards extension and causes a typical "jump."

Tendons

Tendinous "Triad"

If the patient feels pain when the therapist palpates or stretches the tendon, or when he asks for a contraction against resistance, we could be in the presence of a tendon pathology. This can cause instability as it disturbs the activity of the concerned muscle.

The therapist must explore the wrist as a whole and have a good knowledge of the involved anatomical elements.

Cyriax's Criteria

It is a manual muscular test that evaluates the force developed by a maximal contraction, and the pain it produces.

If the developed force is similar to the force on the pain-free healthy side, the tendon is normal.

If the developed force is normal but the contraction is painful, the tendon is pathological.

If the developed force is weak but painless, the motor command is disturbed, which means there is a peripheral or central nervous damage.

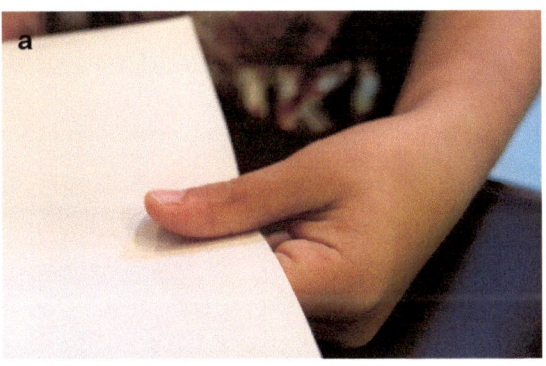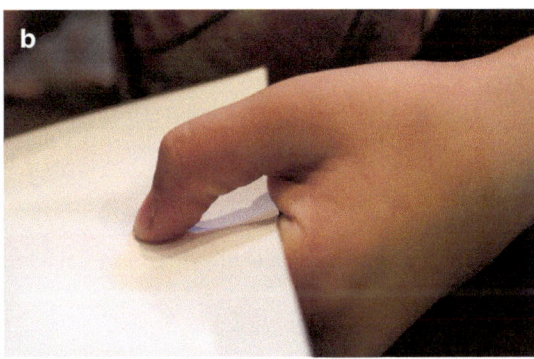

Fig. 1.48 Froment test: holding a paper sheet pulled by the therapist is impossible without compensating with the FPL (innervated by the median nerve) because de adduc-tor pollicis (innervated by the ulnar nerve) is inefficient. (**a**) Negative test, (**b**) Positive test

The test is positive if it reproduces the patient's symptoms (electric shocks, tingling, or other signs of nerve suffering) [62].

Phalen's Test + Compression (Sensitivity 89% and Specificity 96%): Median Nerve

It consists in placing the wrist in maximal flexion during 1 min and checking if this position triggers the patient's symptoms.

The test is positive and more sensitive if it is combined with a compression of the median nerve before it enters the carpal tunnel.

Reversed Phalen's Test + Compression: Ulnar Nerve

It consists in placing the wrist in maximal extension during 1 min and checking if this position triggers the patient's symptoms.

The test is more sensitive if it is combined with a compression of the ulnar nerve at the level of Guyon's canal.

Resisted Supination with Extended Elbow

It consists in asking the patient to do a supination against resistance with his elbow extended. We combine this maneuver with a compression of the radial nerve at the level of the arcade of Fröhse and check if the symptoms occur.

If the symptoms are present, the test is positive and shows a potential compression of the radial nerve at this level.

Scratch Collapse Test

The therapist faces the patient. The patient sits with his arm in adduction, elbows flexed, wrists in a neutral position, and fingers extended. The patient realizes a maximal contraction in external rotation of both shoulders, against the therapist's manual resistance.

The therapist then stimulates the zone of potential nerve compression by scratching the area, and the same test is realized again. If the patient has less strength than the first time, there can be a compression of the stimulated nerve.

This test's validity varies across the studies. As far as we are concerned, its use must be complementary of other specific nerve tests with less contested validity [63–66].

1.3.2.8 Functional Scores

Several functional scores have been described to assess the function of patients with hand pathologies. For example, the DASH and the Quick-DASH (Fig. 1.49) have a comparable excellent validity regarding the patient's self-evaluation.

The 400 points assessment is an objective evaluation of the patient's function by a therapist. It is divided into various categories: mobility, strength, and grabbing with one hand and with two hands [67].

1.3.2.9 Echoscopy

This tool has many advantages and fits right in the hand therapist's tools of choice, whether he

FUNCTIONAL SELF-EVALUATION (Quick DASH)

Answer the questions with the following scoring :
0 = no difficulty   1 = slight difficulty   2 = medium difficulty   3 = important difficulty
4 = impossible

Unscrewing a tightly closed lid	0
Doing heavy cleaning chores (cleaning the floors, walls …)	0
Washing your back	0
Carrying a bag of groceries	0
Cutting food with a knife	0
Doing leasure activities requiring stregth (craft, gardening, tennis …)	0

Answer the question with the following scoring :
0 = not at all   1 = slightly   2 = medium   3 = a lot   4 = extremely

During the last 7 days, has your shoulder, arm or hand bothered you in your interactions with your relatives ?	0

Answer the question with the following scoring :
0 = not at all   1 = slightly   2 = medium   3 = a lot   4 = incapable

Have you been limited in your work or usual daily activities because of your shoulder, arm or hand ?	0

Answer the question with the following scoring :
0 = none   1 = slight   2 = medium   3 = important   4 = extreme

Pain in the shoulder, arm or hand	0
Paintful tingling in the shoulder, arm or hand	0

Answer the question with the following scoring :
0 = no troubled   1 = slightly troubled   2 = moderatly troubled   3 = very troubled   4 = impossible

During the last 7 days, has your sleep been troubled by pain in your shoulder, arm or hand ?	0

Functional impairment / 100	0

Fig. 1.49 Functional self-evaluation (Quick-DASH)

needs it during the assessment or to explain to the patient where his symptoms come from, or even in scientific research.

Assessment

Exploring the area that we want to treat with echoscopy allows a more precise initial evaluation, leading to an adapted rehabilitation proto-col. This imagery technique can also be used at different stages throughout the rehabilitation to check the patient's evolution and judge the effectiveness of the treatment. This way, we can precisely adapt the treatment.

Assessment and Implementation of the Most Adapted Treatment: Case Example 1

The medical diagnosis is a tenosynovitis of the third finger from March 19th. In this case, echoscopy shows an effusion, from which we can conclude that rehabilitation will be focused on drainage to remove the fluid collection. On April 20th, another echoscopy is realized. The effusion has disappeared, and the zone is now more fibrous. The program is adapted and focused on fibrosis and tendon gliding (Fig. 1.50).

Assessing the Treatment Efficiency

Case example 2: Using Doppler mode, we can see if there is hyperemia and follow its evolution. This way, we can compare the hyperemia of the flexor carpi radialis before and after a session to assess the efficiency of our treatment (Fig. 1.51).

Case example 3: In this case, Doppler shows the positive evolution of a tennis elbow, with a hyperemic area declining after 6 days of treatment (Fig. 1.52).

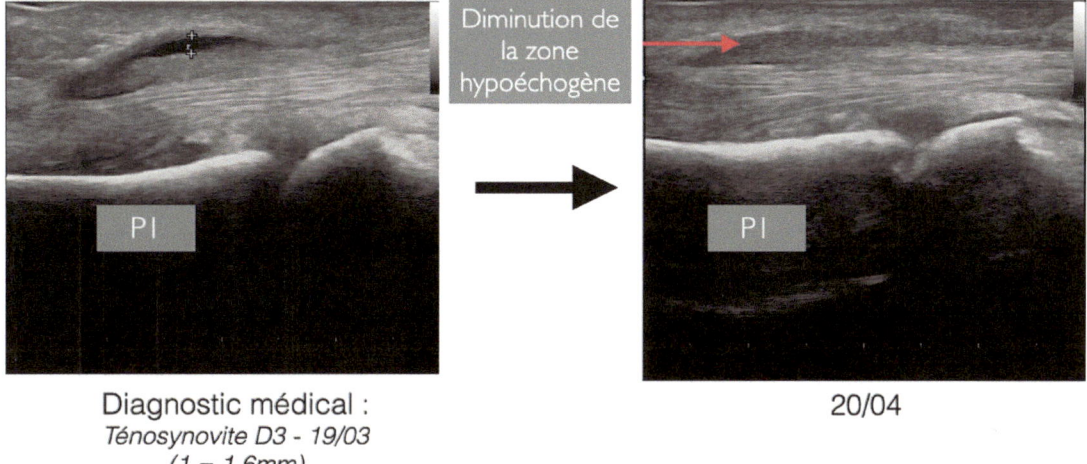

Fig. 1.50 Tenosynovitis in the flexor tendons of the third finger. In rehabilitation, echoscopy allows us to quickly adapt the treatment to histological modifications

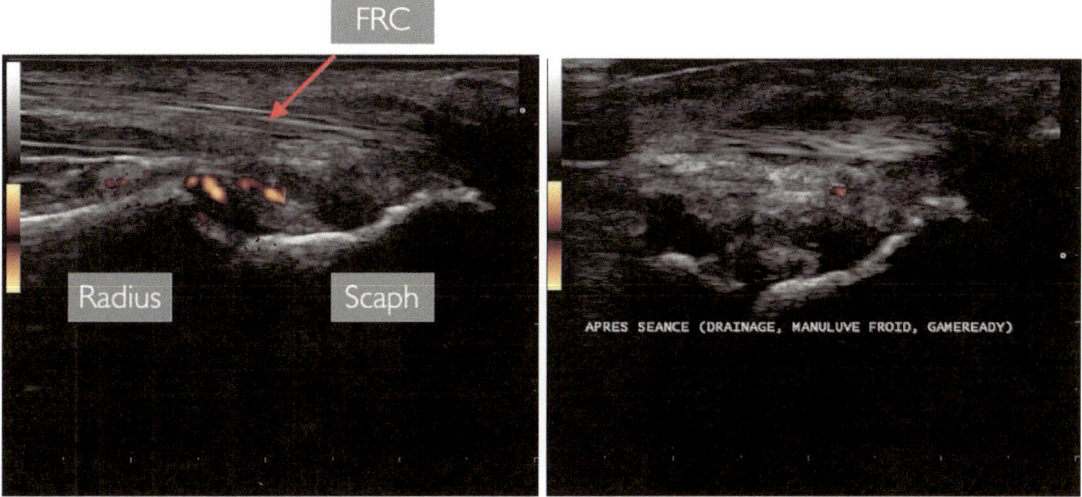

Fig. 1.51 Comparing the hyperemia at the beginning and at the end of the session to verify the short-term effectiveness of treatment

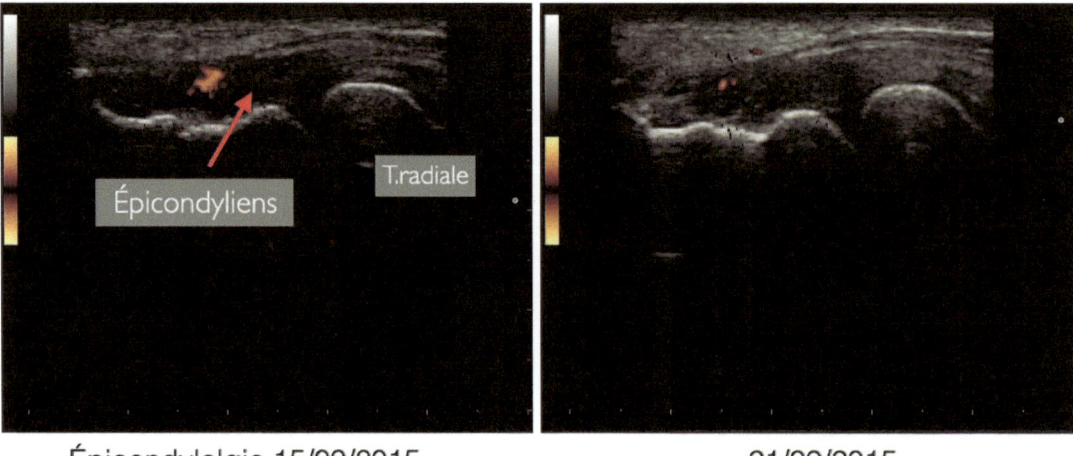

Épicondylalgie 15/09/2015   21/09/2015

Fig. 1.52 Comparing the hyperemia at the beginning of the treatment and 6 days later to verify the effectiveness of treatment

Didactic Aspect

Echoscopy shows symptoms and helps the therapist explain them to the patient with a dynamic visual support. It is most useful in tendon adhesions limiting active mobility.

Scientific Research

Physiotherapists specialize in movement. A dynamic exploration mean is the perfect research tool for this specificity.

References

1. Apard T, Brasseur J. L'échographie pour le chirurgien du membre supérieur. Montpellier: Sauramps Medical; 2019.
2. Le Bars D, Plaghki L. Douleurs: bases anatomiques, physiologiques et psychologiques. Douleurs aiguës, douleurs chroniques, soins palliatifs. Paris: éditins Med-line; 2001. p. 43–82.
3. Woolf C. What to call the amplification of nociceptive signals in the central nervous system that contribute to widespread pain? Pain. 2014;155(10):1911–2.
4. Spallone V, et al. Validation of DN4 as a screening tool for neuropathic pain in painful diabetic polyneuropathy. Diabet Med. 2012;2012(29):578–85.
5. Marquié L, Duarte L, Mauriès V. Les caractéristiques psychométriques du Questionnaire de douleur de Saint-Antoine en consultation d'algologie chez les personnes atteintes de cancer. Douleur Analg. 2008;21:52.
6. Spicher C, Desfoux N, Sprumont P. Atlas des territoires cutanés du corps humain: esthésiologie de 240 branches. Montpellier: Sauramps Medical; 2010.
7. Pellecchia GL. Figure-of-eight method of measuring hand size: reliability and concurrent validity. J Hand Ther. 2003;16(4):300–4.
8. Carrière ME, et al. Des échelles pour évaluer les cicatrices. Rev Francophone Cicatrisation. 2018;2(3):22–5.
9. Girard D, Desmoulière A. Cicatrisation normale et hypertrophique, influence de l'environnement mécanique. Rev Francophone Cicatrisation. 2018;2(3):12–6.
10. Canizares F, et al. Cicatrices cutanées défectueuses. Encycl Méd Chir, Techniques chirurgicales – Chirurgie plastique reconstructrice et esthétique. Paris: Elsevier SAS (tous droits réservés); 2003. p. 45–120.
11. Teot L, et al. Techniques de prise en charge des hypertrophies et congestions cicatricielles. Bulletin d'esthétique dermatologique et de cosmétologie. 2000:229–36.
12. Ferriero G, et al. Validation of a new device to measure postsurgical scar adherence. Phys Ther. 2010;90(5):776–83.
13. Baryza M, Barysa GA. The Vancouver Scar Scale: an administration tool and its interrater reliability. J Burn Care Rehabil. 1995;16(5):535–8.
14. Draaijers LJ, et al. The patient and observer scar assessment scale: a reliable and feasible tool for scar evaluation. Plast Reconstr Surg. 2004;113(7):1960–5. discussion 1966–7.
15. Blancher M-C, Noël L, Liverneaux P. Plaies nerveuses: évaluation et rééducation de la sensibilité. In: La traumatologie des parties molles de la main. Berlin: Springer; 2011. p. 229–47.

16. Dias N. Une pointe ou deux ?: Le destin anthropologique du compas de Weber. Terrain. 2007;49:51–62.
17. Fougeyrollas P. Classification québécoise: processus de production du handicap. Lac-St-Charles, Québec: RIPPH Réseau international sur le processus de production du handicap; 1998.
18. Roudaut Y, et al. Touch sense: functional organization and molecular determinants of mechanosensitive receptors. Channels (Austin). 2012;6(4):234–45.
19. Mabin D. Bilan de la sensibilité: aspects anatomophysiologiques, in Séméiologie de la main et du poignet. Montpellier: Sauramps Medical; 2001. p. 87–96.
20. Noel L, Liverneaux P. Prise en charge et rééducation des lésions nerveuses périphériques. In: EMC - Kinésithérapie - Médecine physique – Réadaptation. Paris: Elsevier Masson; 2013. p. 9 (10).
21. Mackel R, et al. Properties of cutaneous mechanosensitive afferents during the early stages of regeneration in man. Brain Res. 1985;329:49–69.
22. Spicher C, Roll JP. Manuel de rééducation sensitive du corps humain: des troubles de base de la sensibilité cutanée aux complications douloureuses: syndrome loco-régional douloureux complexe, allodynie mécanique, névralgie, lors de lésions neurologiques périphériques [et] cérébrales; 2003.
23. Berthe A, Orset G. Les bilans de la main et du poignet, in Rééducation de la main et du poignet, anatomie fonctionnelle et techniques. Paris: Elsevier Masson; 2013. p. 62–71.
24. Valembois B, et al. Rééducation des troubles de la sensibilité de la main. In: EMC Kinésithérapie - Médecine physique - Réadaptation. Paris: Elsevier Masson; 2006.
25. Moberg E. Objective methods for determining the functional value of sensibility in the hand. J Bone Joint Surg Br. 1958;40-B(3):454–76.
26. Al-Qattan MM. Semmes Weinstein monofilaments versus Weinstein enhanced monofilaments: their use in the hand clinic. Can J Plast Surg. 1995;3(1):51–3.
27. Weinstein S. Fifty years of somatosensory research. J Hand Ther. 1993;6(1):11–22.
28. Chaput E, et al. Evaluation clinique et choix thérapeutique fondés par les données probantes. E-News Somatosens Rehabil. 2007;14(2):55–65.
29. Grobnicu O, et al. Sensibilité de l'hémipulpe radiale de l'index — étude des tests de Semmes-Weinstein versus Cochet-Bonnet chez 25 sujets sains. Hand Surg Rehabil. 2018;37(6):451.
30. Novak CB. Evaluation of hand sensibility: a review. J Hand Ther. 2001;14(4):266–72.
31. Bell-Krotoski J, Weinstein S, Weinstein C. Testing sensibility, including touch-pressure, twopoint discrimination, point localization, and vibration. J Hand Ther. 1993;6(2):114–23.
32. Berquin AD, et al. An adaptive procedure for routine measurement of light-touch sensitivity threshold. Muscle Nerve. 2010;42(3):328–38.
33. Malenfant A, et al. Tactile, thermal and pain sensibility in burned patients with and without chronic pain and paresthesia problems. Pain. 1998;77(3):241–51.
34. Roll JP. Stimulation vibratoire transcutanée et douleur. Douleurs Éval - Diagn - Trait. 2019;20(5):226–31.
35. Purves D, et al. Le système somesthésique: sensibilité tactile et proprioception. Neurosciences (De Boeck Supérieur). 2019:193–211.
36. Jerosch-Herold C. Assessment of sensibility after nerve injury and repair: a systematic review of evidence for validity, reliability and responsiveness of tests. J Hand Surg Br. 2005;30(3):252–64.
37. Pascual-Leone A, et al. The plastic human brain cortex. Annu Rev Neurosci. 2005;28:377–401.
38. Spicher C, et al. La place du test de discrimination de 2 points statiques dans l'examen clinique. Douleur Analg. 2005;18(2):73–8.
39. Quintal I, et al. Méthode de rééducation sensitive de la douleur. In: EMC - Kinésithérapie – Médecine physique - Réadaptation. Paris: Elsevier Masson; 2013.
40. Spicher C. Manuel de rééducation sensitive du corps humain. Genève, Paris: Médecine et hygiène; 2003.
41. Menorca RM, Fussell TS, Elfar JC. Nerve physiology: mechanisms of injury and recovery. Hand Clin. 2013;29(3):317–30.
42. Arnold DMJ, et al. Criteria for symptomatic neuroma. Ann Plast Surg. 2019;82(4):420–7.
43. Marin Braun F. Syndrome douloureux par névrome post-traumatique. In: Lésions traumatiques des nerfs périphériques. Genève, Paris: Elsevier; 2007. p. 144–56.
44. Tubiana R. La main: anatomie fonctionnelle et examen clinique, ed. Paris: Masson; 1990.
45. Debrégeas G, Prevost A, Scheibert J. Toucher digital humain: transduction mécanique de l'information tactile et rôle des empreintes digitales. Images de la Physique; 2009. p. 11–17.
46. Lederman S, Klatzky R. Extracting object properties through haptic exploration. Acta Psychol. 1993;84:29–40.
47. Amirjani N, et al. Normative values and the effects of age, gender, and handedness on the Moberg pick-up test. Muscle Nerve. 2007;35(6):788–92.
48. Amirjani N, et al. Discriminative validity and test–retest reliability of the Dellon-modified Moberg pick-up test in carpal tunnel syndrome patients. J Peripher Nerv Syst. 2011;16:51–8.
49. Baker K. Functional tests for dexterity. In: Rehabilitation of the hand and upper extremity. Paris: Elsevier; 2020. p. 133–40.
50. Rosén B, Lundborg G. A new tactile gnosis instrument in sensibility testing. J Hand Ther. 1998;11(4):251–7.
51. Cooney W, et al. The kinesiology of the thumb trapeziometacarpal joint. J Bone Joint Surg Am. 1981;63:1371–81.
52. Kapandji IA. Physiologie articulaire tome 1 - Membre supérieur. Paris: Maloine; 2005.
53. Carter TI, et al. Accuracy and reliability of three different techniques for manual goniometry for

wrist motion: a cadaveric study. J Hand Surg Am. 2009;34(8):1422–8.

54. Fu E, et al. Elbow position affects distal radioulnar joint kinematics. J Hand Surg Am. 2009;34(7):1261–8.

55. Bain GI, et al. The functional range of motion of the finger joints. J Hand Surg Eur Vol. 2015;40(4):406–11.

56. Brand PW. Mechanical factors in joint stiffness and tissue growth. J Hand Ther. 1995;8(2):91–6.

57. Rayan G, Akelman E. The hand: anatomy, examination, and diagnosis. Philadelphia: Lippincott Williams and Wilkins; 2012.

58. Pratt AL, Ball C. What are we measuring? A critique of range of motion methods currently in use for Dupuytren's disease and recommendations for practice. BMC Musculoskelet Disord. 2016;17:20.

59. Mesplié G. Hand and wrist rehabilitation: theoretical aspects and practical consequences. Cham: Springer; 2015.

60. MacDermid J, Solomon G, Valdes K; American Society of Hand Therapists. Clinical assessment recommendations. 3rd ed. Mount Laurel, NJ: American Society of Hand Therapists; 2015.

61. Goubau JF, et al. The wrist hyperflexion and abduction of the thumb (WHAT) test: a more specific and sensitive test to diagnose de Quervain tenosynovitis than the Eichhoff's test. J Hand Surg Eur Vol. 2014;39(3):286–92.

62. Novak CB, et al. Provocative testing for cubital tunnel syndrome. J Hand Surg. 1994;19(5):817–20.

63. Cheng CJ, et al. Scratch collapse test for evaluation of carpal and cubital tunnel syndrome. J Hand Surg Am. 2008;33(9):1518–24.

64. Hagert E. Clinical diagnosis and wide-awake surgical treatment of proximal median nerve entrapment at the elbow: a prospective study. Hand (N Y). 2013;8(1):41–6.

65. Huynh MNQ, Karir A, Bennett A. Scratch collapse test for carpal tunnel syndrome: a systematic review and meta-analysis. Plast Reconstr Surg Glob Open. 2018;6(9):e1933.

66. Jimenez I, Delgado PJ. The scratch collapse test in the diagnosis of compression of the median nerve in the proximal forearm. J Hand Surg Eur Vol. 2017;42(9):937–40.

67. Bodin A, et al. Est-il nécessaire d'évaluer à la fois les scores QuickDASH et PRWE? Hand Surg Rehabil. 2016;25(6):434.

Clinical Reasoning in the Traumatic and Micro-Traumatic Pathologies of the Hand

2

Grégory Mesplié

A methodological clinical assessment will provide all the clinical elements needed for clinical reasoning and will therefore lead to the most adapted therapeutic orientations.

In traumatic and micro-traumatic injuries of the hand, the patients mostly complain about lack of motion, instability, and pain.

2.1   Lack of Motion

There are many factors responsible for stiffness [1] (Fig. 2.1), so knowing them precisely will allow the physical therapist to optimize the rehabilitation techniques and orthoses he will use. Measuring the lack of motion can be interesting, but a qualitative analysis is key in determining which structures are responsible for this lack of motion, and therefore what techniques will be used to treat it.

The possible etiologies for wrist and finger stiffness are detailed in Table 2.1, but, in any case, the clinical exam helps us identify three categories of lack of motion (Fig. 2.2):

2.1.1   Lack of Motion Depending on the Position of the Upper and Lower Joints

This type of lack of motion is related to the hypo-extensibility or peri-tendinous adhesion of the muscle antagonist to the movement.

Therefore, the treatment will be based on stretching techniques, fighting against peri-tendinous fibrosis (if it exists), and improving tendon gliding.

For example, in case of retraction of the interosseous muscles, the flexion of the interphalangeal joints is possible if the metacarpophalangeal

G. Mesplié (✉)
Institut Sud Aquitain de la Main et du Membre
Supérieur, Biarritz, France

FACTORS CAUSING STIFFNESS		
Factors	Effects	Treatment principles
Bone	Early abutment limiting movement, independent from the position of the next joints and not improving with mobilisation.	Surgery
Integument	Loss of mobility and extensibility of the integuments, limiting antagonist movements.	Specific scar treatment (see chapter : Scar massage and treatment)
Oedèma	Tensioning the integuments while resting. Additional tensioning while moving is impossible	Drainage. Compression bandage. Other specific techniques
Pain	Loss of mobility with no abutment at the end of the movement and no improving with mobilization	Depending of the type of pain (see chapter : Physiology and rehabilitation of sensorial and motor disorders)
Collagen	Stiffness with firm stop progressively improving with mobilization and independent from the position of the next joints	Adapted mobilization. Dynamic orthesis
Muscle	Stiffness when tensioning the hypo-extensible muscle	Stretching. Specific muscle relaxation techniques
Motor pattern	Bad kinematic that can cause a secondary tissue retraction	Re-learning gestures. rebalancing muscular ratios

Fig. 2.1 Factors causing stiffness

Table 2.1 Frequent etiologies for stiffness in fingers and wrist

Clinical signs and etiology for loss of joint mobility in the hand	
Clinical exam, tests	Étiology
Loss of flexion in the wrist	
Stiffness unchanged by the position of the next joints	1. Osteoarticular injuries
	2. Retractile dorsal skin scar
Stiffness more important when the fingers are flexed	Retraction or adhesion of the extensor system
Loss of extension in the wrist	
Stiffness unchanged by the position of the next joints	1. Osteoarticular injuries
	2. Retractile dorsal skin scar
Stiffness more important when the fingers are extended	Retraction or adhesion of the flexor system
Loss of flexion in the metacarpophalangeal joints	
Stiffness unchanged by the position of the wrist and interphalangeal joints	1. Osteoarticular injuries
	Retraction of the collateral ligaments' main bundles
	Retraction of the capsule's dorsal part
	2. Retractile dorsal skin scar
Stiffness more important when the interphalangeal joints are flexed	Adhesion of the extensor tendons in the back of the hand
Stiffness more important when the wrist is flexed	Adhesion of the extensor tendons in the back of the forearm
Loss of extension in the metacarpophalangeal joints	
Stiffness unchanged by the position of the wrist and interphalangeal joints	1. Osteoarticular injuries:
	Retraction of the collateral ligaments' accessory bundles and/or the volar plate
Stiffness more important when the interphalangeal joints are flexed	Hypo-extensibility of the interossei muscles

Table 2.1 (continued)

Clinical signs and etiology for loss of joint mobility in the hand	
Clinical exam, tests	Étiology
Loss of flexion in the proximal interphalangeal joints	
Stiffness unchanged by the position of the wrist and interphalangeal joints	1. Osteoarticular injuries
	Retraction of the collateral ligaments' main bundles
	Retraction of the capsule's dorsal part
	2. Retractile skin scar in the back of the first phalanx
Stiffness decreased when the metacarpophalangeal joint is extended. Stiffness more important when the metacarpophalangeal joint is flexed (Kilgore test)	Retraction or adhesion of the extensor tendon above the metacarpophalangeal joint
Limitation of active extension, active flexion, and passive flexion in the proximal interphalangeal joint	Retraction or adhesion of the extensor tendon in the back of the first phalanx
Stiffness more important when the metacarpophalangeal joint is extended (extrinsic + position) and less important if it is flexed. Finochietto test	Hypo-extensibility of the interossei muscles
No passive stiffness when the interphalangeal joints are flexed and the metacarpophalangeal joints are extended, but the position cannot be maintained actively	Hypo-extensibility of the lumbrical muscles
Paradox finger extension when asking for a finger flexion (Parkes' paradoxical extension syndrome)	
Loss of extension in the proximal interphalangeal joints	
Stiffness unchanged by the position of the next joints	1. Osteoarticular injuries
	Retraction of the collateral ligaments' accessory bundles and/or the volar plate
	2. Dupuytren's disease
	3. Retractile palmar skin scar
Deficit of extension increase when extending the wrist or the metacarpophalangeal joints	Retraction, adhesion, hypo-extensibility of the flexor system
Loss of flexion in the distal interphalangeal joints	
Stiffness unchanged by the position of the next joints	1. Osteoarticular injuries
	2. Adhesion or retraction of the extensor system in zonas 1 and 2
	3. Retractile skin scar in the back of the second phalanx
Passive flexion possible, active flexion impossible	Adhesion of the flexor tendon in its sheath
Stiffness increased when extending the proximal interphalangeal joint (Haines test)	Retraction of the oblique retinacular ligament
Loss of flexion in the distal interphalangeal joints	
Stiffness unchanged by the position of the next joints	1. Osteoarticular injuries:
	Retraction of the collateral ligaments' accessory bundles and/or the volar plate
	2. Retractile palmar skin scar at the level of the second phalanx
Stiffness increased when the proximal interphalangeal joints are extended	Retraction or adhesion of the flexor digitorum profundus

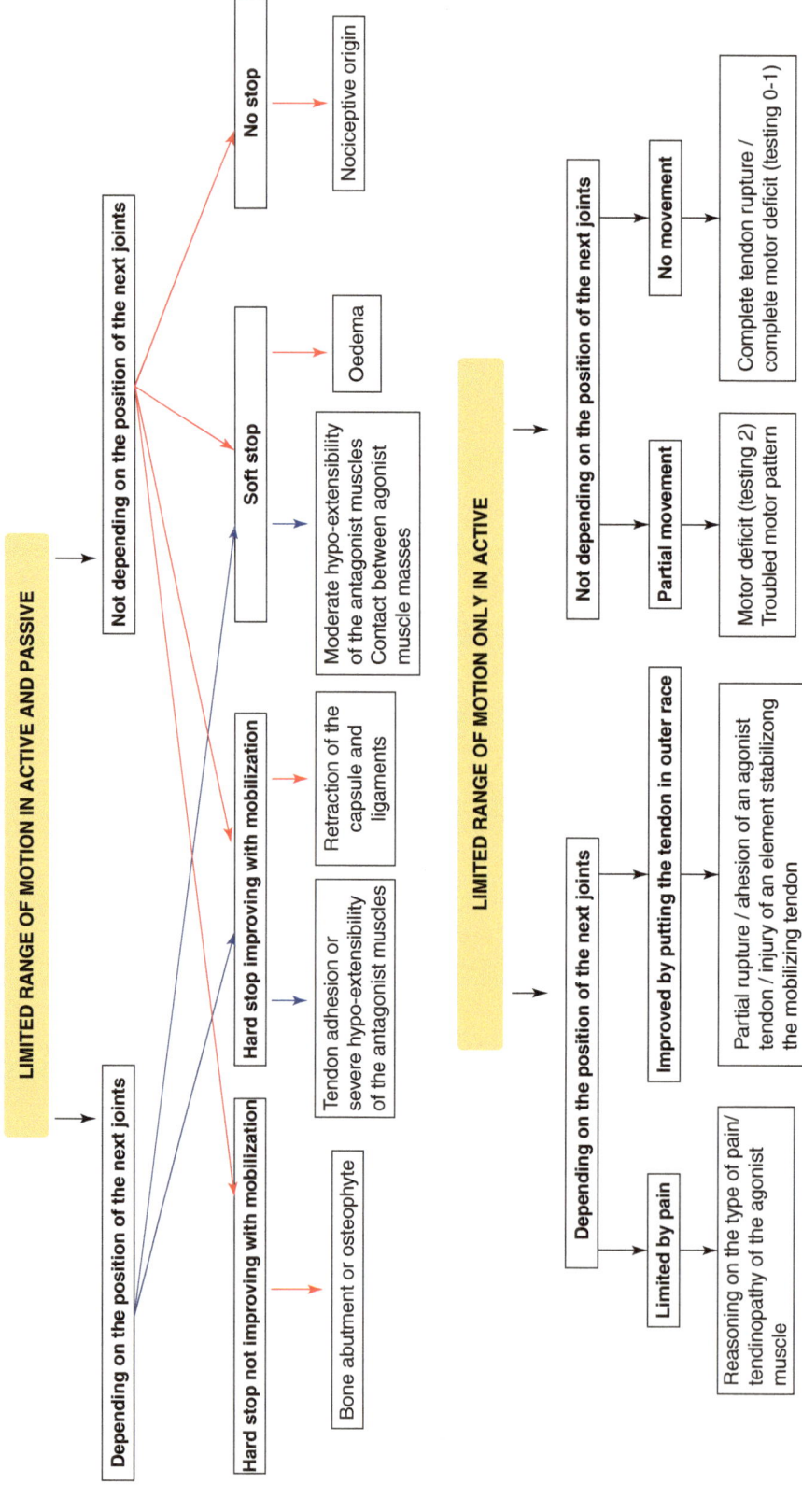

Fig. 2.2 Proposal for a clinical reasoning about the loss of range of motion

joints are flexed, but impossible if those joints are in extension. In this case, the main treatment will be to stretch the interosseous muscles (Fig. 2.3).

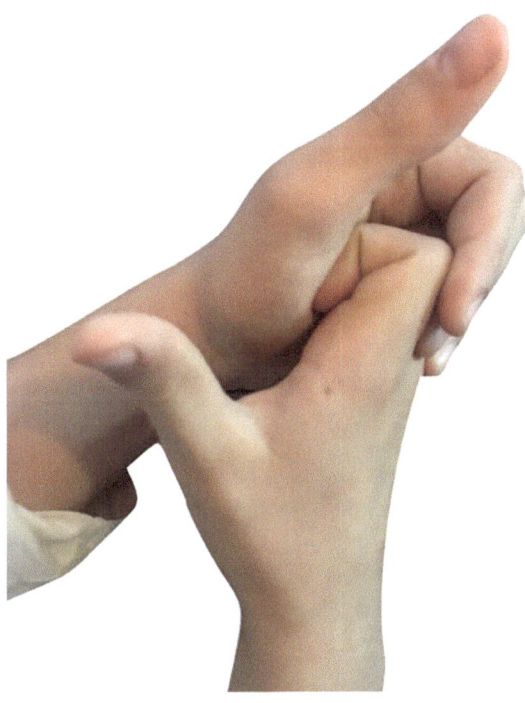

Fig. 2.3 Stretching position for the interossei muscles

On the contrary, if the extensor muscles adhere to the back of the metacarpals, the flexion of the interphalangeal joints will be possible if the metacarpophalangeal joints are in extension, but impossible with these joints in flexion. The main treatment will then be to work on the fibrosis and realize exercises improving the tendon gliding (Fig. 2.4).

2.1.2   Lack of Motion Not Depending on the Position of the Upper and Lower Joints

This kind of stiffness does not depend on the muscle systems. It can come from a joint limitation due to a capsule-ligamentous element (hard stop getting better with mobilization), or an osseous element (hard stop not changing with mobilization).

In case of a limitation due to connective tissue, the rehabilitator will use specific mobilizations and global mobilizations, always respecting the healing process. These mobilizations should be gentle and last long to adapt to the current scientific research regarding the connective tissue's response to stress [2] (Fig. 2.5).

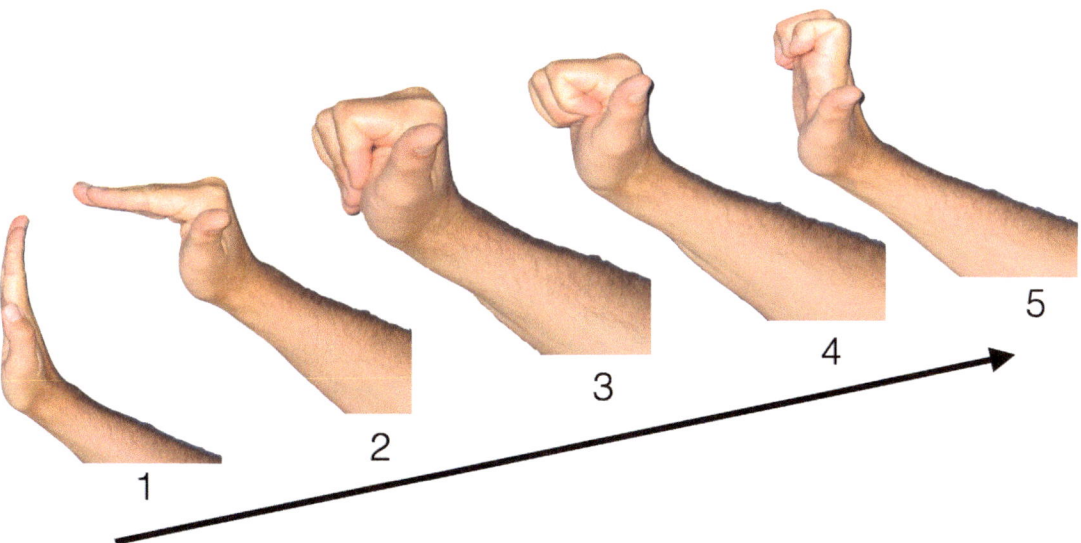

Fig. 2.4 Example for a series of finger movements facilitating extensor tendons gliding in various races. The wrist can also be placed in several positions to vary the difficulty of the exercise

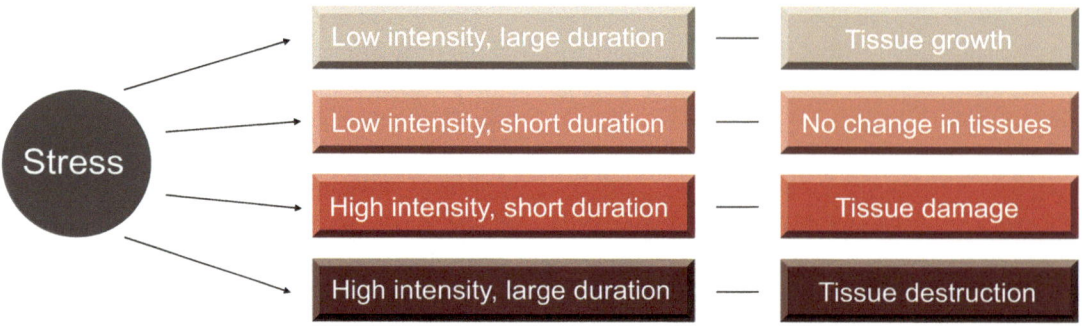

Fig. 2.5 How the connective tissue reacts to stress

Dynamic orthoses can be particularly useful in this type of stiffness [3], but for them to be efficient, they must be made during the second or third month following the injury and worn 6 h a day during at least 8 weeks [4].

If the lack of motion comes from an osseous element (bone or osteophyte), the physical therapist will have an extremely limited effect on it and the solution can be surgery.

An edema can also cause a lack of motion, as it tenses the cutaneous and subcutaneous tissues. In this kind of limitation, any mobilization that is too hard can maintain the trophic disorders, so treating the edema must be the priority to decrease the risk of fibrosis and secondary adhesions.

2.1.3 Lack of Active Motion

This lack of motion does not happen during passive mobilizations. It can be caused by a tendinous break, an injury of a motor nerve, or the injury of one of the elements stabilizing the tendon. In this case, the contraction can be less efficient, or even produce a movement opposed to the normal function.

For example, an injury of the sagittal strip of the extensor tendon at the level of the metacarpophalangeal joint can lead to a luxation of the tendon between the two metacarpals, thus making its contraction useless. If the tendon slips in front of the joint center, it can even flex the metacarpophalangeal joint.

2.2 Instabilities (Fig. 2.6)

2.2.1 Instabilities with Objective Evidence of Damaged Joint

For patients with signs of damaged joint (such as a "click" or cracking when gripping, pain when palpating the ligaments, and positive tests for joint laxity), rehabilitation must at first favor the healing of the damaged capsule-ligamentous elements. It should then concentrate on recovering an optimal neuromuscular function, especially regarding the muscles "protecting" the damaged ligament.

For example, in the metacarpophalangeal joint of the thumb, the adductor pollicis "protects" the ulnar collateral ligament while the abductor pollicis brevis and the flexor pollicis brevis "protect" the radial collateral ligament. In the metacarpophalangeal joints of the fingers, the muscles that play this part are the interosseous muscles homolateral to the injured collateral ligament [5].

2.2.2 Instabilities with No Objective Evidence of Damaged Joint

If the instability is not associated with signs of damaged joint, it can come from a neuromuscular deficit that will be highlighted with dynamometers, or a muscle testing in more severe cases.

Fig. 2.6 Proposal for a clinical reasoning about instability

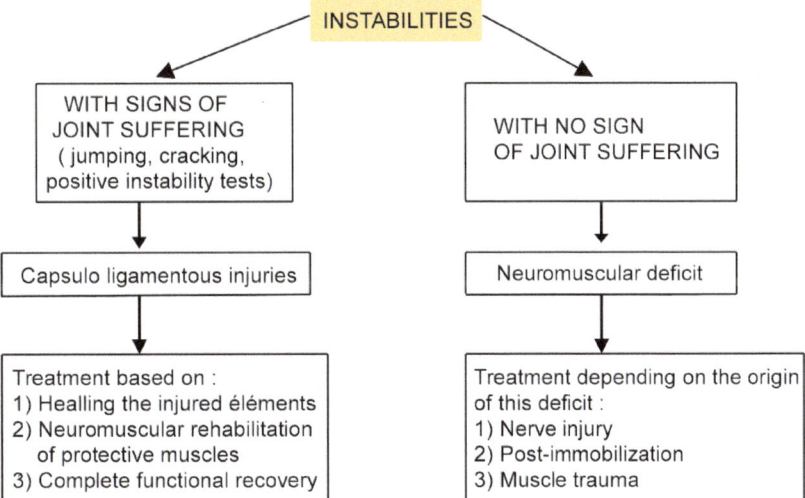

This type of instability can occur after a muscle traumatism, a motor nerve damage, or an immobilization even if it is for a short time. In fact, the first modifications to the motor and premotor cortex happen as early as 5 days after the beginning of the immobilization [6].

If there is an important motor damage with a scoring under 4 in the muscle testing, the protocol will have to be adapted to the stage of the injury (see Chap. 7). If not, the treatment will be a progressive proprioceptive rehabilitation, adapted to the patient's possibilities [7, 8] (see Chap. 8).

2.3   Pain (Fig. 2.7)

It is defined by the International Association for the Study of Pain (IASP) as "an unpleasant sensory and emotional experience associated with, or resembling that associated with, actual or potential tissue damage."

This definition highlights the multifactorial aspect of pain, and the fact that its intensity is not always related to the severity of the tissue injury.

This paragraph is about peripheral pain and does not cover central pain, which is usually treated in specialized centers.

2.3.1   Nociceptive Pain

A nociceptive pain is a sharp pain related to a tissue injury.

In these cases, the injury causing the painful message should be at the center of the treatment. The therapeutic orientation will depend on the other elements of the clinical assessment.

2.3.2   Neuropathic Pain

A neuropathic pain is a chronic pain, where the tissues are no longer the main cause of the problem: the tissue nociception—granted it still exists—is only participating in the clinical picture. Trying to decrease it usually has little positive impact on the patient [9].

The NP4 can be used to determine if the pain we are dealing with is neuropathic or not (sensitivity 80% and specificity 92%) [10]. We can also add other criteria to differentiate a neuropathic pain and a non-neuropathic central sensitization (Table 2.2).

If the neuropathic pain is not a mechanical allodynia, the physical therapist can use every sensorimotor rehabilitation tool, adapted to the patient's somatosensorial capacities. The tech-

Fig. 2.7 Proposal for a clinical reasoning about pain

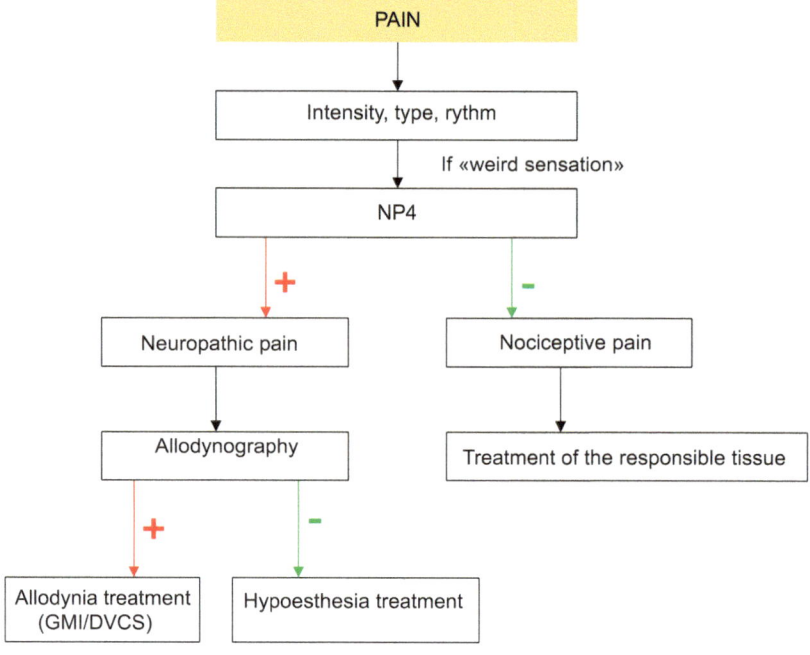

Table 2.2 Criteria participating in differentiating a neuropathic pain and a non-neuropathic central sensitization [11]

Neuropathic pain	Non-neuropathic central sensitization
The patient's history and the related medical diagnoses (stroke, diabetes, cancer, herpes, zoster, etc.) suggest an injury or a disease affecting the somatosensory system	The patient's history and the related medical diagnoses don't suggest a pathology affecting the somatosensory system
There is evidence (clinical/laboratory/imagery) confirming an injury or a disease affecting the somatosensory system	There is no evidence confirming an injury or a disease affecting the somatosensory system
Pain is logical, from a neuro-anatomical point of view	The location of the pain does not match a peripheral nerve territory or the body schema in the central nervous system
The pain is typically described as burning, throbbing, and tingling	The pain is mostly described as dull and diffuse
Sensory dysfunctions (hypoesthesia, allodynia) are found in the symptomatic area	Sensory dysfunctions are found outside and far away from the symptomatic area

niques used (touch exercises) must not trigger pain and can help improve the symptoms as they influence brain plasticity (see Chap. 7).

If the neuropathic pain is a mechanical allodynia (pain triggered by a usually non-painful stimulus), the physical therapist must not touch the concerned area; otherwise, he would increase the symptoms [12]. The treatment will be based on specific techniques such as progressive motor imagery [13], hypnosis, or distant vibrotactile counter-stimulation [14], as well as protecting the allodynic area in daily activities (see Chap. 7).

2.4 Conclusion

In conclusion, the treatment for traumatic and micro-traumatic injuries of the hand can only be optimal if realized after a thorough clinical assessment, leading to the selection of rehabilitation techniques adapted to the physiological origins and possible fears of our patients.

This clinical reasoning requires a good knowledge of the biomechanics and physiopathology of the hand, as well as a precise methodology when conducting the clinical examination.

References

1. Delprat J, et al. Rééducation des raideurs posttraumatiques des doigts. In: Encycl Méd Chir. Kinésithérapie-Médecine physique-Réadaptation, vol. 26-220-A-13; Paris: Masson; 2003. 16 p.
2. Nguyen T, et al. Effects of cell seeding and cyclic stretch on the fiber remodeling in an extracellular matrix-derived bioscaffold. Tissue Eng Part A. 2009;15(4):957–63.
3. Glasgow C, et al. Dynamic splinting for the stiff hand after trauma: predictors of contracture resolution. J Hand Ther. 2011;24(3):195–205; quiz 206.
4. Valdes K, et al. Efficacy of orthotic devices for increased active proximal interphalangeal extension joint range of motion: a systematic review. J Hand Ther. 2019;32(2):184–93.
5. Mesplié G. Sprains of the metacarpophalangeal joint of the thumb. In: Hand and wrist rehabilitation. Cham: Springer; 2015. p. 173–88.
6. Roll R, et al. Illusory movements prevent cortical disruption caused by immobilization. NeuroImage. 2012;62(1):510–9.
7. Hagert E. Proprioception of the wrist joint: a review of current concepts and possible implications on the rehabilitation of the wrist. J Hand Ther. 2010;23(1):2–16; quiz 17.
8. Mesplie G, et al. Rehabilitation of distal radioulnar joint instability. Hand Surg Rehabil. 2017;36(5):314–21.
9. Woolf C. What to call the amplification of nociceptive signals in the central nervous system that contribute to widespread pain? Pain. 2014;155(10):1911–2.
10. Spallone V, et al. Validation of DN4 as a screening tool for neuropathic pain in painful diabetic polyneuropathy. Diabet Med. 2012;29(5):578–85.
11. Mesplié G. Raisonnement clinique dans les pathologies traumatiques et micro-traumatiques de la main. Kinésithérapie, la revue. 2020;20(222):69–77.
12. Mesplié G. Rééducation de la main - Bilan diagnostique, techniques de rééducation et poignet traumatique, vol. Tome 1. Montpellier: Sauramps Médical; 2011.
13. Moseley GL. Graded motor imagery for pathologic pain: a randomized controlled trial. Neurology. 2006;67(12):2129–34.
14. Packham TL, et al. Somatosensory rehabilitation for allodynia in complex regional pain syndrome of the upper limb: a retrospective cohort study. J Hand Ther. 2018;31(1):10–9.

Part II

Rehabilitation Tools and Techniques

Grégory Mesplié

3.1 Cryotherapy

The etymology of the word "cryo" comes from the Greek "crio," meaning "cold" or "frost."

The "cryo-therapy" is, therefore, a therapy based on using cold temperatures according to specific modalities guaranteeing efficiency and safety for the patients.

3.1.1 Local Effects When Applying Cold

Applying cold locally can help with the tissue healing process. Here are the steps of this process:

- **Vascular and exudative phase**: Healing cells arrive on the area and an edema occurs. The interest of this phase is to destroy the causal agent and to clean up the injured area to allow the activation of the healing process.
- **Granulomatous phase**: A hyper-vascularized connective tissue burgeons.
- **Remodeling phase** for the connective bourgeon.

By applying cold, we optimize the healing process, fight against pain, and avoid complica-

tions related to the vicious circle "Pain-Stiffness-Edema."

The vasomotor reaction we get when applying cold locally is complex:

- **Vasoconstriction** of the vessels, thus limiting heat distribution and leading to the tissues getting colder and the cell metabolism slowing down.
- **Vasodilatation**, which is paradoxical, happens after about 10 min.

If the cold application is maintained, these two phases keep occurring according to the "Hunting-reaction" [1] or Lewis's reaction, that is to say with from 1 to 3 cycles every 30 min.

When the cold application is stopped, a vasodilatation occurs. Its intensity depends on the vasomotor state when the application is stopped.

The effects we are looking for are:

- **Anti-inflammatory**, thanks to the vasomotor and metabolic consequences of the cold application [1]. The vasoconstriction decreases the blood flow and minimizes the formation of the edema, while the slowdown of the cell metabolism limits the inflammatory mediators release (amines and peptides). Some authors say that the anti-edema effect is due to the alternance between vasoconstriction and vasodilatation, which would have a "pumping" effect on the arterial and venous systems.

G. Mesplié (✉)
Institut Sud Aquitain de la Main et du Membre
Supérieur, Biarritz, France

Objective	Mechanism	Method
Reducing the secondary hypoxic injuries	Decreasing the enzymatic metabolism	<11°C
Fighting against pain	Gate control Decreasing the conduction speed in Aδ and C fibers Decreasing the enzymatic metabolism	<13,6°C <12,5°C <11°C
Limiting the formation of oedema	Vasoconstriction Decreasing the capillary permeability	Gradual cooling to reach a skin temperature of aprrroximately 14,3°C
Encouraging arteriovenous exchanges	Vasodilatation Increasing the capillary permeability	Fast cooling during 3 min to reach a skin temperature of approximately 7°C

Fig. 3.1 Application modalities and objectives of cryotherapy [3]

- **Anti-hemorrhagic**, thanks to the vasomotor phenomenon related to cold.
- **Muscle relaxant** because of the inhibition of the gamma motoneurons causing the muscle tone to drop.
- **Analgesic,** thanks to the anti-inflammatory effects, because the conduction decreases in nociceptive fibers and the nociceptors become less excitable when applying cold [2].

3.1.2   Application

To get the effects described in the previous paragraph, we should lower the skin temperature under 15 °C. However, the temperature should not be under 7 °C, or else we run the risk of tissue injury (in the nerves in particular). The temperature should be adapted to the primary objectives [3] (Fig. 3.1).

Moreover, it appears that the anti-edema effect would be substantially improved if combined with a compression [4].

3.1.3   Ice Bag and Similar Techniques

Applying cold on tissues is a technique that has been used for many years, with ice bags or other

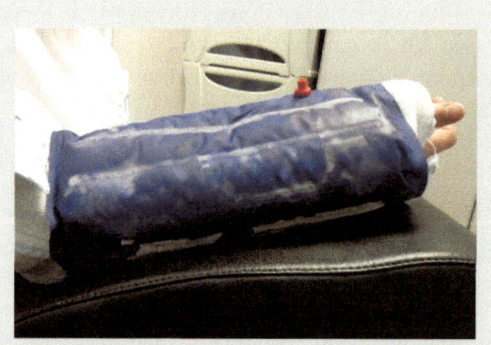

Fig. 3.2 The anti-edema trio: cold-compression-elevation

It should be noted that there are some systems that combine the application of cold and a compression. This, combined with an elevation of the limb, helps implementing the anti-edema trio: Cold-compression-elevation (Fig. 3.2).

similar techniques with a temperature of −0.5 °C. These techniques are easy to implement and low cost, and allow reducing the skin temperature to less than 15 °C. We usually advise an application lasting 15–20 min, two to three times a day.

Using a cloth can be helpful to avoid burns. It is better if the cloth is humid, so it does not decrease the intensity or the duration of the lowering of the temperature.

3.1.4 Immersion

It is a technique which mostly has a myo-relaxing effect and is therefore ideal in spastic patients.

The hand is placed in a water at 7 °C during no longer than 4–5 min.

On the contrary, for a shorter exposition to a cold temperature, the muscle tone increases.

3.1.5 Gaseous Cryotherapy

There are devices expelling CO_2 at a temperature of −78 °C, and others with compressed air that expel air at a temperature of −50 °C (Fig. 3.3).

The application modalities can change depending on the device, but the principle stays: lower the skin temperature to 7 °C (30 s–1 min), then maintain it at 10 °C for 10 min using the same device or with ice bags.

Using a laser thermometer helps following these modalities (Fig. 3.4).

It seems that this technique is the most efficient on all the factors described earlier, especially if it is combined with a compression and a position with the limb elevated [5].

3.1.6 System Combining Compression and Cryotherapy

Some modern devices associate a controlled compression with cryotherapy. The temperature can be controlled as well, so we can get an interesting analgesic and trophic effect (Fig. 3.5).

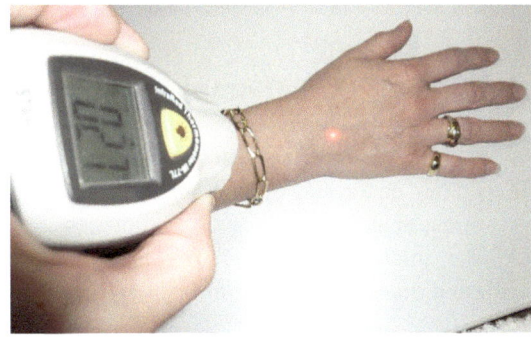

Fig. 3.4 Laser thermometer controlling the protocol as well as possible

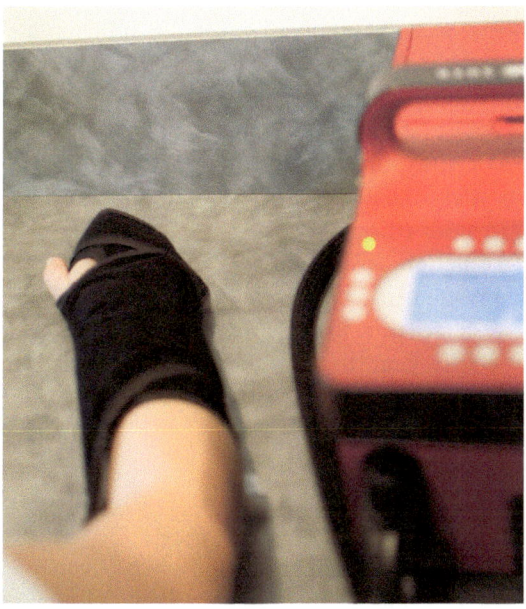

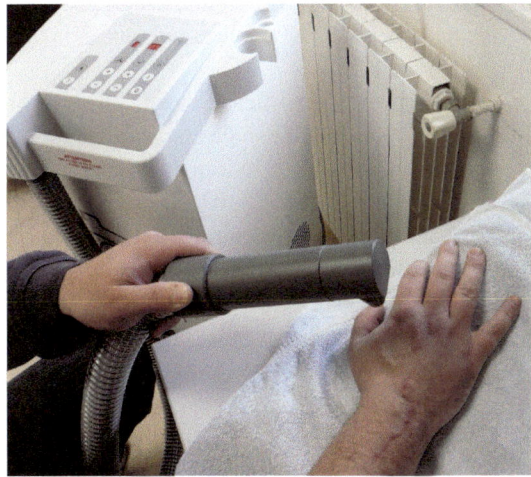

Fig. 3.3 Air-compression device expelling air at approximately −50 °C

Fig. 3.5 System combining cryotherapy and pressotherapy, with settable values

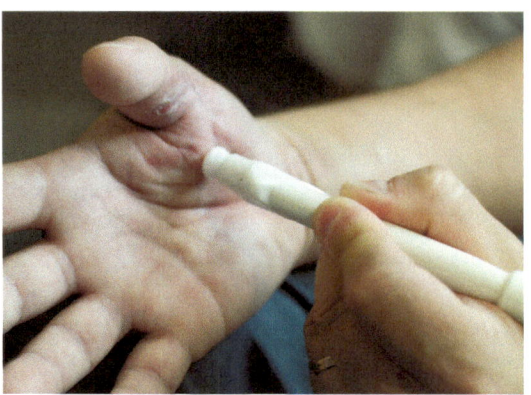

Fig. 3.6 Use on a non-inflammatory scar

3.2 Depresso-Therapy

It is a device creating a localized depression, depending on the size of the used head. It helps in scar treatment, softening and draining them.

The intensity and type of suction can be adjusted depending on the indications:

- **Pulse mode and/or low suction intensities** when the scar is still inflammatory, moving the head far from the scar. Like this, we can mobilize and drain the tissues close to the scar without maintaining its inflammatory state. This state can be assessed by diascopy, with a recoloring of the scar faster than 2 s (see Chap. 1).
- **Continuous mode and/or higher intensities** when the scar is not inflammatory anymore (diascopy > 2 s—see Chap. 1). The suction is applied directly on the scar to soften it and speed up its evolution by decreasing the edema, as it stimulates the angiogenesis and the granulation tissues (Fig. 3.6).

3.3 Electrotherapy

Electrostimulation consists of a production of action potentials on excitable cells (nerve or muscle) using an electric current.

3.3.1 Essential Notions

The work of Weiss and Lapicque helps us understand better the essential rules of electrostimulation and draw therapeutic applications.

The main formula from their work is:

$$Q = q + I \cdot t$$
where Q is the quantity of current needed to reach the threshold
t is the duration of the current impulse
I is the impulse intensity
Q is a coefficient experimentally determined, corresponding to the intersection between the curve and the ordinate axis

The curve Intensity-Duration helps defining two essential electrostimulation notions (Fig. 3.7):

- **Rheobase**: Minimal stimulation intensity, even with a long impulse duration.
- **Chronaxie**: Minimal application duration for a current which intensity is twice the rheobase, to get a stimulation.

The optimal current (production of an action potential and optimal comfort) must meet several criteria:

- Current impulses (constant current generator).
- Rectangular shape for a fast efficiency and a reduction of the application duration and intensity.
- Bipolar with a zero mean to avoid burns due to polarization (even if some applications require polarized currents, like ionophoresis).
- Impulse duration equal to the chronaxie of the structure we want to stimulate, thus reducing the electric energy we use.

3.3.2 Practical Impact: Striomotor Currents

This type of current produces a muscle contraction and has several therapeutic interests:

Fig. 3.7 Intensity-duration curve

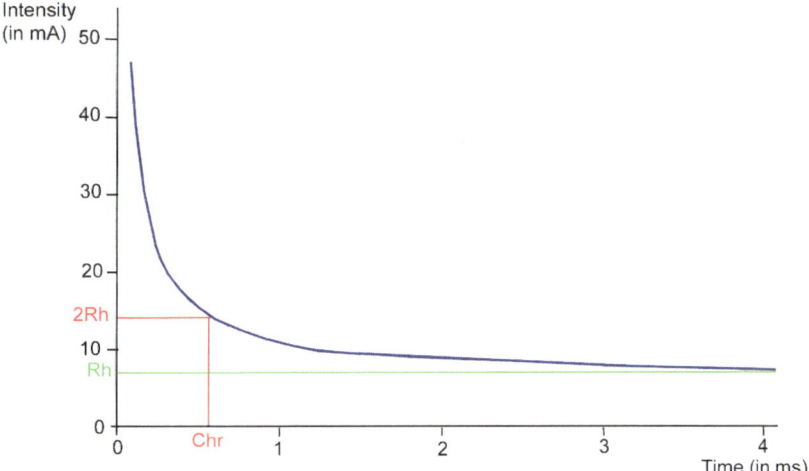

- Improving the muscle trophicity.
- Sensorimotor effect.
- Analgesic effect (gate-control).
- Improving the synchronization between motor units.

Using striomotor currents alone only affects muscle trophicity as there is no motor command. If we combine it with an active muscle contraction, we can get a better coordination at the intramuscular (synchronizing the muscle motor units) and extra-muscular (synchronizing with the other muscles) level. This way, we can optimize all the elements identified earlier.

An electrically induced contraction results in a higher energetic stimulation than the one required with a voluntary muscle contraction—with the same developed force.

Therefore, these currents can be used when working on muscle reinforcement, with several goals: analgesic, proprioceptive, or to improve joint amplitudes.

The motor unit is made of the neuron (anterior horn of the spinal cord), the axon, the neuromuscular synapse (motor plate), and the corresponding muscle fibers. We can get a muscle contraction when stimulating these elements, knowing that the nerve cells are more excitable than the muscle cells. The innervation rate corresponds to the number of muscle fibers innerved by a motoneuron (the smaller it is, the greater the precision of the contraction).

3.3.2.1 Innervated Muscles

The characteristics will depend on the location and the type of motor unit. We want to stimulate the nerve cells that are easier to stimulate than the muscle cells.

For the upper limb, the ideal impulse width is 200–400 ms [6].

For type 1 motor units (type I muscle fibers, aerobic chain), the ideal frequency is between 20 and 30 Hz. For type 2 motor units (type IIa and IIb muscle fibers, anaerobic lactic and alactic chains), the ideal frequency is between 30 and 80 Hz. Higher frequencies are above the physiological frequencies, they can produce muscle tetany [6] and are therefore of no interest for this kind of stimulation.

A wide majority of electrostimulation devices use rectangular biphasic currents with a zero mean, for the reasons mentioned in the previous chapter (Fig. 3.8).

When there is an active muscle contraction, there is a "turn-over" between the motor units, limiting the fatigue and making the contraction more synchronized during the electrostimulation (even more so as the intensity of the stimulation increases) [7] (Fig. 3.9).

This physiological difference leads to an increased fatigability during an electrostimulation, which must be compensated for by rest periods between the electric stimuli. The best ratio between rest periods and stimulation periods is 1:5.

Location	Type of concerned motor unit	Pulse width	Frequency
Superior limb		200 to 400 µs	
	Type I, aerobic way		20 to 30 Hz
	Type IIa and IIb, lactic anaerobic way and alactic anaerobic way		30 to 80 Hz

Fig. 3.8 Types of currents used for innervated muscles in the superior limb depending on the targeted motor units

Fig. 3.9 Increase of the number of muscle fibers requested when increasing the intensity of the electric current

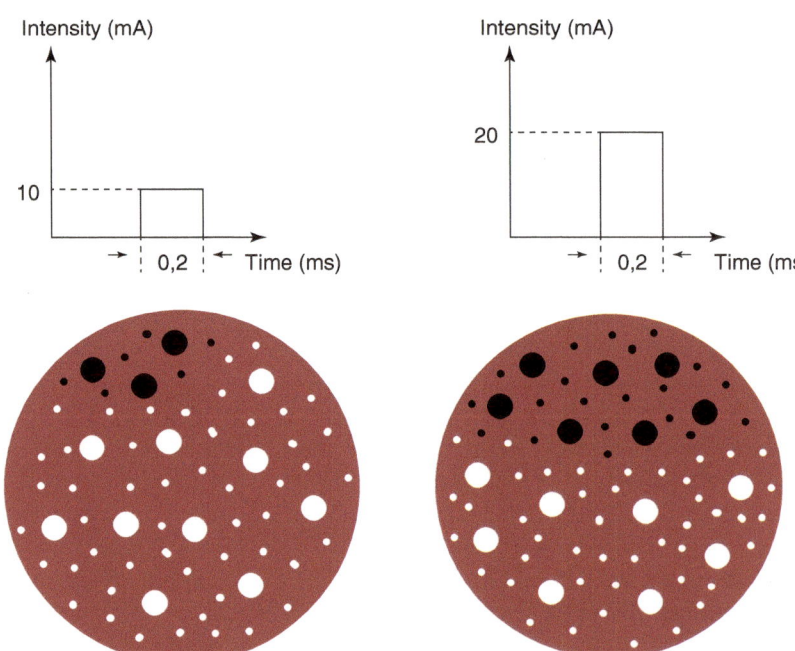

In practice, we ask the patient to participate in the contraction produced by the electric impulse to maintain the intentional control. Each contraction period is followed by an associated rest period, with low frequency currents (not tetanizing).

The electrodes are placed according to the muscle we want to stimulate. The proximal electrode is placed at the level of the nerve trunk corresponding to the muscle we want to stimulate, and the distal electrode is placed at the level of its motor point. Placing the electrodes is not always easy, as the density of motor points is particularly high in the forearm and the hand [8] (Fig. 3.10).

3.3.2.2 Denervated Muscles

Electrical stimulations can help in promoting nerve regeneration [9] after surgery.

When the muscle is completely denervated, the electric currents must stimulate the muscle fiber directly, which is less excitable than the motor nerve.

When the muscle is partially denervated, the currents can stimulate the motor nerve to act on the muscle fibers that are still innervated, or directly on the muscle fiber.

These stimulations help preventing muscle atrophy and fibrosis related to muscle disuse.

Muscle action	Proximal electrod placement	Distal electrod placement	Position of the wrist and forearm	Image
Flexer digitorum superficialis	Median nerve/ medial epicondyle	For the 3rd, 4th and 5th fingers : in the middle of the anterior part of the forearm. More external for the index finger	Supination or reference position. No wrist extension.	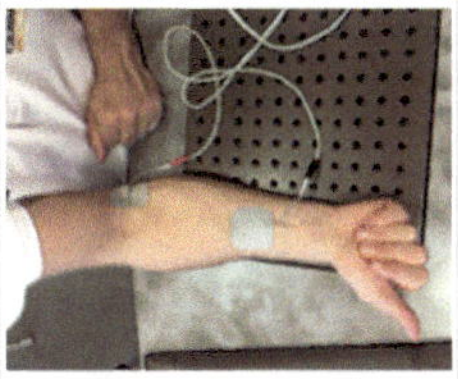
Flexer digitorum profundus (ulnar)	Ulnar nerve above the elbow.	In the middle of the posterior part of the forearm, on the internal side of the ulna.	Supination or reference position. No wrist extension	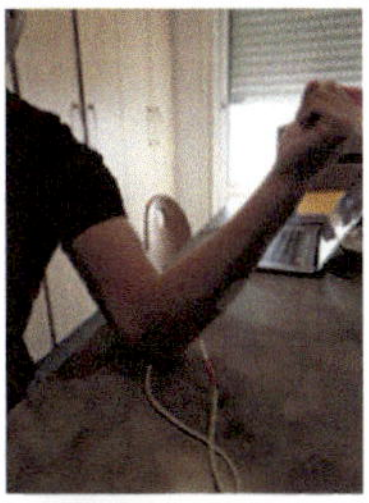
Flexer digitorum profundus (radial)	Median nerve above the elbow	Between the radius and the ulna on the posterior side of the forearm	Pronation or reference position. No wrist extension	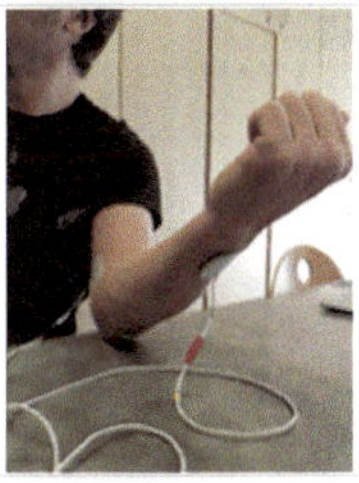
Global fingers flexion	Nerve trunks. Internal part of the arm between the biceps and triceps	At the elbow crease, medial to the biceps tendon	Reference position. No wrist extension.	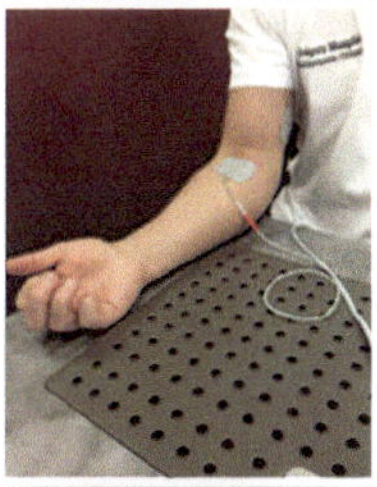
Flexer pollicis longus	Median nerve above the elbow	Between the inferior 1/3 and the middle 1/3 of the forearm, on the anterior and external part.	Supination. No wrist extension	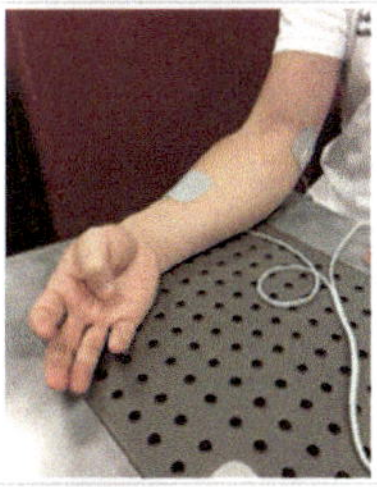
Wrist and fingers extension	Radial nerve above the elbow	Posterior side of the middle 1/3 of the forearm	Pronation	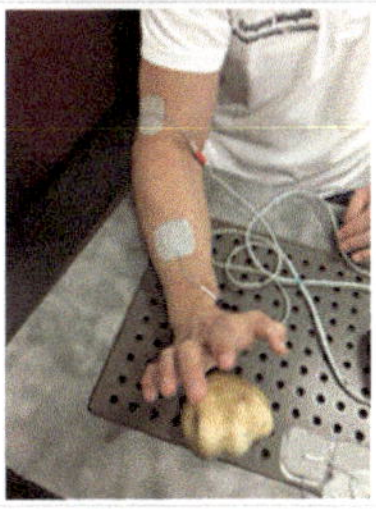

Fig. 3.10 Electrode placement

Muscle action	Proximal electrod placement	Distal electrod placement	Position of the wrist and forearm	Image
Thumb extension and abduction	Radial nerve above the elbow	Posterior external side of thesuperior 1/3 of the forearm	Pronation	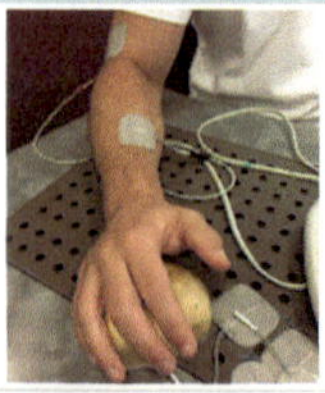
Index extension	Radial nerve above the elbow	Posterior external side of the middle 1/3 of the forearm	Pronation	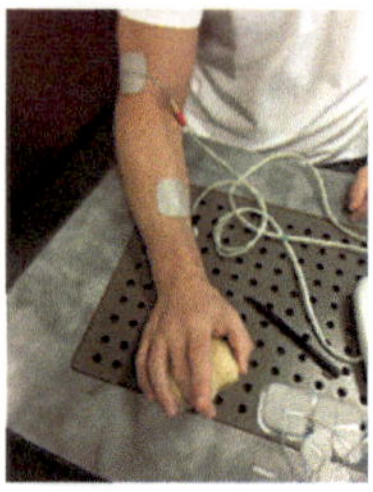
5th finger extension	Radial nerve above, the elbow	Posterior, internal side of the middle 1/3 of tthe forearm	Pronation	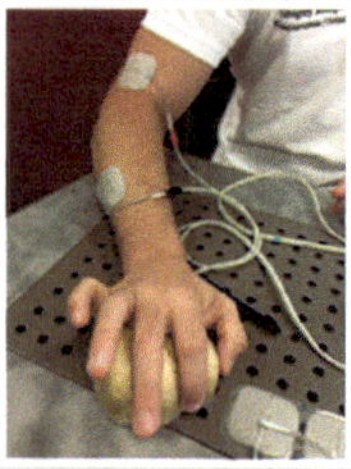
Extensor carpi radialis (brevis and longus)	Radial nerve above the elbow	Posterior side of the superior 1 /3 of the forearm	Pronation	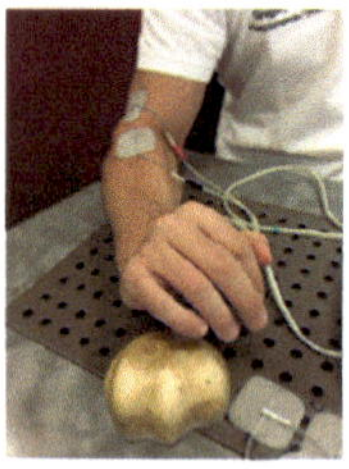
Extensor carpi ulnaris	Radial nerve above the elbow	Posterior, internal side of the middle 1/3 of the forearm, medial to the ulnar ridge	Pronation	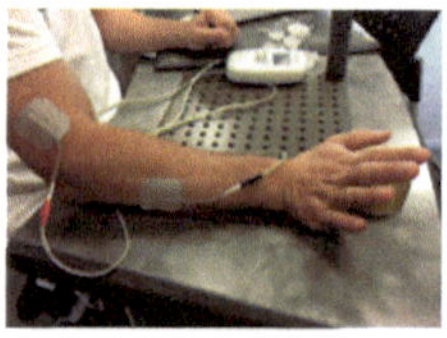
Flexer carpi radialis	Median nerve above the elbow	Anterior external side of the proximal middle 1/3 of the arm	Supination	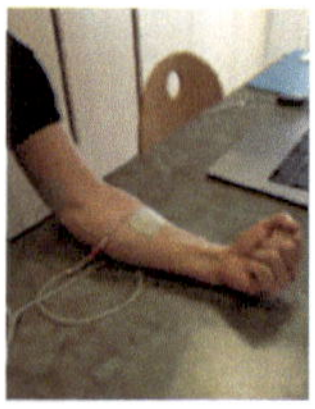

Fig. 3.10 (continued)

Muscle action	Proximal electrod placement	Distal electrod placement	Position of the wrist and forearm	Image
Flexor carpi ulnaris	Ulnar nerve above the elbow	Anterior internal part of the forearm, at 1/2	Supination	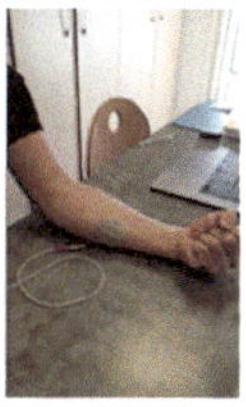
Pronator quadratus	Median nerve (anterior interosseous)	Between the radius and tthe ulna on the posterior side of the forearm	Supination	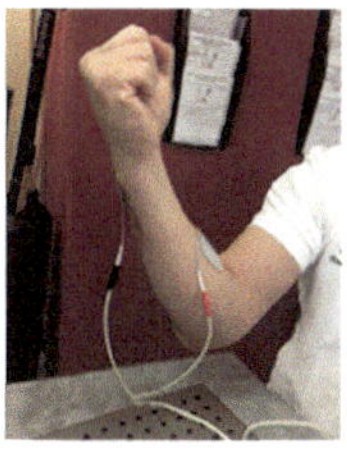
Pronator teres	Median nerve above the elbow	At the elbow crease, medial to the biceps'tendon	Supination	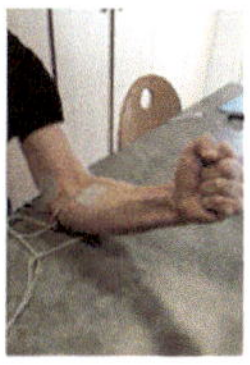
First dorsal interosseous	Ulnar nerve between the medial epicondyle and the olecranon	At the level of the first dorsal interosseous	Pronation	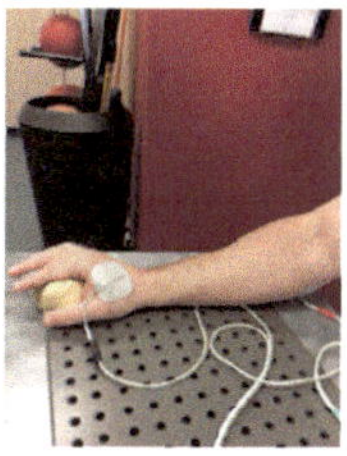

Fig. 3.10 (continued)

In practice, we use several types of electric current depending on the nerve injury. In case of neurapraxia, we use the same currents as the ones for innervated muscles.

In case of neurotmesis with complete denervation and a surgical repair, we use a unidirectional impulse with fixed or alternating polarity, rectangular, separated with rest periods lasting at least 1 s, and with an impulse width of 0.1 ms. The ideal frequency seems to be 20 Hz, applied continuously during an hour [9]. The intensity must produce a muscle contraction, and the electrodes are placed next to the nerve we want to stimulate [10].

This last application can be combined with passive mobilizations of the concerned joint and imagined movements to maintain the patient's motor pattern.

3.3.3 Practical Impact: Analgesic Currents

The analgesic effect of electrostimulation can be achieved with low frequency (2–8 Hz) [7] or high frequency (25–150 Hz) currents. Their actions are complementary and take part in peripheral and central pain regulation, thanks to

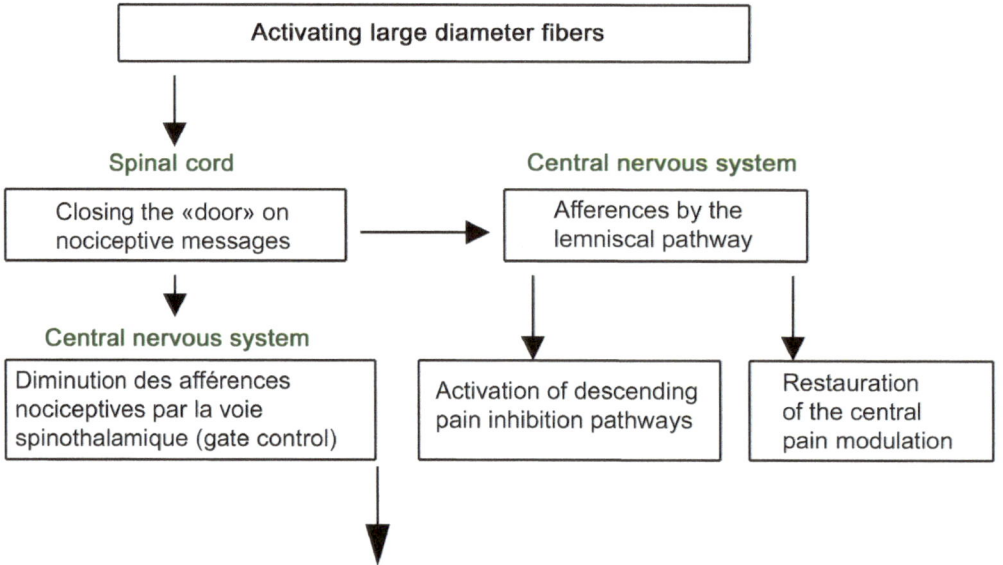

Fig. 3.11 Physiological effects of analgesic currents

their effects on neurotransmitters (beta-endorphin, methionine-enkephalin), central excitability, and various peripheral mechanisms (lowering the level of substance P, gate control) [11] (Fig. 3.11).

For both these analgesic currents, a daily use is a significant efficiency factor [12].

3.3.3.1 High Frequency TENS

We use currents with an impulse width of 40–75 ms, and a frequency wobbled between 25 and 150 Hz (the wobble is the variation of the frequency, lessening the habituation without increasing the intensity). We use bipolar currents with a zero mean.

We place two same-sized electrodes around the painful area or proximally to it, depending on the concerned nerve path (Fig. 3.12).

The intensity must be one where the patient feels intense "tingling," but still comfortable for the concerned area. The current is applied for 30 min.

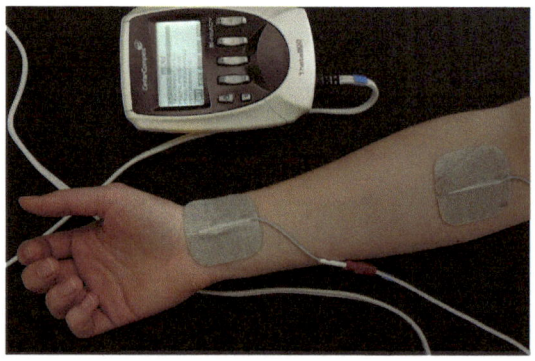

Fig. 3.12 Electrodes placement for high-frequency TENS on the median nerve territory

3.3.3.2 Low Frequency TENS

We use currents with and impulse width of 150–250 ms and a frequency between 2 and 8 Hz. The currents are bipolar with a zero mean.

We place two large electrodes (at least 150 cm^2) on the spine and/or on the painful area.

The intensity must produce fasciculations on the stimulated area.

3.3.3.3 Mixed Currents

We use two different generators to combine the effects of the two types of currents.

This protocol is particularly useful in CRPS.

3.3.4 Practical Impact: Tonolysis

Applying an electrostimulation with extremely low frequency leads to muscle relaxing.

We use stimulations with an impulse width of 150 ms for the upper limb (200 for the trunk and 250 for the lower limb), and a frequency of 1 Hz.

We place the active electrode (anode) on the contractured area, and a bigger one anywhere else (Fig. 3.13).

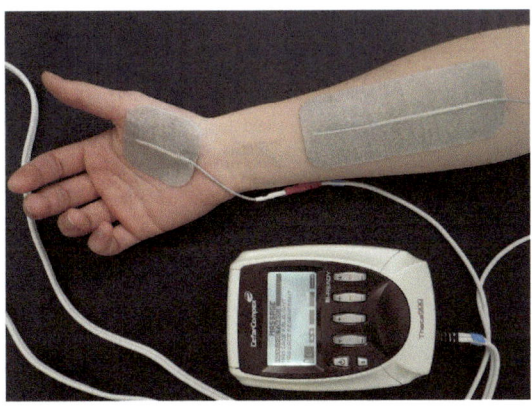

Fig. 3.13 Tonolysis current for thenar muscles. The large electrode is placed wherever, and the smaller (active) one is placed on the treated area

The intensity must provoke a "twitch" in the concerned muscle.

3.3.5 Practical Impact: Ionophoresis

We use a galvanic (polarized) current to ionize drug substances so that they penetrate the tissues better.

Positive drug substances will be attracted towards the cathode (negative electrode) and pushed away from the anode (positive electrode), and vice versa.

One electrode is the "active" one and is soaked in the drug substance depending on its ionization (the anode for positive substances and the cathode for negative substances).

The application duration depends on the treatment.

The ideal intensity is 0.1 mA/cm^2 on the active electrode.

3.4 Fluidotherapy and Thermotherapy

3.4.1 Fluidotherapy

Using hot water or air (Fig. 3.14), we obtain a relaxation of the tissues as their viscoelasticity increases, thus helping improve joint motion [13].

These techniques combine mechanical (buoyancy or displacement resistance), thermic (warming up), and physical (emollient) effects.

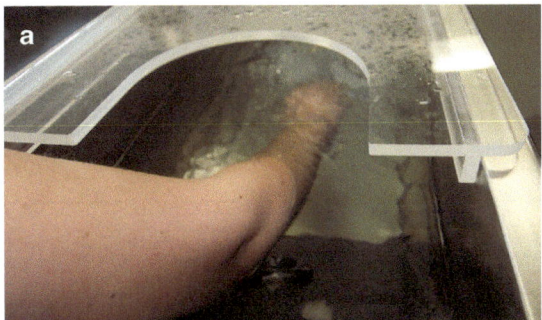 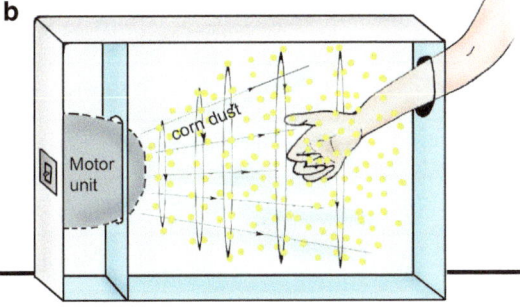

Fig. 3.14 Device allowing the hand to be immersed in hot water and massaged by jets (**a**), and dry fluidotherapy system combining a hot air flow with corn dust (**b**)

The immersion lasts approximately 20 min, the patient stays still or realizes slow pain-free movements.

These techniques can only be used if there is no wound to avoid any septic risk.

Some devices combine the effect of heat with a mechanical stimulation with sawdust or marbles (glass, steel, or ceramic). They have an analgesic effect and improve local trophicity, sensitivity, or even the scar (Fig. 3.15).

Immersion in hot baths can be more useful than applying hot packs for improving joint motion [13].

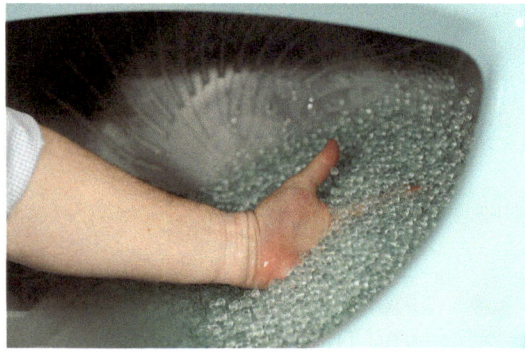

Fig. 3.15 Wet fluidotherapy combined with a massage by small glass marbles

3.4.2 Heat

We can use heated materials that match the shape of the hand or forearm to improve the viscoelasticity of tissues, relax the muscles and enhancing gliding between the different layers of tissues.

It can be hot packs such as cherry pit heat pillows or paraffin baths. They can have an opposite or similar effect to the application of cold (Table 3.1).

With cherry pit heat pillows, we can ask the patient to move slowly for a global warm-up of the hand or wrist. This exercise lasts 20–30 min (Fig. 3.16).

For paraffin baths, the patient can leave his hand resting, or take a position with maximal amplitudes so that the posture is tolerated better, or even easier thanks to the heat. The ideal temperature seems to be 50 °C [14].

The patient realizes 10 baths (lasting a few seconds), leaving a layer of paraffin between each bath. He then keeps the paraffin "glove" for 15 min before taking it off (Fig. 3.17).

Paraffin baths seem to be particularly interesting in scleroderma [15] and arthrosis, with significant results after 3 months [14] if the

Table 3.1 Compared physiological effects between heat and cold

	CRYOTHÉRAPIE	THERMOTHÉRAPIE
Pain	▼	▼
Blood flow and metabolic activity	▼	▲
Nerve conduction velocity	▼	▲
Muscle spasms	▼	▼
Elasticity and extensibilityof muscles and tissues	▼	▲
Tissue healing	▲	▲
Heart rate	▲	▲
Blood pressure	▲	▼

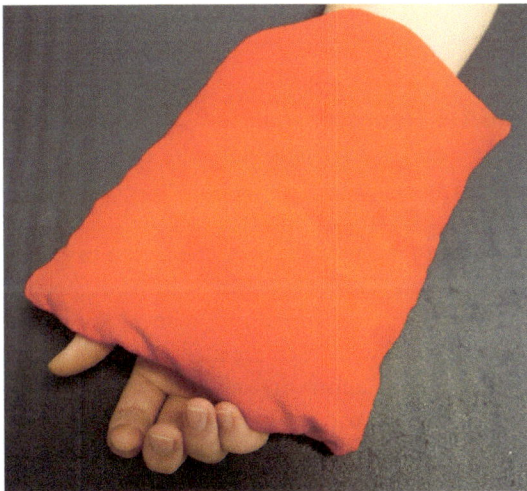

Fig. 3.16 Cherry pit heat pillows have a good capacity of preserving heat

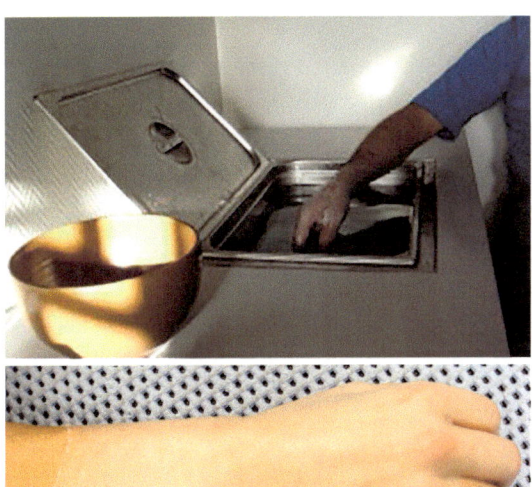

Fig. 3.17 Paraffin baths

patients are treated five times a week for 3 weeks.

We do not realize these exercises on inflammatory areas, as it could get worse. A proximal application can be realized, as there is an arterial and venous collapse proximally to the edematous area in inflammatory phases.

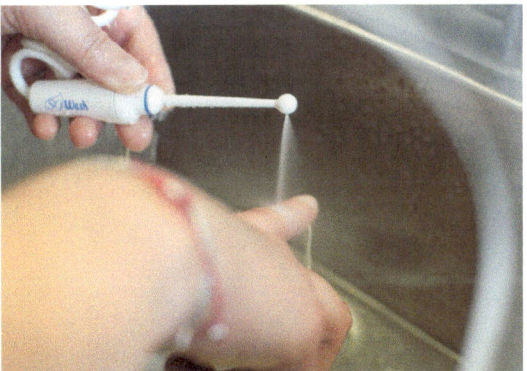

Fig. 3.18 Using a high-pressure water jet with trophic, analgesic, and sensorial purposes

3.5   High-Pressure Water Jet

Using an adjustable high-pressure water jet (maximum 3 bar) precisely stimulates the concerned area with an adjustable temperature water.

This exercise creates an analgesic effect by stimulating the gate control and a trophic effect (vasodilatation with hot water or vasoconstriction with cold water).

Using it on or around a scar (if the wound is closed) helps desensitizing it (Fig. 3.18).

3.6   Mechanical Waves

Vibrators produce longitudinal mechanical waves oscillating in their spreading direction.

There effects can be quite different and depend on how they are applied. They can be analgesic, vasomotor, muscle relaxing, or proprioceptive.

3.6.1   Transcutaneous Vibratory Stimulations (Fig. 3.19)

With a low frequency (50–100 Hz) and a low amplitude (<1 mm), they can help in treating:

3.6.1.1 Pain
The device's head is applied on the painful area and along the sensory nerve concerned by this

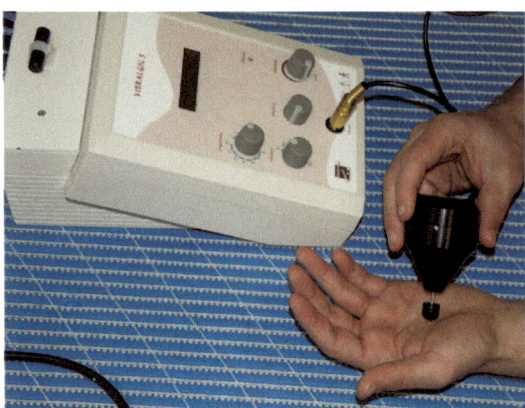

Fig. 3.19 Example of device that can produce vibrations with settable frequency and amplitude

area. If the contact is painful, the head will be applied far from the painful area but always on the nervous pathway.

The ideal frequency seems to be 100 Hz and the analgesic effect appears to be related to the gate control described in the Sect. 3.3.

The treatment is inefficient before 10 min of stimulation and after 20–25 min. The pain relief can last 3–6 h.

3.6.1.2 Proprioception

An 80 Hz [16] stimulation applied on a tendon provokes a contraction of the antagonist muscle and create and illusion of movement. This has a great proprioceptive interest, particularly during immobilization [17].

The stimulation lasts about 30 min.

3.6.1.3 Skin Sensitivity

These waves can also be used when working on sensitivity as they stimulate some mechanoreceptors that are sensitive to vibrations.

When there is no injury, the receptors at the fingertips can feel mechanical waves up to a frequency of 1000 Hz.

After a nerve injury causing anesthesia or hypoesthesia, the first perceived frequencies are low frequency vibrations (<100 Hz).

After nerve suture, vibrations should be applied distally, with no direct contact for 3 weeks.

Applying these waves must be completely pain-free.

3.6.1.4 Neuroma

These waves also help with the desensitization that is realized after an amputation or a painful scar (see Chap. 7).

During the first sessions, the stump or painful scar (where a nerve branch can be trapped in fibrosis) will be stimulated with slow circular movements, with high frequencies (>200 Hz if the generator allows it) and very low intensities adapted to the patient's pain threshold.

The habituation effect allows the patient to tolerate more intense stimulations, with high intensities and low frequencies. The treatment lasts 20 min. This protocol seems to significantly decrease the perceived pain [18].

It should be noted that these techniques are interesting to treat neuromas but must not be used on a nerve regeneration site if it is healthy, as it could disturb the regrowth process.

3.6.2 Infrasounds (Fig. 3.20)

Infrasounds are mechanical waves with a frequency lower than 20 Hz and an amplitude higher than 1 mm. They fight against pain, create a reflex muscle relaxation, and improve the local trophicity. They are applied perpendicularly on the area to be effective at a deep level.

If the device's amplitude is higher than 5 mm, it must not be used on healing fractures.

3.6.3 Ultrasounds (Fig. 3.21)

They are mechanical high frequency vibrations (0.5–3 MHz) induced by a quartz or a piezoelectric ceramic. It can have a thermic or a fibrinolytic effect depending on hox it is applied.

The devices we use in physical therapy usually allow to choose between a frequency of

If the developed force is weak and painful, the origin can be mixed or related to a peripheral or central pain.

Eichhoff's Test (Sensitivity 89%, Specificity 14%)

It is less known than Finkelstein's test but has a greater level of validity.

The patient places his thumb in the palm of his hand and the therapist places the wrist in ulnar inclination, causing the patient to feel the described pain [61].

This test can be combined with the WHAT test (Wrist Hyperflexion and Abduction of the Thumb). In this test, pain is produced by the muscle contraction. If it is positive, it helps refine the diagnosis (sensitivity 99%, specificity 29% if both tests are positive).

Extensor Carpi Ulnaris Instability

This test allows to differentiate the types of pain of the medial part of the wrist: Those related to a tenosynovitis of the extensor carpi ulnaris and those related to a tendon instability when its insertion on the dorsal retinaculum loosens.

It consists in applying a maximal forearm supination: This movement will create pain, or even a "jump" of the tendon. In the case of a tenosynovitis, this test will not create pain.

Nerves

These signs show nerve damages causing a loss of motricity and/or sensitivity.

Wartenberg's Sign

The patient cannot bring his fourth and fifth fingers together because of the weakness of the fourth palmar interosseous muscle that cannot compensate the abduction realized by the extensor digiti minimi (Fig. 1.47).

Froment's Sign

It is characterized by a flexion of the thumb's interphalangeal joint when pinching a piece of paper. This compensation is due to the contraction of the flexor pollicis longus (median nerve) that makes up for the weakness of the adductor pollicis (ulnar nerve) (Fig. 1.48).

Ulnar Claw

It appears in the two ulnar fingers in active extension. The metacarpophalangeal joints are in hyperextension while the interphalangeal joints stay in flexion. It is related to a motor deficit in the interossei muscles (ulnar nerve) that cannot compensate the action of the extensor digitorum muscle (radial nerve).

"Monkey" Hand

The patient's thumb is in extension and adduction because the external thenar muscles (median nerve) are weak while the adductor pollicis (ulnar nerve) and thumb extensor muscles (radial nerve) have a normal activity.

"Falling" Hand

The hand and wrist "fall" because their extensor muscles are weak. This posture can correspond to a radial nerve damage.

Pseudo-Tinel (Sensitivity 70% and Specificity 98%) [62]

It consists in tapping the areas of potential nerve compression, depending on the assessed nerve (*see "Entrapment Syndromes" in Volume 3*), from distal to proximal.

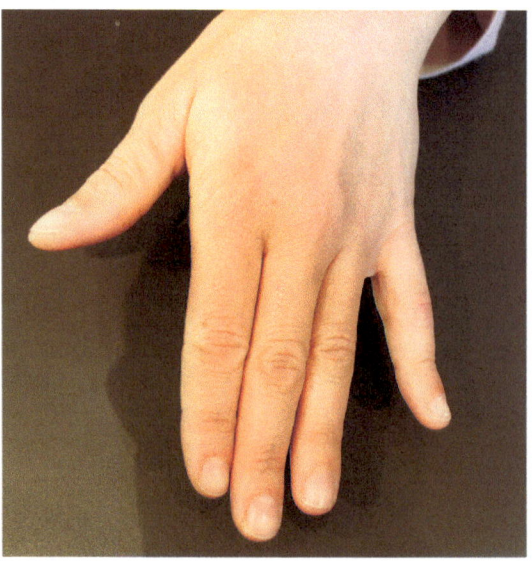

Fig. 1.47 Wartenberg sign, meaning the fourth palmar interosseous muscle is weak, which is compatible with an ulnar nerve injury

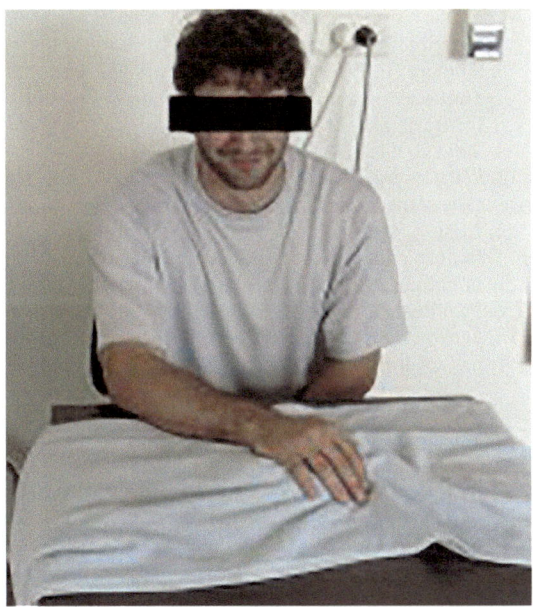

Fig. 3.20 Device producing vibrations with low frequency and high amplitude

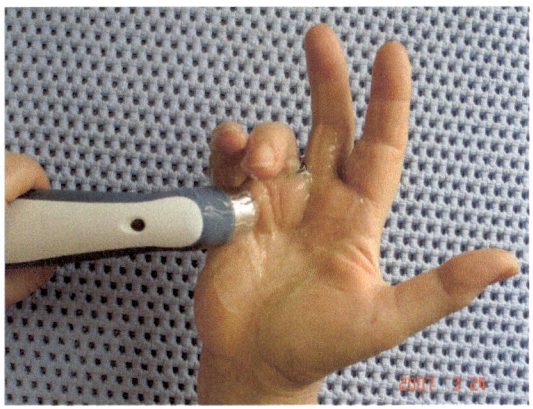

Fig. 3.21 Ultrasound device

1 MHz and a frequency of 3 MHz, and between two modes (continuous or pulse).

The choice of the frequency determines the treatment's depth: up to 3 cm with 1 MHz and up to 0.5 cm with 3 MHz.

With the pulse mode we will work on the fibrinolytic aspect of the treatment, while the continuous mode favors thermic effects.

The level of evidence for using ultrasounds is quite low [19].

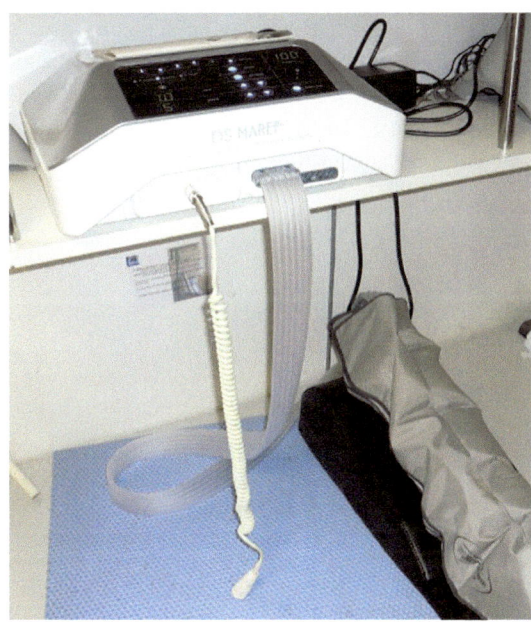

Fig. 3.22 Pressotherapy device creating pressure from distal to proximal or from proximal to distal

3.7 Pressotherapy

It is a pneumatic device producing compressions from distal to proximal, or the other way around depending on the indications (Fig. 3.22).

From distal to proximal, it drains the upper limb globally, with significant effects on posttraumatic edemas of the hand [20]. The protocol consists in 30 min sessions with a 40 mmHg pressure, and periods of compression/loosening of 20/40 s.

From proximal to distal, it creates a blood flow towards the distal extremity of the upper limb, which can be interesting in ischemic pathologies.

3.8 Scottish Baths

They appear to create a vasomotor effect that can be useful in case of edema, even if there is a low level of evidence [21].

Several protocols have been described [21], and the ratio 3:1 between hot bath (40 °C) and cold bath (15 °C) seems to be the most effective [22]:

- Use two tanks, bowls, buckets, basins, etc.
- Fill one with hot tap water (between 38 and 40 °C) and the other with cold tap water (between 12 and 15 °C).
- Put the hand in the hot water for 3 min, and immediately after that put the hand in the cold water for 1 min.
- Repeat four times. The session lasts 16 min.
- End with the cold bath.

References

1. Quesnot A, Chanussot J, Corbel I. La cryothérapie en rééducation: revue de la littérature. Kinésithér Scient. 2001;412:39–48.
2. Chatap G, et al. Les douleurs du sujet âgé. Évaluation prospective de l'antalgie par cryothérapie gazeuse hyperbare au dioxyde de carbone (neurocryostimulation). Rev Rhum. 2007;74:1289–94.
3. Bellot F. Cryothérapie post-traumatique entre pratique et théorie. Kinésithér Scient. 2015;0570: 31–6.
4. Cohn B, Draeger R, Jackson D. The effects of cold therapy in the postoperative management of pain in patients undergoing anterior cruciate ligament reconstruction. Am J Sports Med. 1989;17:344–9.
5. Mourot L, Cluzeau C, Regnard J. Physiological assessment of a gaseous cryotherapy device: thermal effects and changes in cardiovascular autonomic control. Ann Readapt Med Phys. 2007;50(4): 209–17.
6. Crépon F. Électrostimulation musculaire: critères de choix des paramètres de stimulation. Kinésithér Scient. 2013;541:43–5.
7. Crépon F, et al. Electrothérapie. Electrostimulation. In: EMC kinésithérapie – médecine physique – réadaptation. Paris: Masson; 2007.
8. Thomas D. Electrostimulation des muscles fléchisseurs des doigts et du poignet: proposition d'une nouvelle cartographie. Cah Kinésithér. 1996;178:37–42.
9. Gordon T, English AW. Strategies to promote peripheral nerve regeneration: electrical stimulation and/or exercise. Eur J Neurosci. 2016;43(3):336–50.
10. Ahlborn P, Schachner M, Irintchev A. One hour electrical stimulation accelerates functional recovery after femoral nerve repair. Exp Neurol. 2007;208(1):137–44.
11. GT Vance C, et al. Using TENS for pain control: the state of the evidence. Pain Manag. 2014;4(3):197–209.
12. Kong X, Gozani SN. Effectiveness of fixed site high-frequency transcutaneous electrical nerve stimulation in chronic pain: a large-scale, observational study. J Pain Res. 2018;11:703–14.
13. Szekeres M, et al. The short-term effects of hot packs vs therapeutic whirlpool on active wrist range of motion for patients with distal radius fracture: a randomized controlled trial. J Hand Ther. 2018;31(3):276–81.
14. Dilek B, et al. Efficacy of paraffin bath therapy in hand osteoarthritis: a single-blinded randomized controlled trial. Arch Phys Med Rehabil. 2013;94(4):642–9.
15. Mancuso T, Poole JL. The effect of paraffin and exercise on hand function in persons with scleroderma: a series of single case studies. J Hand Ther. 2009;22(1):71–77; quiz 78.
16. Crépon F. Stimulation Vibratoire Transcutanée: Rééducation proprioceptive vibratoire de la motricité. Kinésithér Scient. 2015;566:47–53.
17. Roll R, et al. Illusory movements prevent cortical disruption caused by immobilization. NeuroImage. 2012;62(1):510–9.
18. Spicher C, Kohut G. Rapid relief of a painful, long-standing posttraumatic digital neuroma treated by transcutaneous vibratory stimulation (TVS). J Hand Ther. 1996;9(1):47–51.
19. Robertson VJ, Baker KG. A review of therapeutic ultrasound: effectiveness studies. Phys Ther. 2001;81:1339–50.
20. Griffin JW, et al. Reduction of chronic posttraumatic hand edema: a comparison of high voltage pulsed current, intermittent pneumatic compression, and placebo treatments. Phys Ther. 1990;70(5):279–86.
21. Breger Stanton DE, Lazaro R, Macdermid JC. A systematic review of the effectiveness of contrast baths. J Hand Ther. 2009;22(1):57–69; quiz 70.
22. Stanton DB, et al. Contrast baths: what do we know about their use? J Hand Ther. 2003;16(4):343–6.

Rémy Dehez

4.1 Integumentary Physiology

4.1.1 Skin Anatomy

The skin is the largest organ in the human body, making 15% of an adult's weight. It is the structure that protects internal tissues from mechanical damage, microbial infection, ultraviolet light, and extreme temperatures. It is organized in three layers that are the epidermis, the dermis, and the hypodermis (from superficial to deep) [1].

The epidermis is the most external layer of the skin. It is also the most biologically active as the basal layer of the epithelium is constantly renewed.

It is a coating epithelium, not vascularized but innervated, and made of four types of cells:

- Keratinocytes (90%) that migrate from the deepest layer towards the surface area.
- Langerhans cells, Merkel cells, and melanocytes.

The junction between the dermis and the epidermis is a complex basal membrane that plays the part of a mechanical support in the adhesion between the dermis and the epidermis. It also regulates the exchanges of metabolic products between the two compartments.

The dermis is a supporting, compressible, and elastic connective tissue that protects the epidermis and the neurovascular plexus that go through it.

The hypodermis is an adipose tissue that makes up the deepest layer of the skin, separating is from the underlying aponeuroses or the periosteum. It plays an important part in thermoregulation, isolation, energy supply, and protection against mechanical injuries (Fig. 4.1).

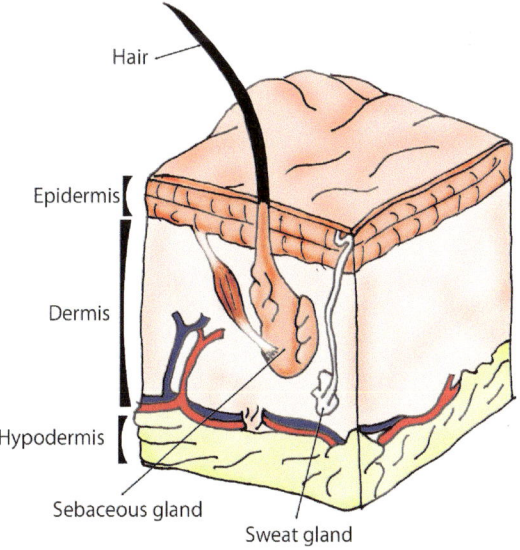

Fig. 4.1 The different layers of the skin: epidermis, dermis, hypodermis

R. Dehez (✉)
Institut Sud Aquitain de la Main et du Membre Supérieur, Biarritz, France

Cap Kiné, Capbreton, France

4.1.2 Palmar Skin

The palmar skin is the functional part of the hand, allowing a good grip efficiency.

Its integumentary physiology is like one of the other cutaneous parts; however, it has some characteristics of its own.

It is made of a thick stratum corneum (Fig. 4.2) (up to 1–2 mm) [2] that is very resistant as it is well hydrated by sweat glands.

It is relatively flexible but not very mobile as it is anchored to the deep layer to stabilize the grips.

This palmar skin is full of mechanoreceptors and organized in friction ridges. This organization helps optimizing the vibrotactile abilities as perpendicular pressures stimulate the ridge and the receptor within as well as receptors in nearby ridges (Fig. 4.3).

On a macroscopic level, the friction ridges correspond to fingerprints and help stabilizing grips as well.

The palmar side of the hand also has numerous fat pads that increase the congruence between the hand and the object. They are bounded by a system of fibrous tracts that attaches the skin to the different aponeurotic planes:

- **The thenar pad** covers the internal part of the thenar muscles.
- **The hypothenar pad** covers the hypothenar muscles and the internal side of the hand.
- **The metacarpophalangeal pad** stretches transversally from the ulnar side to the radial side of the hand, at the level of the metacarpophalangeal joints, it is thicker in the interdigital spaces.
- **In the fingers**, there also is a pad on each phalanx.

4.1.3 Dorsal Skin

The dorsal skin is the social side of the hand. Unlike the palmar skin, this part is very extensible and mobile with respect to the underlying tissue. When

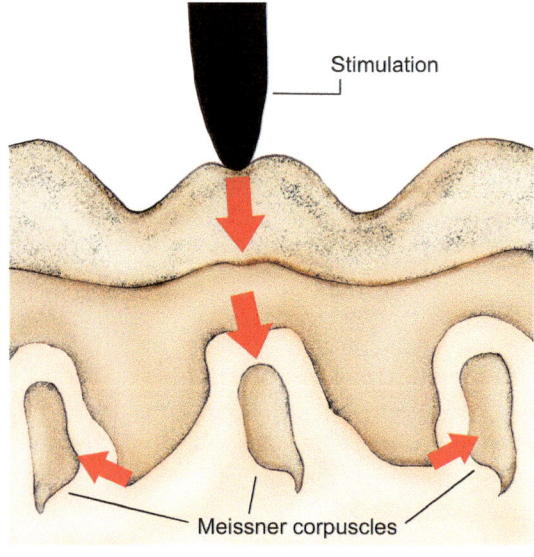

Fig. 4.3 The papillary dermis' organization optimizes cutaneous sensitivity

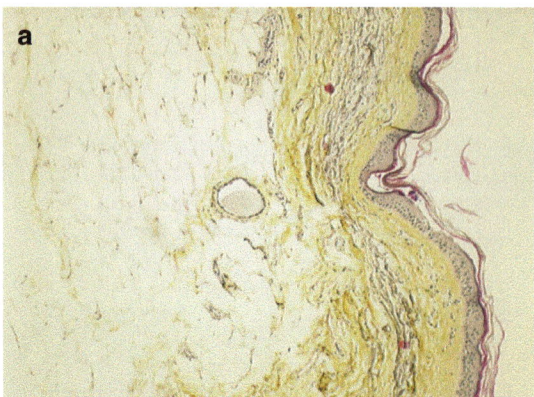 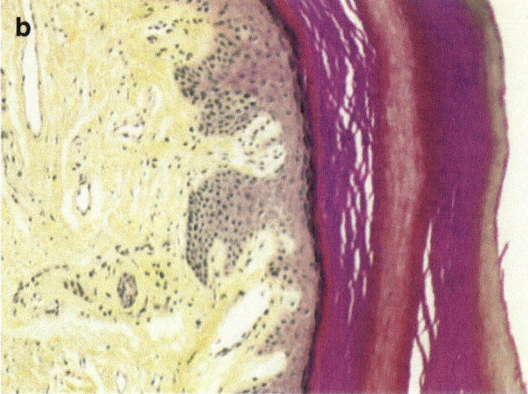

Fig. 4.2 Comparison between two cross sections of dorsal and palmar hand skin. Dorsal skin (**a**) has a thin stratum corneum (superficial layer), does not have friction ridges, and is very mobile. Palmar skin (**b**) has a thick stratum corneum and friction ridges and is attached to deep tissues (Photo form Pr Casoli's laboratory, Bordeaux)

flexing the fingers, its length increases by 20% in comparison with its rest position. On the back of the metacarpophalangeal joints, this extensibility and mobility allow the joint flexion, while on the back of the interphalangeal joints the flexion is allowed by "excess" cutaneous tissue (Fig. 4.4).

The dorsal skin's layers are like the palmar skin's layer; however, its stratum corneum is much thinner (0.02 mm).

Regarding the nails, they serve as an abutment to keep the pulp from gliding when gripping an object. They also optimize the vibrotactile abilities by reflecting the waves created when touching.

4.1.4   Dorso-Palmar Partition

The partitioning between the palmar and dorsal skins is materialized by a deep connective sys-tem, making them independent from one another. It is well visible in the interdigital commissures and on the ulnar side of the hand. In the fingers, this connective system stabilizes the skin regard-ing the bone and avoids the skin envelope to move as a "glove finger" regarding the motor system.

4.1.5   Functional Units

Described by Micron, the functional units are delimited by the most mobile areas in the cuta-neous tissue. The surgeon must not go through these zones to avoid adhesive or hypertrophic scars. If it is not possible, a Z-shaped inci-sion will be realized around the unit (Figs. 4.5 and 4.6).

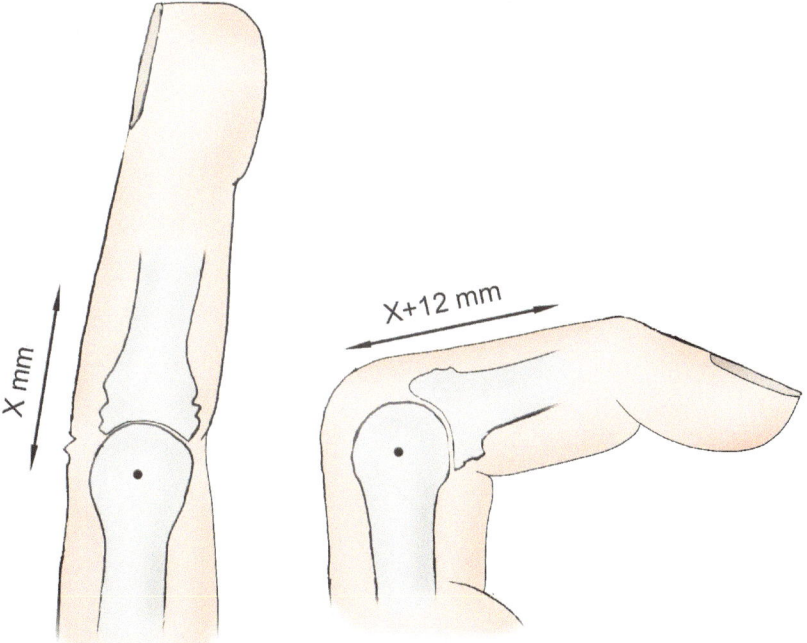

Fig. 4.4 "Excess" cutaneous tissue at the level of the interphalangeal joints allows flexion in these joints

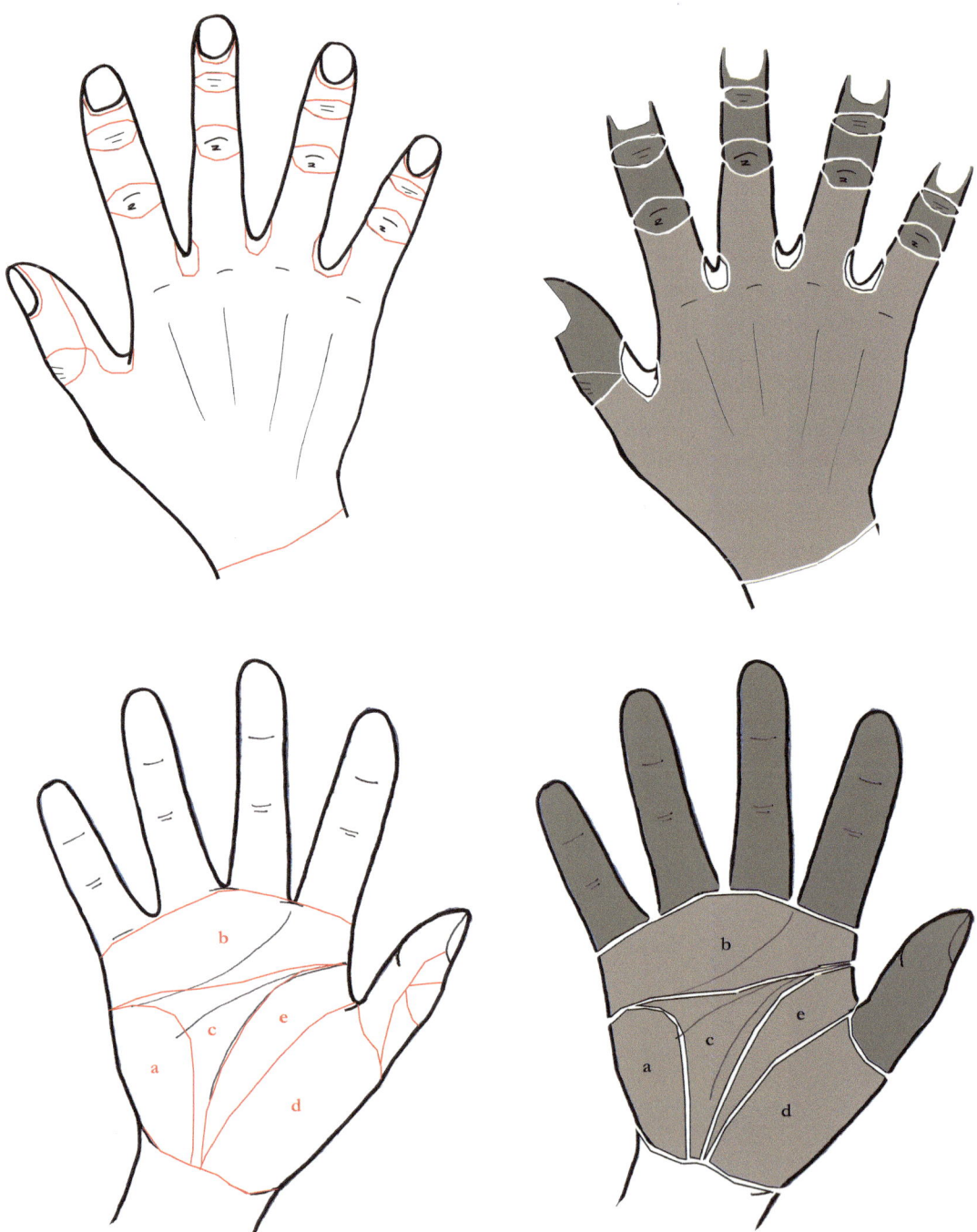

Fig. 4.5 Cutaneous functional units in the hand

Fig. 4.6 Surgical incisions must avoid going through these zones. If it cannot be avoided, a Z-shaped incision will be realized

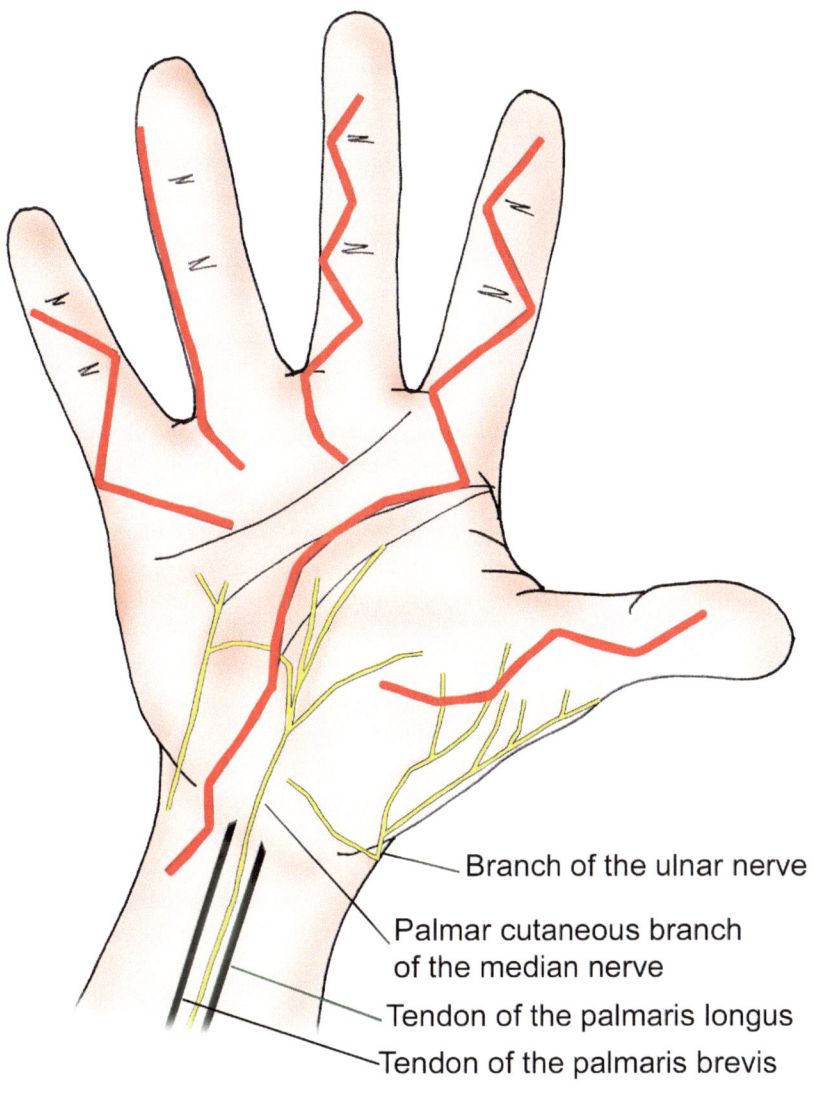

Branch of the ulnar nerve

Palmar cutaneous branch of the median nerve

Tendon of the palmaris longus

Tendon of the palmaris brevis

PALMAR INCISIONS

4.2   Healing Process

The healing process after an injury with skin damage is complex, with several mechanisms depending on the stages: hemostasis, inflammation, angiogenesis, growth, re-epithelialization, and remodeling [3, 4] (Fig. 4.7).

4.2.1   Hemostasis

Hemostasis is the first step of the healing process, stopping the bleeding after a vascular injury. It happens in three steps: vasoconstriction, primary hemostasis, and secondary hemostasis.

	Dermal healing	Epidermal healing
Vascular inflammatory phase 1st hour ⟶ 3rd day	Role of patelets producing growth factors Role of polynuclears and macrophage monocytes secreting proteolytic enzymes.	Keratinocytes actively migrate from the injury site, early since the 6th hour.
Proliferative or granulation phase 3rd day ⟶ 12th day	Role of fibroblasts (retraction and contraction) Role of neovessels bringing oxygen that is essential in tissue healing	The multiplyinng of keratinocytes is stimulated, mostly by the epidermal growth factor.
Remodeling or maturation phase 12th day ⟶ 2nd year	Simultaneous destruction of neocollagen and permanent synthesis of mature collagen.	Epidermal maturation with restoration of structures from the periphery towards the middle of the wound

Fig. 4.7 Healing timeline

The cell implied in the process is the platelet. When there is no injury, the platelets are protected against an inadvertent activation by a single layer of healthy endothelial cells. In non-injured skin, the platelets are not attached to the vessel walls and do not aggregate.

The matrix component implied in the process is the fibrinogen, an essential component of the blood clot.

When the skin is injured, the immediate response to stop the bleeding is vasoconstriction. Then primary hemostasis and secondary hemostasis occur through two competing paths that are mechanically intertwined.

The primary hemostasis includes platelet aggregation and the formation of homeostatic plugs caused by the exposure to collagen in the subendothelial matrix.

The secondary hemostasis is the activation of the coagulation cascade, where the soluble fibrinogen is converted in insoluble strands that make up the fibrin mesh.

The homeostatic plug and the fibrin mesh combined form the thrombus. It stops the bleeding, releases supplements and growth factors, and provides a temporary scaffold to infiltrate the cells needed for wound healing.

4.2.2 Inflammatory Phase

As wound healing implies several steps, it is important to understand the first signals that activate the inflammatory response in the injured tissue. It takes time to activate the transcription process, so the wound goes through quicker paths, including the increase of intracellular Ca^{2+}. It happens on the wound edges during the first

minutes after wounding and spreads towards the center of the wound. The DAMPs (Damage-Associated Molecular Patterns) include DNA, peptides, ECM components, ATP and uric acid, hydrogen peroxide (H_2O_2), and lipid mediators.

The chemokines released by the injured cells also give signals for recruiting inflammatory cells.

The neutrophiles are immediately recruited in the clot as a first line of defense. The monocytes are recruited in the 48–96 h after the injury and transform into macrophages, activated by the tissues on the site of the injury. The adaptive immune system includes Langerhans cells, dermal dendritic cells, and T-cells. It is also activated.

The activated inflammatory cells are:

- **Neutrophiles**. They are usually not seen in normal skin and are produced in the bone marrow. On the day after the injury, they represent 50% of the wound cells. They destroy infectious threats by releasing toxic granules, producing an oxidative explosion, starting phagocytosis, and generating Neutrophil Extracellular Traps (NET).
- **Macrophages**. They come from monocytes. They accumulate during the first 24–48 h at the level of the wound. They are essential for a normal healing and tissue regeneration. Pro-inflammatory macrophages recognize and engulf pathogens. In addition to being bactericidal, the macrophages are essential to eliminate the neutrophiles used during the 3–4 days following the injury. It is an important role as an incomplete neutrophile clearance leads to a persistent inflammation. When the inflammation is resolved, the inflammatory macrophage's phenotype changes and it becomes a type of anti-inflammatory cell. Those anti-

inflammatory macrophages contribute to the formation of new vessels. The macrophages can also transform into fiber cells and contribute to the scar formation.

- **Mastocytes**. In the skin, they essentially act as effectors for allergic reactions. These cells also contain several mediators in their granules. Immediately after an injury, the mastocytes release factors including inflammatory cytokines, vasodilatation agents, vascular permeability factors, and proteases. All these factors improve the immune cells recruitment in the wound.
- **Dendric cells**. They present antigens that take part in starting the response of T-cells. In the epidermis, they manifest as Langerhans cells. They are in lymph nodes draining the skin when there is a skin infection.
- **T-cells**. They are in the dermis and epidermis and facilitate the re-epithelialization of the wounds. They can also be found in lymph nodes draining the skin and increasing the neutrophiles recruitment after infection.

4.2.3 Granulation Tissue and Neovascularization

During the proliferative phase of wound healing, new connective tissue (or granulation tissue) develops, at the same time as other healing processes such as re-epithelialization, neovascularization, and immunomodulation.

The granulation tissue is mainly made of activated fibroblasts that synthetize extracellular matrix and help contracting the wound after differentiating into myofibroblasts. It also acts as a scaffold for other cells and components, including the new extracellular matrix, the new blood vessels, and the inflammatory cells. In the end, the granulation tissue is replaced by normal connective tissue during the wound remodeling.

The neovascularization is essential for an efficient healing. It is necessary for the supply of nutrients to maintain the oxygen homeostasis and to allow cell proliferation and tissue regeneration. The formation of new blood vessels in adults occurs mostly through angiogenesis.

The angiogenesis process includes the proliferation, the migration, and the ramification of endothelial cells to create new blood vessels.

Alongside the proliferation of endothelial cells, the pericytes (cells embedded in the cell membrane) within the basal lamina are activated and give a structural integrity to the endothelial cells. In addition to the local cells, progenitor cells that circulate in the bone marrow support the formation of new blood vessels during the healing process. The formation of new blood vessels implies several cell types, with the major cellular diversity occurring in the perivascular space.

4.2.4 Re-Epithelialization

It happens simultaneously and involves the proliferation of unipotent epidermal stem cells of the basal lamina, as well as the dedifferentiation of differentiated epidermal cells in terminal phase.

The repair of the epidermal layer also involves reconstruction of the cutaneous appendages. Stem cells have also been discovered in sebaceous glands, sweat glands, and hair follicles. They could also activate the local repair of the appendages. These epidermal stem cells are mostly unipotent in homeostasis, but they become highly plastic in case of injury and can engender other types of cells to quickly repair the epidermis.

4.2.5 Tissue Maturing and Remodeling

In most clinical contexts, the moment the acute and chronic wounds close is considered the end of the wound healing. However, a remodeling or tissue maturing can occur during several months, if not years. The remodeling phase consists of the decrease of neovascularization, a periodic deposit on the extracellular matrix, and an ulterior reconstitution of the granulation tissue into scar tissue.

The granulation tissue is mainly composed of type III collagen which is partly replaced by stronger type I collagen as the wound remodeling progresses. This process is the result of a type I collagen synthesis and a type III collagen lysis, followed by the reorganization of the extracellular matrix.

4.3 Pathological Scars

The repair of cutaneous tissue can result in a wide range of pathological scar types like hypertrophic, keloid, adhesive, and retractile scars [5].

Table 4.1 describes the main differences between a hypertrophic scar and a keloid scar.

4.3.1 Hypertrophic Scars

Hypertrophic scars are the result of a prolonged inflammatory response. The formation of collagen increases, as well as its adhesiveness and its contractile strength, leading to vascular scars that are red, thick, and not mobile.

They are described as firm scars that remain at the limits of the original wound. Hypertrophic scars can create functional limits, mainly because of the reduced range of motion. They gradually heal in 12–18 months and are most frequent in young, light, and dark skins, as they are more sensitive [6].

4.3.2 Keloid Scars

Compared with hypertrophic scars, keloid scars gradually spread towards the surrounding healthy skin. They can be particularly pejorative on an aesthetic and emotional plan. They develop in areas with important arterial tension, for example, the pre-sternal area and the earlobe. There is a high incidence in people of African, Caribbean, or Asian origin, suggesting a genetic predisposition. They are rare in the hand [6].

4.3.3 Adhesive Scars

They are depressed scars, forming adhesions with adjacent tissues such as fasciae, muscles, and bones. They impede gliding between the various structures and the planes underneath. They can be permanent or appear only with movement [7].

4.3.4 Retractile Scars

Retraction is a constant physiological phenomenon in the healing process. These scars are only considered pathological if they are uncomfortable for the patient on a functional or aesthetic level. There are flat retractile scars and raised retractile scars (also called bands) [7].

4.3.5 Burn Scars

Burn scars are generally large, leaving a fragile, dry, thin skin that can be hyposensitive or hypersensitive. They lead to a risk of retractions, especially at the level of Langer's lines (described in 1861) (Fig. 4.8).

Table 4.1 Main differences between hypertrophic and keloid scars

Hypertrophic scar	Cicatrice Chéloïde
Remains within the limits of the initial injury	Expands beyond the limits of the initial injury
Does not depend on ethnic characteristics	More frequent in people with pigmented skin
Often in areas subjected to stress	Can appear in areas that are not under stress
Spontaneously improves with time	Little or no improvement with time (inflammatory decrease only)
Few recurrences after surgical excision	Many recurrences after surgical excision

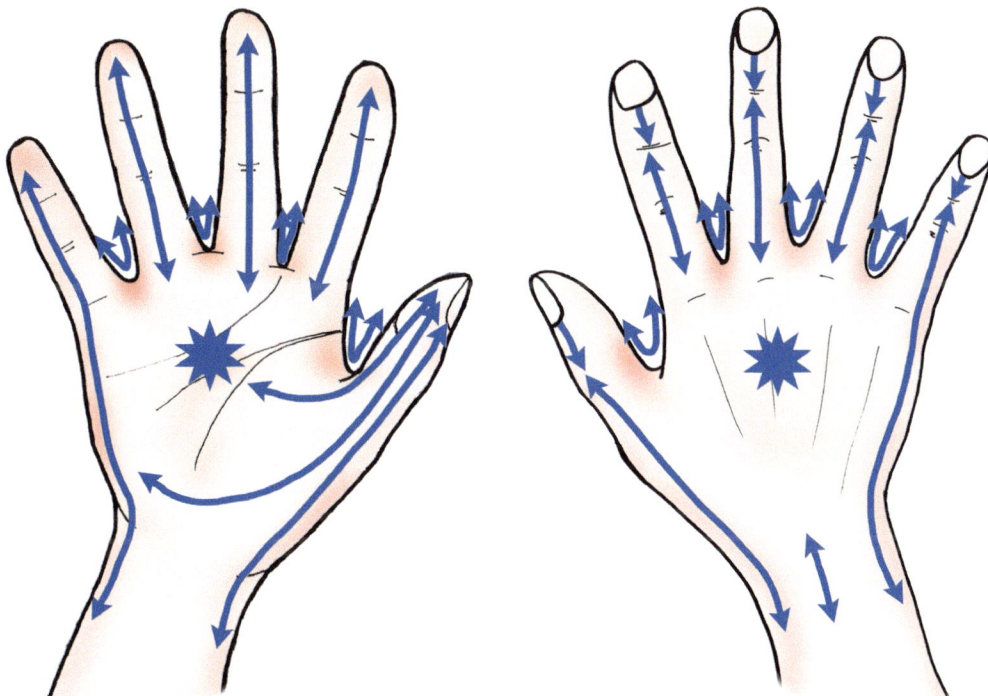

Fig. 4.8 Predictable bands locations

4.4 Factors Influencing Healing [8, 9]

The healing process depends on several local and general factors, which explains the significant differences observed within their evolution (Table 4.2).

4.4.1 Local Factors

- **Tissue oxygenation**: Oxygen is important to cellular metabolism and is essential to almost every wound healing process. It prevents wound infections, induces angiogenesis, increases the keratinocytes' differentiation, migration, and re-epithelialization, improves fibroblast proliferation and collagen synthesis, and favors wound contraction [10].
- **Wound orientation**: It affects the scar evolution. If the wound is oriented in parallel with the collagen fibers, the healing will be easier with less risk of retraction.

- **Wound edges**: They must be sharp, and the stitches should be reduced to a minimum.
- **Wound location**: It is important as some areas (shoulders, thorax) often heal in an abnormal way. Healing is better in thin skin.
- **Presence of foreign bodies**.
- **Ethnic origin or skin color**: African and Asian populations are more likely to develop keloid scars.
- **Presence of infection**: An infection in the wound lengthens the inflammation process and block the healing process (staphylococcus, for example).

4.4.2 General Factors

- **Age**: Aging slows the wound healing process but does not really alter the quality of healing. It is also interesting to note that exercising improves cutaneous wound healing in the elderly [11].
- **Sexual hormones in older people**: They play a role in the healing deficit in older people. It

Table 4.2 Mostly observed quantitative scar evolutions (according to Morel-Fatio)

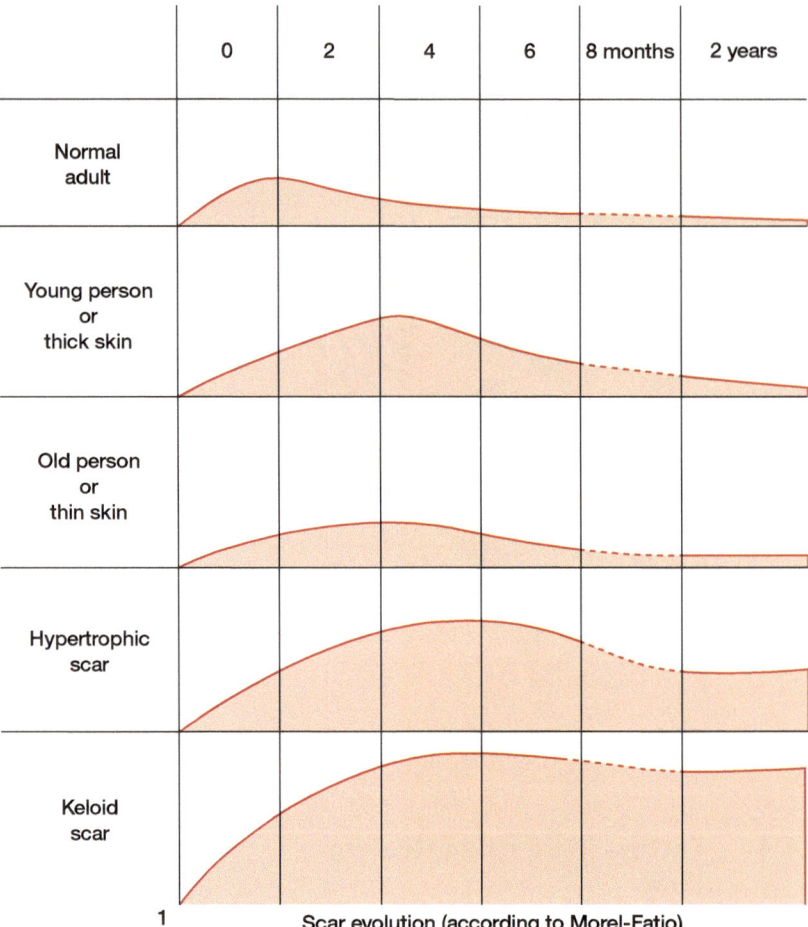

	0	2	4	6	8 months	2 years
Normal adult						
Young person or thick skin						
Old person or thin skin						
Hypertrophic scar						
Keloid scar						

Scar evolution (according to Morel-Fatio)

has been proven that older men have a slower acute wound healing that older women [12].

- **Stress**: Stress disturbs the neuroendocrine immune system's balance. This, combined with the psychological aspect (depression, anxiety), slows the healing process down.
- **Diseases**: Diabetes, keloids, fibrosis, hereditary healing disorders, jaundice, and uremia all disturb the healing process.
- **Obesity**: Obese people often face complications in wounds, for example, skin infections, dehiscences, hematomas and seromas, pressure ulcers, and venous ulcers [13].
- **Alcohol**: Consuming alcohol interferes with wound healing and increases the risk of infection by decreasing the rate of recruited neutrophiles.
- **Tobacco**: Smoking causes hypovascularization in the wound through several mechanisms (including nicotine). It promotes

arteriopathies, as well as carboxyhemoglobinemia that limits hemoglobin's capacities for transporting oxygen.

- **Nutrition**: It is a particularly important factor in wound healing. Malnutrition and specific nutritional deficiencies can clearly have a deep impact on wound healing after trauma or surgery. Protein, carbohydrate, arginine, glutamine, polyunsaturated acid, vitamin A, vitamin C, vitamin E, magnesium, copper, zinc, and iron all play and important role. A lack of any of these elements can disturb the wound healing process. The mechanisms connecting nutrition and healing are yet to be explored.
- **Medical treatments**: The healing process can be disturbed by glucocorticoid steroids, non-steroidal anti-inflammatory drugs, and chemotherapy.

4.5   Scar Treatment (Table 4.6)

4.5.1   Noninvasive Methods

4.5.1.1 Preventive Treatment

Priorities for proper healing are fast wound closure, early dead tissue debridement, preventing or treating inflammation and infection, and providing adequate dressings to create a humid healing environment. When applying a dressing on the hand, it is also important to find a good balance between wound protection and freedom of movement, as a dressing covering too much of an area can keep the hand from moving and create important stiffness and/or the functional exclusion of a finger.

General preventive measures are sun protection, hydrating creams, using dressings keeping the scar humid (like silicone gel). It has been discovered that trans-epidermal water loss is increased in hypertrophic and keloid scars. Hydrating agents rise the skin's water content or humidity, while silicone-based dressings help reducing water evaporation through the skin and restoring the barrier function of the skin [14, 15].

4.5.1.2 Compressive Treatment

There are more and more proofs supporting the use of a compressive treatment in scar management [6, 15, 16]. It can be used on hypertrophic scars, keloid scars, and especially on burn scars. Pressotherapy should be applied only when the wound is closed, and the patient can tolerate the pressure. It can help relieving edema, itching, and pain.

If we compare several types of pressure, it seems that a pressure of at least 15 mmHg is required. For burn scars, a pressure between 24 and 40 mmHg is ideal. Studies show that compressive treatments improve the aspect and the size of the scar with no influence on the healing time [17].

Table 4.3 describes hypotheses for action mechanisms of compressive treatments [17].

In the hand and fingers, a compressive treatment can be applied using elastic bandages, contention gloves, or tube-shaped elastic dressings.

Table 4.3 Compression applied on a scar: effects and mechanisms hypotheses

Effect	Mechanisms hypotheses
Blood flow decrease	1. Decreases the alpha-macroglobulin (inhibitor of collagenase) which increases degradation of collagen by collagenase
	2. Excessive hypoxia that induces a fibroblastic degeneration with an increased collagen degradation
Hydration	Stabilizes the mastocytes, reduces the development of neovessels and the production of extracellular matrix

4.5.1.3 Occlusive Treatment with Silicone

Recent guidelines recommend silicone as a frontline prophylactic option for hypertrophic and keloid scars [6, 14, 18]. In fact, among all the noninvasive treatment options, silicone is universally considered as the gold standard in scar treatment. Compared with invasive treatments, silicone is interesting as it is easy to use and has only minor potential side effects (pruritus, contact dermatitis, dry skin). This therapy prevents and treats scars by occluding and hydrating scar tissue.

Silicone can be found in film form or in gel form. Silicone films must be worn on the scar during 12–24 h a day, for 3–6 months. The composition of these silicone films varies considerably: some only contain medical silicone while some contain silicone and polytetrafluoroethylene that reinforces the film so that it can be thin, durable, flexible, and breathable. In hand therapy, we can also use silicone paste or silicone plates in orthoses.

Many explanations have been proposed regarding the action mechanisms of silicone products:

- Increasing the skin's surface temperature, which can increase the collagenase activity and lead to a faster collagen degradation.
- Creating a negative static electric field between the silicone and the skin, causing the collagen to realign and the scar to shrink.

The occlusion and hydration of the stratum corneum are now considered the main mechanisms in silicone action. The silicone sheets

Table 4.4 Silicon applied on a scar: effects and mechanisms hypotheses

Effect	Mechanisms hypotheses
Hydration	Decrease the capillary activity and the collagen production by inhibiting the fibroblastic proliferation. The hydration can be caused by occlusion
Temperature	Increasing the temperature raises the collagenase, so the application of silicon reduces hypertrophic scars by decomposing collagen
Polarization	The negative charge in silicon polarizes the scar tissue, leading to an involution of the scar
Oxygenation	After a silicon application, the hydrated stratum corneum is more permeable to oxygen: the oxygen pressure in epidermis and dermis increases
	An increased oxygen pressure inhibits the tissue's hypoxia signal
	Hypoxia stimulates angiogenesis and tissue growth in healing wounds, so suppressing this phenomenon stops tissue growth and avoids excessive scar formation
	The opposite phenomenon has also been described in the mechanisms of compressive treatment
Mastocytes	Some studies show that silicon increases the concentration of mastocytes in the scar's cellular matrix, with an ulterior accelerated tissue remodeling
	However, this is a very controverted information

decrease skin's water evaporation and increase the stratum corneum's hydration. Reducing transepidermal water loss decreases the stimulation of keratinocytes, so they stop producing cytokines. Therefore, fibroblasts are not activated, which prevents the formation of excessive scars. Occlusion is also an important element of the silicone products' action mechanism [17].

Table 4.4 describes hypotheses for action mechanisms of silicone [17].

4.5.1.4 Manual Techniques

Before starting other treatments like manual techniques, depresso-therapy, or physiotherapy, it is important to realize a diascopy test to evaluate cutaneous inflammation [9].

It consists in applying a pressure on the scar during a few seconds with a transparent glass plate until the scar whitens, and then taking it off. The more inflammatory the scar, the less time it takes it to recolor. The normal recoloration time is around 3 s. When it is under 2 s, it is not recommended to do massages and depresso-therapy.

Other criteria must be analyzed during the rehabilitation sessions or in self-rehabilitation to avoid negative side effects [16, 19] (Table 4.5).

Manual Lymphatic Drainage (MLD)

MLD can be realized from the first weeks after healing. The main goal is to drain the postoperative or post-traumatic edema as it can slow the healing process down.

Table 4.5 Contraindication to scar massage

Contraindications	
Formal	Relative
– Diascopy test < 2 s	– Localized or generalized eczema
– Skin cancer	– Psoriasis
– Malignant dyskeratoses	– Pruritus
– Cutaneous tuberculosis	– Scars in contact with osteosynthesis elements
– Lymphoma cutis	
– Large bullous dermatosis in inflammatory stage in adults (herpes, zoster)	
– Any inflammatory and/or infectious skin diseases	
– Skin conditions in general	

MLD is described in several steps [20]:

- **Emptying of the lymph nodes**, draining the scar: The lymph node should be isolated with the ulnar side of the fifth finger, stretching the skin, and lowering the hand. The pressure should be soft and prolonged to empty the lymph node.
- **Maneuvers between the scar and the lymph node**: The radial side of the index meets the skin and slightly stretches it. Then the other fingers and the palm of the hand successively contact the skin. This movement is realized with large elbow and shoulder movements (abduction and adduction).

- **Resorption maneuver on the scar**: Always directed towards the lymph nodes, we circle around the scar with one or several fingers. These pressures are realized with a circular wrist movement, and adduction and abduction movements in the shoulder and elbow.

Massages

Few studies exist compared to the wide range of massage techniques, so we cannot determine their real efficiency. However, various techniques are used in the global treatment of a pathological hand.

- **Effleurage**: The therapist's hand glides along the patient's skin without pressuring or stretching it. The movement can be longitudinal if the therapist's hands are parallel to the massaged segment, transversal when they are perpendicular to the massaged segment, or oval when they are side by side or realize circular movements. With this technique, the therapist intends to get the first contact with the patient and to have a sedative and pleasant effect (Fig. 4.9).
- **Deep gliding pressures**: The movement is like the effleurage, with a more important pressure to have more impact on the elements underneath the stratum corneum. With this technique, the therapist intends to relax the muscles and to improve the venous return when the massage is realized slowly and from distal to proximal. It is not recommended in case of a fragile veinous system [21, 22].

Digital gliding pressures are realized with one or several fingertips on narrow and precise areas. Along the fingers, the technique is realized with the thumbs' pulps placed on the ulnar or radial side of a finger, and the pulps of the second and third fingers placed on the opposite side to improve the veinous return in the finger: this way, the massage is realized along the collateral veins (Fig. 4.10).

- **Static pressures (reflex points)**: The therapist applies a local pressure without gliding, contacting slowly with the skin and releasing it progressively. With this technique, the therapist intends to improve the blood circulation if it is realized from distal to proximal, to relax muscle contractures, and to have an analgesic effect by promoting the secretion of endorphins [21, 22].
- **Superficial kneading or "palpate and roll" technique**: The therapist lifts the skin to create a skin fold and kneads it between his thumb and his four other fingers or between his thumb and his index finger to massage the narrow areas in the hand and fingers. With this technique, the therapist intends to pull the skin from the underlying plan [21, 22]. In hand rehabilitation, it is used to massage the scars that can be adhesive and limit the skin's mobility—and therefore the fingers' mobility. The therapist's fingers can be placed in the same direction as the scar, perpendicularly, or obliquely (Fig. 4.11).

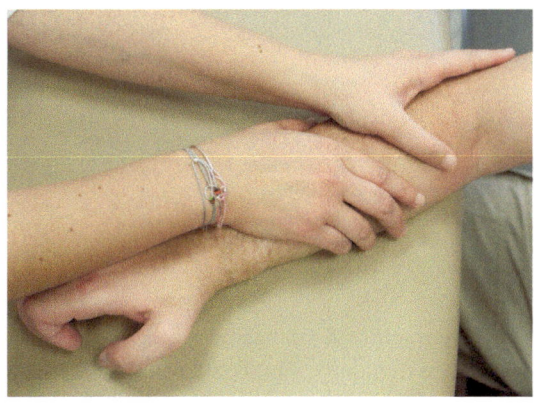

Fig. 4.9 Effleurage

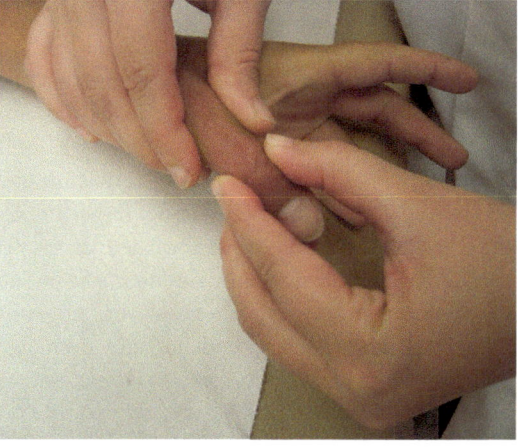

Fig. 4.10 Massage to drain thXe edema

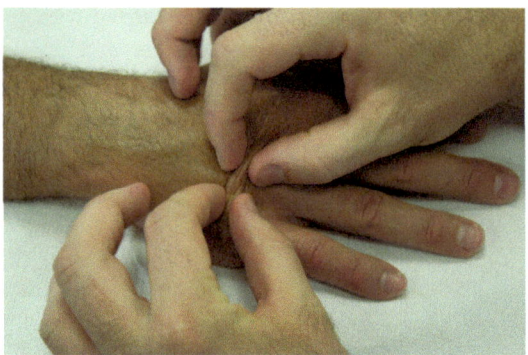

Fig. 4.11 Superficial kneading to improve the mobility of the skin envelope

- **Deep kneading**: The therapist lifts the muscular tissue and moves the muscles with respect to each other, applying pressure, torsion, and elongation. The movement can be transversal or longitudinal depending on the position of the hands in relation to the muscle fibers. With this technique, the therapist intends to maintain and improve the muscles properties (elasticity and extensibility) and to relax the muscle [21, 22] (Fig. 4.12).
- **Frictions**: The therapist mobilizes the layers in relation to one another. His hands remain fixed to the cutaneous plan, moves it, and mobilizes it with respect to the deep plan (muscle, fascia, or ligament) (Fig. 4.13). With this technique, the therapist intends to fight against scar fibrosis [21, 22].
- **Deep transverse massage (DTM)**: This technique is described by Cyriac and is intended to be used on ligaments and tendons after traumatic injuries. The friction is realized with the index fingertip—with or without the third fingertip—placed on the tendon in its maximal stretch position. The fingers move quite quickly (3–4 frictions/s) during a few minutes, until the pain decreases. The fingertips are placed transversally to the treated fibers [21, 22]. With this technique, the therapist intends to treat tendinopathies. However, no study proves its efficiency, and it could even have negative effects according to some authors [23, 24] (Fig. 4.14).
- **Vibrations**: A series of vibrations transmitted to the tissues without losing contact with the

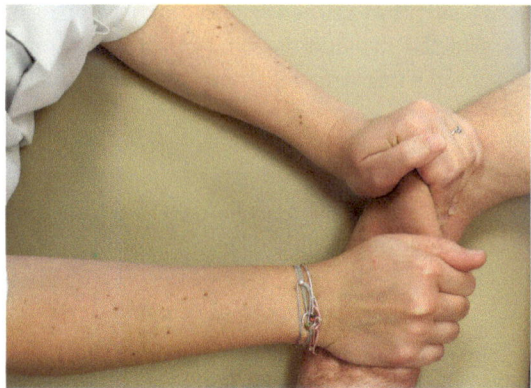

Fig. 4.12 Deep kneading on the forearm posterior muscles

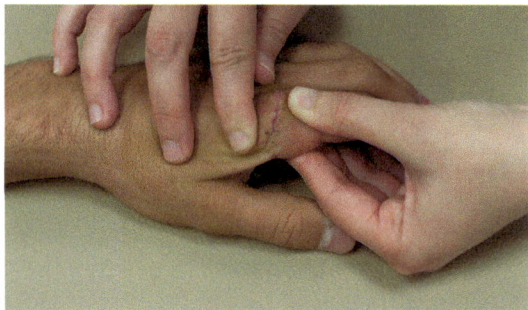

Fig. 4.13 Friction to mobilize the tissues around the scar

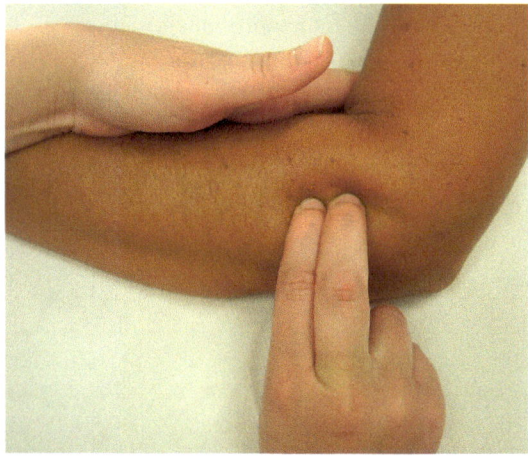

Fig. 4.14 Deep transverse massage (DTM)

integuments. This technique is difficult to realize manually. Physiotherapy devices seem more efficient, and they allow the therapist to adjust the vibration frequency. With this technique, the therapist intends to have a sedative, circulatory, and sensory effect [21, 22].

- **Jacquet-Leroy's plastic massage**: The therapist pinches and kneads the integuments while avoiding stretching them and progressively increasing the duration and intensity of the massage. With this technique, the therapist intends to reduce the scar adhesions [9, 20].
- **"Clamp and rotate" technique**: The therapist pinches the skin between his fingertips and lifts it while rotating it quickly (snapping his fingers). With this technique, the therapist intends to reduce fibrosis [9, 20].

Physiotherapy
- **Depresso-therapy**: This technique uses a depresso-therapy device that allows the therapist to adjust the strength and mode of suction. Some systems combine depresso-therapy and a "palpate and roll" technique. With this system, all the body parts can be treated, even the ones that are hard to reach. The described physiological aspects are hypervascularization and hyperoxygenation, defibration and tissue flexibility, tissue and lymphatic drainage, toning, and skin lifting [25]. Using this system is not recommended before the 40th day, some anti-inflammatory programs can be used but the diascopy test must be above 2 s [9].
- **Ultrasounds**: They are often used in all sorts of rehabilitation protocols. In scar treatment, some old studies show that they stimulate the synthesis of growth factors and increase the resistance to traction and the elasticity of the treated collagen. These studies are from the 1980s and have been contested since [6]. The current literature does not prove the effectiveness of ultrasounds in scar treatment [6].
- **Cryotherapy**: This technique is used on hypertrophic and keloid scars. It is sometimes combined with other treatments like corticosteroids. Cryotherapy can be less supported by some patients than by others as it can cause pain, cutaneous atrophy, and hypopigmentation, especially with surface techniques because of the high frequency of treatment [16].
- **Micro-needling**: This technology is not very invasive and can be used to treat various skin conditions. The device looks like a derma-roller with tiny needles. Modern devices have multiple needles from 0.5 to 1.5 mm long. The roll is applied on the skin to create micro-perforations in the stratum corneum and the papillary dermis. These micro-injuries trigger a release of growth factors, thus leading to the formation of collagen and elastin in the dermis. Micro-needling can also be used for a transdermal drug delivery as it creates pores in the stratum corneum. The applications of micro-needling have expanded over the last decades and now include the treatment of acne vulgaris, scars, facial rejuvenation, dyspigmentation, alopecia, hyperhidrosis, and trans-epidermal drug delivery. Using micro-needling on hypertrophic scars has proven to be effective, notably by normalizing the collagen-elastin extracellular matrix in the reticular dermis of burn patients [26]. This device is recommended at the end of the inflammatory phase, twice a week during 1–2 months [9].

4.5.2 Invasive Treatments

4.5.2.1 Corticosteroids
An intralesional injection of corticosteroids can help reducing hypertrophic scars. These injections can be used on their own or combined with other therapies (silicone gel, for example).

Corticosteroids can also be delivered topically. However, due to the tissues' poor absorption, they are likely to be efficient only on relatively superficial injuries. The most common side effects include hypopigmentation, skin atrophy, subcutaneous fat atrophy, telangiectasia, rebound effect, and inefficiency.

The injections objectively reduce the volume of hypertrophic and keloid scars. They also improve their flexibility, size, and symptoms such as pruritus.

The three involved mechanisms are:

- **Suppression of inflammation**: Through the inhibition of the leucocytes and monocytes migration.
- **Vasoconstriction**: It can reduce the oxygen and nutrients supply to the wound site.

- **Antimitotic effect**: It inhibits the keratinocytes and fibroblasts and slows the re-epithelialization and the formation of new collagens down. The inhibition of the fibroblasts' proliferation by corticosteroids can be dose-dependent and might not be observed with low doses, as shown in studies on tissue cultures [17].

4.5.2.2 Laser

Advances made in laser technology have triggered evolutions in the treatment of various skin conditions. The developments in this technology can be very promising in the improvement of skin scars. It has been claimed that an appropriate laser choice and use can significantly improve most scars. However, despite promising first results, scar laser treatment does not look so efficient over time, with a high relapse rate.

The erbium laser has become a valuable tool for improving light burn scars that can be disturbing on an aesthetic level. It seems to be particularly interesting when treating specific areas like the fingers and the eyes, nose, and lips contours. However, the long-term benefit has not been proven by well controlled comparative studies. Several laser types have been tried, including pulsed laser deposition (PLD) and long pulsed

dye laser (LPDL). None of these laser techniques is efficient enough to be a part of the actual gold standard for scar treatment [17] (Table 4.6).

4.5.2.3 Surgery

The decision to have surgery on hypertrophic scars is based on several parameters such as the age of the scar, its location, its size, its cause, the inefficiency of conservative treatments, the patient's expectations, and the surgeon's expertise. The scar's appearance must be critically assessed as there are many hypertrophic scars diagnosed as keloid scars and the relapse rate is high for surgically removed keloid scars.

The surgeon can bring several solutions to improve hypertrophic scars. The healthy skin surrounding the hypertrophic scar can be used to cover it. Z-plasty has proven effective too. It is based on the principle of converting the scar direction from vertical to parallel to the minimal tension lines. Tissue expansion and surgical flaps are also quite common solutions. Using skin substitutes in reconstructive surgery also improves the results of wound healing.

As there is a high hypertrophy relapse rate, other therapies are recommended after surgery such as compression, silicone application, intralesional corticosteroids, or radiotherapy [17].

Table 4.6 Gold standard for scar treatment depending on the scar type and the timeline

Scar type	At the beginning	After 3 months	After 6 months	After 12 months
Linear scar (post-surgery or traumatic)	Avoid sun exposure Preventive treatment: – Hydration – Taping – Silicon – Compression? Always reevaluate the scar after 6 months	Normal maturation of the scar: stop the treatment at 3 months Beginning of hypertrophy: – Continue or intensify the treatment as long as needed – Pressotherapy	Late maturation of the scar: continue with the silicon as long as needed Hypertrophy: – Continue the previous treatment – Send to a specialist for corticosteroid injections – Consider surgery	Differential diagnosis between permanent hypertrophic scar or not – Send to a specialized surgeon – Continue the preventive treatment (pressotherapy, silicon, etc.)

Table 4.6 (continued)

Scar type	At the beginning	After 3 months	After 6 months	After 12 months
Hypertrophic extensive scar (after prolonged healing)	Avoid sun exposure Preventive treatment: – Silicon + compression – Hydration Always reevaluate the scar after 6 weeks	Normal maturation of the scar (rare): Stop the treatment at 3 months Beginning of hypertrophy: – Custom-fit compressive clothing – Corticosteroid injections with a specialist – Surgery if needed	On hypertrophy: continue or intensify the treatment – Custom-fit compressive clothing + silicon – Send to a specialist for corticoid injections – Surgery if needed	Permanent hypertrophic scar: – Send to a specialized surgeon – Continue the preventive treatment (pressotherapy, silicon, etc.)
	At the beginning	**From 1 to 6 months**		**After 12 months**
Keloid scar	Avoid sun exposure Starting keloid: – Silicon + compression – Hydration	Evolving keloid: – Silicon + compression – Send to the specialist for corticosteroid injections		If no improvement: send to a specialized surgeon (scar excision)

References

1. Khavkin J, Ellis DA. Aging skin: histology, physiology, and pathology. Facial Plast Surg Clin North Am. 2011;19(2):229–34.
2. Gosain A, DiPietro LA. Aging and wound healing. World J Surg. 2004;28(3):321–6.
3. Rodrigues M, et al. Wound healing: a cellular perspective. Physiol Rev. 2019;99(1):665–706.
4. Witte M, Barbul A. General principles of wound healing. Surg Clin North Am. 1997;77(3):509–28.
5. Bayat A, McGrouther A, Ferguson M. Skin scarring – clinical review. Br Med J. 2003;326:88–92.
6. Jones L. Scar management in hand therapy – is our practice evidence based? Br J Hand Ther. 2005;10(2):40–6.
7. Chaput B, et al. Anomalies de la cicatrisation. EMC - Techniques chirurgicales - Chirurgie plastique reconstructrice et esthétique. 2012;7(2):1–12.
8. Guo S, Dipietro LA. Factors affecting wound healing. J Dent Res. 2010;89(3):219–29.
9. Vancoppenolle E. La prise en charge des cicatrices. Mémoire du diplôme inter-universitaire de rééducation et d'appareillage de la main; 2015.
10. Rodriguez PG, et al. The role of oxygen in wound healing: a review of the literature. Dermatol Surg. 2008;34(9):1159–69.
11. Keylock KT, et al. Exercise accelerates cutaneous wound healing and decreases wound inflammation in aged mice. Am J Physiol Regul Integr Comp Physiol. 2008;294(1):R179–84.
12. Hardman MJ, Ashcroft GS. Estrogen, not intrinsic aging, is the major regulator of delayed human wound healing in the elderly. Genome Biol. 2008;9(5):R80.
13. Wilson J, Clark J. Obesity: impediment to postsurgical wound healing. Adv Skin Wound Care. 2004;17:426–35.
14. Meaume S, et al. Management of scars: updated practical guidelines and use of silicones. Eur J Dermatol. 2014;24(4):435–43.
15. Monstrey S, et al. Updated scar management practical guidelines: non-invasive and invasive measures. J Plast Reconstr Aesthet Surg. 2014;67(8):1017–25.
16. Atiyeh BS. Nonsurgical management of hypertrophic scars: evidence-based therapies, standard practices, and emerging methods. Aesthet Plast Surg. 2007;31(5):468–492; discussion 493–4.
17. Bloemen MC, et al. Prevention and curative management of hypertrophic scar formation. Burns. 2009;35(4):463–75.
18. Berman B, et al. A review of the biologic effects, clinical efficacy, and safety of silicone elastomer sheeting for hypertrophic and keloid scar treatment and man-

agement. Dermatol Surg. 2007;33(11):1291–1302; discussion 1302–3.

19. Xhardez Y, et al. VADE-MECUM de Kinésithérapie et de Rééducation fonctionnelle. Paris: Maloine; 2013.

20. Marchi-Lipski F. Possibilité de la kinésithérapie dans les cicatrices. In: EMC Kinésithérapie-Médecine physique-Réadaptation. Paris: Masson; 1998.

21. Dufour M. Massages. EM consulte; Elsevier, 1996.

22. Dufour M. Massage et massothérapie, effets techniques et applications. Paris: Maloine; 1999.

23. Loew LM, et al. Deep transverse friction massage for treating lateral elbow or lateral knee tendinitis. Cochrane Database Syst Rev. 2014;11:CD003528.

24. Trudel D, et al. Rehabilitation for patients with lateral epicondylitis: a systematic review. J Hand Ther. 2004;17(2):243–66.

25. Vergereau R, Cumin M. LPG System et Dermatologie en particulier cicatrices. Groupe de Réflexion en Chirurgie Dermatologique; 1996. p. 27–29.

26. Hou A, et al. Microneedling: a comprehensive review. Dermatol Surg. 2017;43(3):321–39.

Hand and Wrist Mobilizations

Romain Prolonge

5.1 General Background

A normal function of the hand implies that all wrist and hand joints are free to move normally. Any disorder or restriction leads to hand dysfunctions from slight compensation mechanisms to heavy impairments according to the disorder's significance.

After injury, hand and wrist could suffer from several types of mobility loss. Facing these different origins, the therapist needs to lead a precise clinical reasoning (see Chap. 2) to use the most suitable treatments and techniques. Loss of mobility can come from a loss of muscular extensibility, pain, trophic disturbances, cutaneous scars, disturbances of the osteoarticular kinematics or of the motor control.

The use of wrist and hand joints mobilizations is a useful tool to treat mobility disorders. However, before describing mobilization techniques, it is interesting to talk about kinematic notions.

5.1.1 Osteoarticular Kinematics

A normal osteoarticular kinematics relies on three complementary motions:

- Firstly, there are the motions that produce the oscillatory movements of the two bones in relation to each other. They are behind voluntary movements.
- Secondly, there are the accessory motions that occur between joint surfaces. They cannot be performed voluntarily but are necessary for a normal joint mobility. They can be divided into five types: rolls, spins, slides, distractions, and compressions [1].
- Finally, there are movements of ligaments and capsular elements. Lateral structures should be able to slide freely, following the oscillatory movement. Anterior and posterior structures need to be able to fold and unfold freely.

Any disorder in the osteoarticular kinematic leads to a mechanical loss of mobility which will naturally evolve in stiffness if nothing is done to improve joints mobility.

5.1.2 An Early Mobilization

After injury, tissue repair often predisposes hand and wrist joints to reduce their range of motion [2]. Three successive phases can be observed in tissue repair:

R. Prolonge (✉)
Institut Sud Aquitain de la Main et du Membre
Supérieur, Biarritz, France

- **The acute inflammatory response**, with its pain and edema may reduce the joint full range of motion.
- **The cell proliferation phase** (from the third/fourth day to the eighth week) marks the beginning of histological changes. From now, joint immobilization will cause detrimental joint changes. Indeed, new collagen deposited during fibroplasia will create disorganized interfibrillar crosslinks. As a result, joint key elements (such as collateral ligaments, capsule, volar plate) will shorten and thicken.
- **The remodeling phase** (from the eighth week to several years) is the last tissue repairing phase. Collagen fibers are reorganized according to physical constraints. At this point, if the joint is not mobilized through its full range of motion, joint structures made of collagen fibers will remain in a shortened state prohibiting achieving a normal range of motion.

Therefore, within the limits of post-surgical instructions, it is essential to begin the earliest fit joint mobilization, to prevent joint stiffness. Indeed, the best way to deal with joint stiffness is, when possible, to prevent it in the first place.

5.1.3 A Mobilization at the Right Dose

Dosing mobilization is a way to achieve the best results. The dosing principles rely on the ability of connective tissues to be remodeled according to constraints placed on them [3]. Therefore, a mobilization correctly dosed allows good results. Nevertheless, an incorrectly dosed manipulation is counterproductive. On the one hand, if the mobilization is too light, injured tissues will not be remodeled enough, leading to stiffness and a loss of mobility. On the other hand, a too intense mobilization will be perceived as a physical aggression. As a result, an acute inflammatory response will occur leading to a loss of mobility. Joint mobilization is applying the right amount of stress, in intensity and duration, allowing a successful remodeling of injured tissues [2].

Therefore, a therapist needs to adapt his mobilization techniques to achieve the best result.

The application of physical constraints to connective tissues induces viscoelastic changes in the extracellular matrix. According to the intensity of the applied stress, connective tissue response can be divided into four phases [2]:

- **Phase 1**: For low stress levels, under tension areas initiate movements within the extracellular matrix allowing collagen fibers to unfold.
- **Phase 2**: As stress levels increase, movements within the extracellular matrix increase as well. Collagen fibers slide in relation to each other allowing fibers realignment and overall tissue elongation.
- **Phase 3**: Stress levels have increased and reached the point where collagen fibers sliding is no longer possible. From now on, they will stiffen.
- **Phase 4**: If stress levels are too high, connective tissues cannot manage them and will fail. The subsequently inflammatory response will induce a scar tissue production, increasing the risk of stiffness. In the end, applying too high stress levels can lead to diametrically opposed results from the initial objective.

Dosing joint mobilizations between phase 2 and phase 3 is the best method to be efficient. Indeed, this dose allows joint structures to hold their elastic behavior while getting close to its yield point (Fig. 5.1).

A joint mobilization applied at the right dose allows closing the gap between the current joint mobility and its desired goal. Dosing a mobilization and the search for an optimal stress load need to be repeated each time since it depends on the daily patient's condition, his progression, or the stage of healing. Moreover, some patients have low irritable tissues and can tolerate a wide range of applied constraints (Fig. 5.2a). On the contrary, other patients have an important tissues irritability, prompt to develop an early inflammatory syndrome. In this case, it could be challenging to find the right dose of mobilization to apply (Fig. 5.2b) [3].

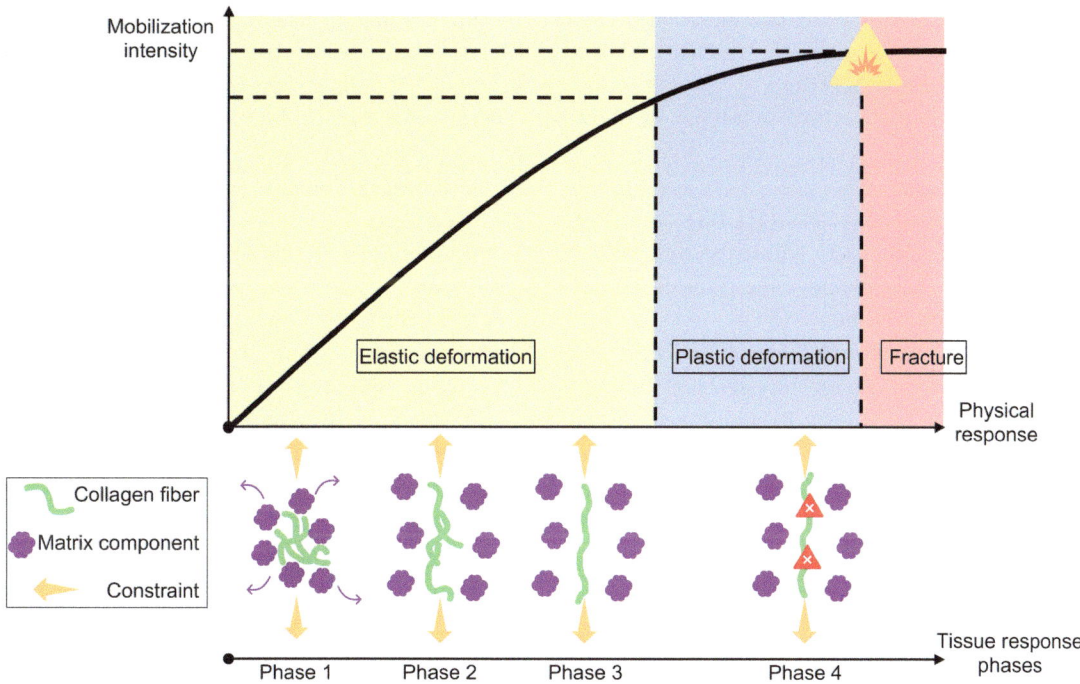

Fig. 5.1 Physical response and tissue response phases according to the intensity of the mobilization

Fig. 5.2 Search for an optimal stress load. (**a**) Patient with low irritable tissues tolerating a wide range of applied constraints. (**b**) Patient with high tissues irritability imposing a reduced stress load

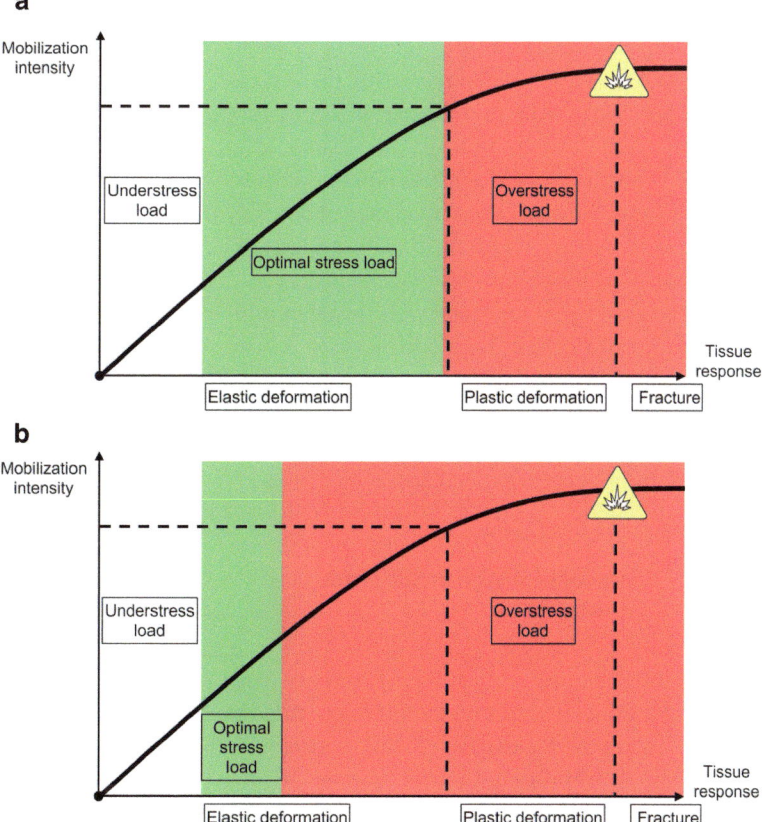

To adjust the right dose, two factors need to be taken into consideration: the intensity and the duration of the applied stress.

These two factors allow two types of mobilizations [2]:

- **High load brief stress (HLBS) techniques** allow the therapist to adjust the right amount of stress load to achieve the right dose over a short period of time.
- **Low load prolonged stress (LLPS) techniques** allow, with low physical constraints, to achieve the right dose by holding these constraints over a long period of time.

Passive mobilizations or active exercises belong to the HLBS techniques whereas splinting to increase range of motion belongs to the LLPS techniques.

Using HLBS techniques is controversial and there is a lack of evidence on this matter. Advocates of these techniques stand up that the induced inflammatory response and the scar tissue formation can be managed. Therefore, a controlled stimulation could lead to physiological responses allowing tissues to lengthen, preventing long-term stiffness. Detractors of these techniques suggest that the induced inflammatory response will lead to fibrosis, increasing joint stiffness. The lack of consensus upon these divergent theories shows a lack of evidence and justify the need of further research to truly understand stress-induced tissue response mechanisms [2].

In conclusion, an early and well-dosed mobilization could prevent joint stiffness to occur. Nevertheless, in everyday clinical practice, hand and wrist joint stiffness is still a reality. Therefore, the therapist needs to have techniques at his disposal to fight against joint stiffness.

5.1.4 The Total End Range Time Theory

The total end range time (TERT) theory suggested by Flowers relies on the principle that the improvement in passive range of motion of a stiff joint is proportional to the amount of time the joint is held at its end range. This constraint dictates how connective tissue is remodeled affecting its final length and strength [4]. Therefore, the more time the joint spends under appropriate tension at the end of available range of motion, the more passive range of motion will increase [2].

According to the TERT concept, the greatest results are obtained not by increasing the technique intensity but by increasing its duration. This statement shows the dominant place of mobilizing splinting to fight against stiffened joints since splinting techniques allow to hold a joint at its end of available range of motion for a long period of time.

Nevertheless, a stiffened joint could come from various osteoarticular structures disruptions. Moreover, it could be difficult to deal with all these disruptions, at the same time, with only one splint. In this case, additional joint mobilization techniques could be useful to recover a normal range of motion.

5.1.5 Different Approaches in Joint Mobilization

Joint mobilizations are manual techniques focusing on synovial joints. These techniques are used to increase range of motion, decrease pain, and improve patient's functional abilities.

Joint mobilization techniques rely on two types of motion. On the one hand, there are repetitive passive movements in different part of the range of motion, known as oscillatory joint mobilizations. On the other hand, there are the accessory movements. Depending on the case, the therapist can focus his technique on a simple oscillatory mobilization or combining oscillatory and accessory mobilization according to biomechanical principles.

5.1.5.1 Kaltenborn's Approach
Kaltenborn developed passive joint mobilizations based on biomechanical principles [5]. His techniques rely on joint tractions and accessory mobilizations. Kaltenborn's mobilization is described as a three-part grading scale:

- **Grade 1**: Joint traction is used alone to suppress compressive forces in the joint.
- **Grade 2**: Joint traction is paired up with accessory sliding motions. The goal is to tighten and get rid of the slack in the connective tissues around the joint.
- **Grade 3**: As in grade 2, joint traction and accessory sliding motions are paired up. Nevertheless, the desired result is to stretch the connective tissues.

The overall goal of Kaltenborn's techniques is a return to normal joint biomechanics.

5.1.5.2 Maitland's Approach

While Kaltenborn's techniques are based on joint biomechanics, Maitland's techniques are passive mobilizations based on the perception of symptoms, such as pain or stiffness.

These techniques use oscillatory mobilizations, varying amplitude, and speed according to the patient's tolerance [6]. Maitland's mobilization is described as a five-part grading scale [1]:

- **Grade 1**: Small amplitude and slow oscillatory mobilizations at the beginning of the range of motion. The goal is to reduce the pain.
- **Grade 2**: Large amplitude and slow oscillatory mobilizations within the available range of motion. The goal is also to reduce the pain.
- **Grade 3**: Large amplitude and slow oscillatory mobilizations between the middle and the end of the range of motion. The goal is to increase the range of motion.
- **Grade 4**: Small amplitude and slow oscillatory mobilizations at the end of the available range of motion. The goal is also to increase the range of motion.
- **Grade 5**: Small amplitude and high velocity thrust at the end of the available range of motion.

Choosing which one of Maitland's techniques to use is dictated by the patient's perception of symptoms. The overall goals of Maitland's techniques are to decrease the pain and increase the range of motion.

5.1.5.3 Mulligan's Approach

The Mulligan's techniques mix a passive mobilization made by the therapist with a patient's active movement allowing to manage joint "positional fault." Just as in Maitland's technique, Mulligan's techniques are based on patient's perception of symptoms. In the first place, the therapist needs to find the painful movement. Then, he needs to find which accessory mobilization can reduce the pain [7]. Therefore, the therapist makes a passive accessory mobilization while the patient makes the active painful oscillatory movement. If patient's symptoms do not decrease, the therapist needs to find another accessory mobilization. Once identified, he mobilizes the joint in this direction to correct the positional fault occurred after injury of the joint [8].

5.1.5.4 From Theories to Practice

Even though there are multiple approaches of joint mobilizations, they share the same base. Indeed, a joint mobilization is always an association of oscillatory and accessory mobilizations aiming for the return of a normal joint's mobility.

5.2 Mobilization Techniques

When mobilizing hand and wrist joints, for oscillatory mobilizations as much as accessory mobilizations, the therapist must have efficient holds, without inserting an intermediate joint. Therefore, his holds should be close to the joint, especially for accessory mobilizations. Then, he performs the mobilization according to the joint biomechanics. Finally, a good joint mobilization is a well-dosed and painless mobilization.

5.2.1 The Convexity and Concavity Rules

From the moment a joint is not perfectly conforming, any oscillatory motion from a bone in relation to another produces an accessory motion of translation. According to the joint anatomical structure, this accessory motion occurs in a specific direction [9].

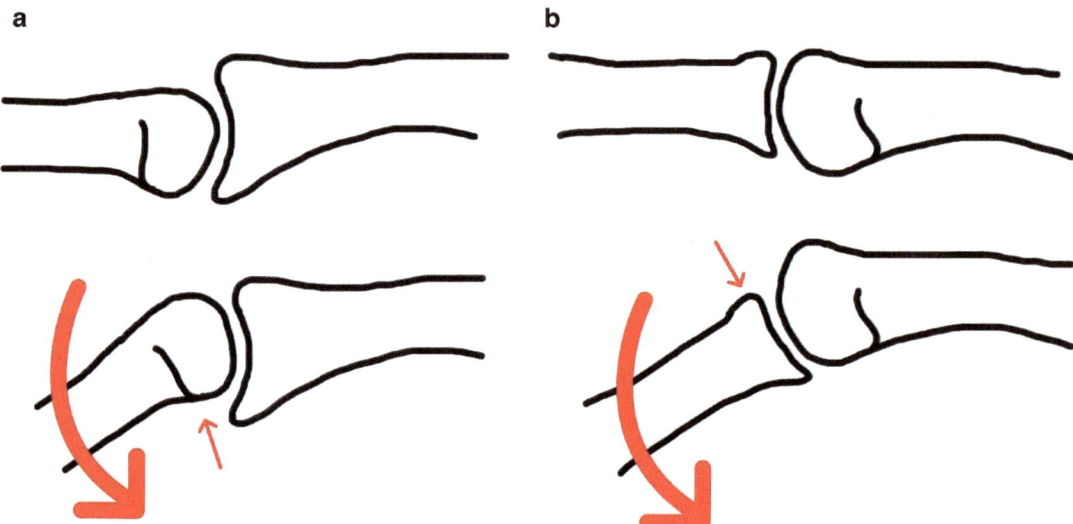

Fig. 5.3 (**a**) Convexity rule: a convex structure in relation to a concave structure requires a translation in the opposite direction. (**b**) Concavity rule: a concave structure in relation to a convex structure requires a translation in the same direction

Mobilizing a convex structure in relation to a concave structure follows the convexity rule. The oscillatory motion and the accessory translation occur in an opposite direction (Fig. 5.3a).

Mobilizing a concave structure in relation to a convex structure obeys the concavity rule. The oscillatory motion and the accessory translation occur in the same direction (Fig. 5.3b).

5.2.2 How to Use Mobilization Techniques

There are different ways to mobilize a joint. There are techniques focusing only on oscillatory movements, others focusing only on accessory movements while others combine oscillatory and accessory movements. There are types of mobilization that can be performed within all the joint available range of motion whereas other types focus on a specific part of this range of motion. Finally, joint mobilizations can be done at various, from low to high velocity [9].

For low velocity mobilization, the amount of stress applied on the joint is slowly and gradually increased until reaching the pathological restriction. It is the setup phase. Then, the mobilization continues further, without any twitch and without triggering painful symptom. It is beyond restriction phase. Finally, and in the same way, the stress is slowly and gradually untightened. It is the release phase. For this type of mobilization, the amount of time spent in each of the three phases is the same.

For high velocity mobilization, first, the therapist gradually increased the stress in the joint until reaching the pathological restriction. From then on, he realizes a short thrust in a small range of motion and in the way of the mobilization. As an example, in a flexion-extension mobilization in the sagittal plane, the thrust is executed in an anteroposterior axis. At the end, the stress is released.

5.2.3 The Radioulnar Unit Mobilization

The radioulnar unit is responsible for the mobility and the stability of the forearm during pronation and supination movements. This motion's kinematics is complex. It requires the participation of the radius, the ulna, the proximal and distal radioulnar joints, and the interosseous membrane.

5.2.3.1 The Proximal Radioulnar Joint

The proximal radioulnar joint is one of the joints of the elbow unit. It shares his capsule with the humeroulnar and humeroradial joints. It is a trochoid joint between the head of the radius and the radial notch of the ulna, stabilized by the annular and quadrate ligaments. During pronation and supination movements, the head of the radius not only rotates but also has an anteroposterior translation along the radial notch of the ulna [10]. With pronation, the radial head makes an internal rotation and translates anteriorly. On the contrary, with supination, the radial head makes an external rotation and translates posteriorly [9] (Table 5.1).

Regarding anteroposterior translation motions, some authors dispute the ability to manually obtain such translations [11] especially in supination.

In addition, there is a lack of evidence on the influence of the flexion-extension position of the elbow upon the pronation and supination mobility in the proximal radioulnar joint. Therefore, for convenience purpose, the forearm pronation is realized with an extended elbow and the forearm supination is realized with a flexed elbow.

To mobilize the proximal radioulnar joint in pronation, the therapist holds, with one hand, the lower third of the forearm, with the elbow in extension and mobilizes the joint toward pronation. Moreover, with his other hand, the therapist puts his thumb in

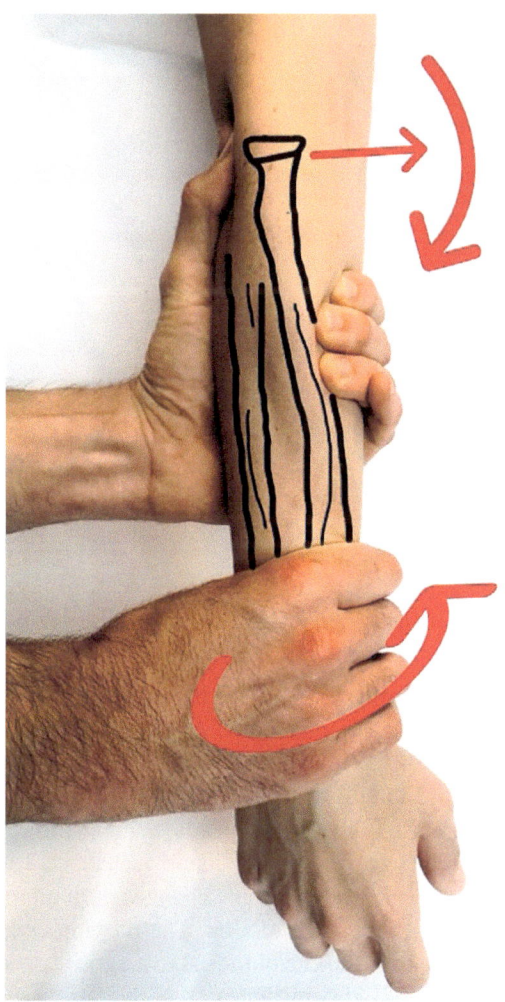

Fig. 5.4 Mobilization of the proximal radioulnar joint in pronation and anterior translation, elbow in extension

front of the dorsal face of the radial head and makes anterior push to realize the translation (Fig. 5.4).

On the contrary, mobilizing the proximal radioulnar joint in supination, the therapist holds the elbow in flexion. With one hand, he grasps the lower third of the forearm and mobilizes the joint toward supination. With his other hand, the therapist surrounds the proximal extremity of the radius and pulls it posteriorly, to realize the posterior translation (Fig. 5.5).

Table 5.1 Summary of motions in relation to proximal radioulnar joint mobilization

	Mobilization in pronation	Mobilization in supination
Elbow's position	Extension	Flexion
Radial head translations	Anterior	Posterior

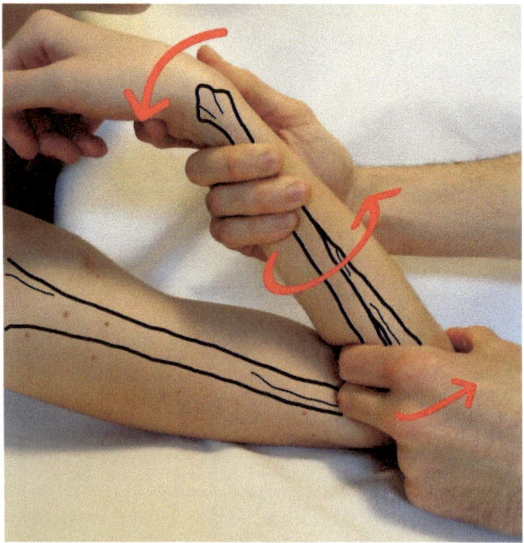

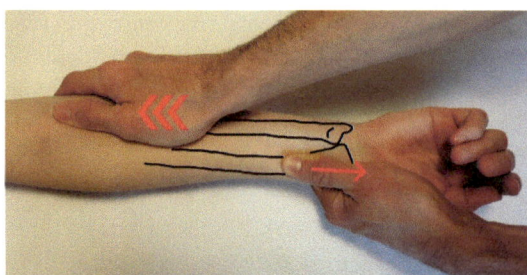

Fig. 5.6 Mobilization of the interosseous membrane by an axial pull of the radius

Fig. 5.5 Mobilization of the proximal radioulnar joint in supination and posterior translation, elbow in flexion

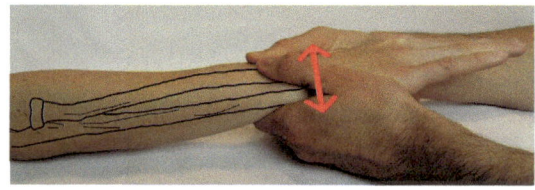

Fig. 5.7 Anteroposterior mobilization of the distal part of the interosseous membrane in pronation

5.2.3.2 The Interosseous Membrane

The interosseous membrane of the forearm is a fibrous sheet of crossed connective tissues between the radius and the ulna. Therefore, the membrane mobilization depends on the mobilization of the two bones in relation to each other. The tension inside the membrane changes during pronation and supination motion. The proximal part of the interosseous membrane is in a tense state in pronation. The intermediate part of the membrane is in a tense state in an intermediate position between pronation and supination. The distal part of the interosseous membrane is in a tense state in supination. In this way, the therapist can choose the level of tension inside the membrane through the pronation and supination position.

Mobilizing the radius in relation to the ulna allows a mobilization of the interosseous membrane:

- **Mobilization by pulling in the radius axis**: The therapist holds, from one hand, the lower extremity of the radius and pulls it in the axis of the bone whereas, from the other hand, he holds in place the anterior surface of the forearm (Fig. 5.6).
- **Anteroposterior mobilization**: The therapist holds the ulna in place with one hand whereas he holds, with the other hand, the radius and

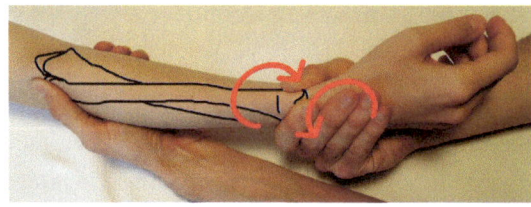

Fig. 5.8 Mobilization of the interosseous membrane with pronosupination motion of the forearm

shifts it through an anteroposterior axis. This mobilization can be done in all parts of the interosseous membrane (Fig. 5.7).
- **Pronation and supination mobilization**: Mobilizing the forearm from pronation to supination automatically changes the tension state within the membrane, taking part in its mobilization. The therapist holds the patient elbow in flexion and grasps the proximal and distal radioulnar joints. Then, the therapist mobilizes the forearm within all the pronation and supination range of motion available (Fig. 5.8).

5.2.3.3 The Distal Radioulnar Joint

Pronation and supination motion is a relatively circular movement of the radius and the ulna around their own rotational centers. Through all the motion, the ulna only rotates within a range of

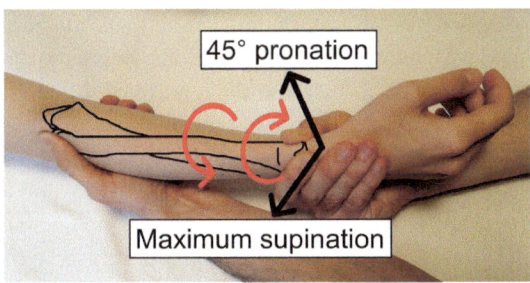

Fig. 5.9 Mobilization of the distal radioulnar joint from maximum supination and 45° pronation

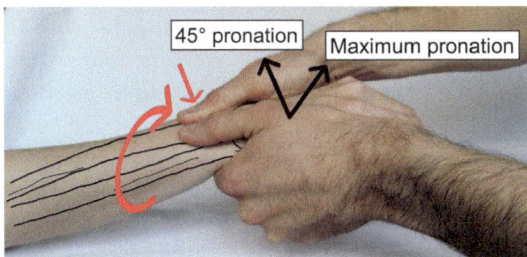

Fig. 5.10 Mobilization of the distal radioulnar joint from 45° pronation to maximum pronation, with a palmar translation

6°. However, the radius mobility in rotation is much more significant. From maximum supination to 45° pronation, the radius goes over almost all its rotational motion and rotates within a range of 140°. Then, from 45° pronation to maximum pronation, the radius stops its rotational motion and allows a palmar translation.

This translation may be caused by the morphology of the distal radioulnar joint and the contraction of the pronator quadratus [12]. As a result, the passive distal radioulnar joint mobilization needs to take this characteristic into account.

- **From maximum supination to 45° pronation**: The patient's elbow is held in a 90° position. The therapist grasps distal and proximal radioulnar joints. His proximal hand is fixed whereas his distal hand moves the forearm within maximum supination and 45° pronation (Fig. 5.9).

    From 45° pronation to maximum pronation: The patient's elbow is held in a 90° position. The therapist holds from one hand the lower extremity of the radius and from his other hand, he grasps the ulnar head. The ulna remains fixed

whereas the radius is mobilized, from 45° pronation to maximum pronation, with a palmar translation (Fig. 5.10).

5.2.4 Wrist Mobilizations

5.2.4.1 Radiocarpal Joint

Biomechanical Reminder

The radiocarpal joint is an ellipsoid joint between the forearm and the wrist. Its proximal part is made of the carpal articular surface of the lower end of the radius and the triangular fibrocartilage complex. The distal part of the radiocarpal joint is made of the proximal row of carpal bones, acting as a carpal condyle. The carpal articular surface of the radius is articulated with the scaphoid bone and the lateral part of the lunate bone. The triangular fibrocartilage complex is articulated with the medial part of the lunate bone and the triquetrum bone [9].

In a sagittal plane, the radiocarpal joint allows flexion-extension motion. In a frontal plane, it allows radial-ulnar deviations. Automatic pronation-supination motions of the proximal row of carpal bones in relation to the radius can be observed in the transverse plane although the range of motion is much lower.

Out-of-plane carpal motion combines, with different ranges of motion, movements in the radiocarpal joint in sagittal, frontal, and transverse planes [13] (Table 5.2).

During flexion and extension of the wrist, the main part of the radiocarpal joint occurs in the sagittal plane whereas frontal and transverse parts of the movement are of a lower importance. Nevertheless, frontal and transverse mobilities are essential to obtain a complete and harmonious motion.

During wrist deviations, the frontal and sagittal components of the movement have an equivalent significance. Therefore, ulnar deviation of the wrist is composed of an ulnar deviation in the frontal plane and an extension in the sagittal plane with an equivalent significance. Likewise, the radial deviation of the wrist is composed of a radial deviation in the frontal plane and a flexion in the sagittal plane. Wrist deviations allow a much lower amount of pronation-supination of the proximal row, in the transverse plane.

Regarding accessory motions, the convexity rule is applied. Wrist flexion comes with a posterior translation in the radiocarpal joint. On the contrary, wrist extension comes with an anterior translation in the joint. Wrist ulnar deviation is associated with a radial translation whereas radial deviation is associated with an ulnar translation in the radiocarpal joint. Finally, a study showed that during a wrist extension, a radial translation also occurs in the joint [14] (Table 5.3).

Mobilization Techniques

To realize radiocarpal joint mobilizations, the therapist holds, from one hand, the proximal row of carpal bones and, from the other hand, immobilizes the lower end of the radius respecting the slope of the bone facing downward and toward the outside in the frontal pane (Fig. 5.11). The distal hand of the therapist mobilizes the joint and realizes the accessory motions. In practice, to simplify and to increase the control of the mobilizations, it seems to be interesting to mobilize an association of two components, according to the combinations shown in Tables 5.2 and 5.3, and to vary the association (Figs. 5.12, 5.13, and 5.14).

For example, searching for mobility in wrist extension needs to seek associated motions (in this case, radial deviation et pronation-supination) as well as accessory motions (in this case, anterior and radial translation). In this way, wrist extension mobilization can be decomposed, with the radiocarpal joint point of view, in four manual mobilization techniques. The first combines extension with radial deviation. The second combines extension with pronation and supination of the proximal row of carpal bones. The third technique combines extension with accessory anterior translation. Finally, the fourth technique combines extension with accessory radial translation.

In practice, accessory mobilizations need to respect the anatomy of the lower end of the radius. That is to say, radial, and ulnar translations need to follow, in the frontal plane, the oblique nature of the radius slope downward and toward the outside. In the same way, anterior and posterior translations need to respect, in the sagittal plane, the radius slope downward and backward.

Within the radiocarpal unit, the radioscaphoid joint is one the main actors in the flexion-extension motion of the wrist. To restore this mobility, a specific mobilization of the translations between the scaphoid and the radius can be required. From one hand, the therapist immobilizes the lower end of the radius. From the other hand, he grasps the scaphoid through its tubercle and dorsal surface, between his thumb and index finger. Finally, the therapist realizes the antero-posterior translation of the scaphoid (Fig. 5.15).

A traction force can be used to reduce constraints upon articular surfaces while making

Table 5.2 Summary of associated motions of radiocarpal joint according to wrist's movement

	Sagittal plane	Frontal plane	Tranverse plane
Wrist's flexion	Flexion	Slight ulnar deviation	Scaphoid and triquetrum: slight pronation
			Lunate: slight supination
Wrist's extension	Extension	Slight radial deviation	Scaphoid and triquetrum: slight supination
			Lunate: slight pronation
Wrist's ulnar deviation	Extension	Ulnar deviation	Scaphoid and lunate: slight pronation
			Triquetrum: slight supination
Wrist's radial deviation	Flexion	Radial deviation	Slight supination

Table 5.3 Summary of associated motions according to radiocarpal joint mobilization

	Mobilization in flexion	Mobilization in extension	Mobilization in ulnar deviation	Mobilization in radial deviation
Anteroposterior translations	Posterior	Anterior	–	–
radioulnar translations	Insignificant	Radial	Radial	Ulnar

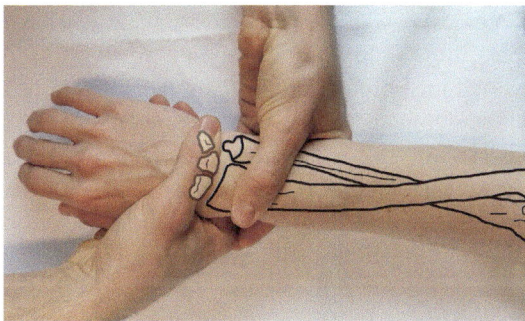

Fig. 5.11 Therapist's hands position respecting the slope of the radius in the frontal plane

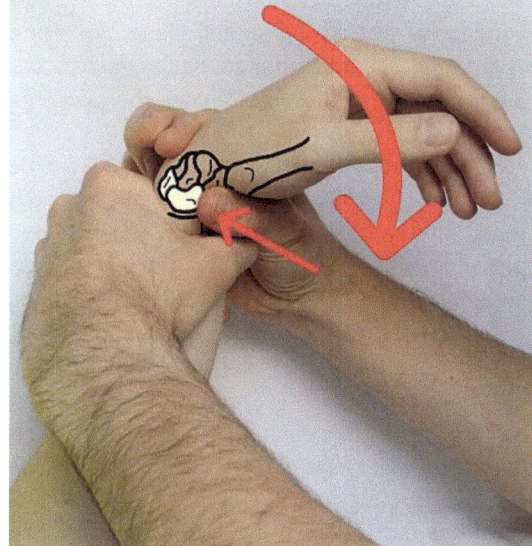

Fig. 5.12 Mobilization of the radiocarpal joint in flexion and posterior translation

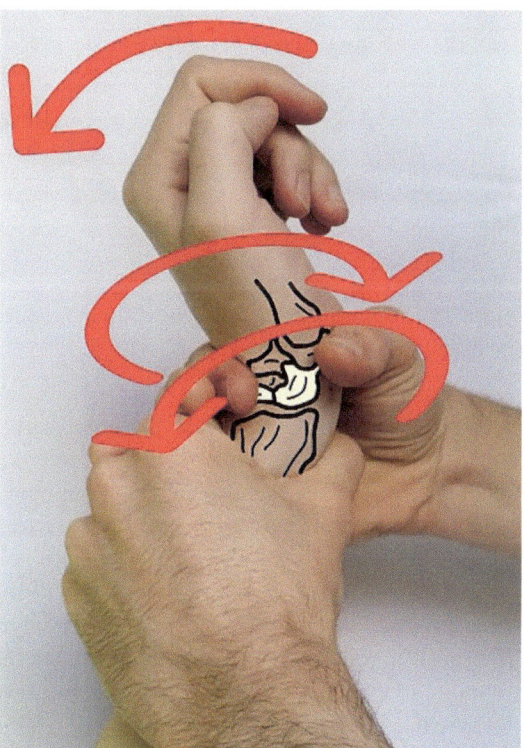

Fig. 5.13 Mobilization of the radiocarpal joint in extension and pronosupination

translation mobilizations. To maintain the traction force while mobilizing, the use of finger traps can be useful. According to the case, it is more useful to focus the traction the radial or the ulnar side. In the first case, finger traps will be placed on the index and middle fingers. In the second case, finger traps will be placed on the ring and little fingers [15].

5.2.4.2 Midcarpal Joint

Biomechanical Reminder

Carpal bones have, at the same time, a great mobility, and a great stability. Facing the com-

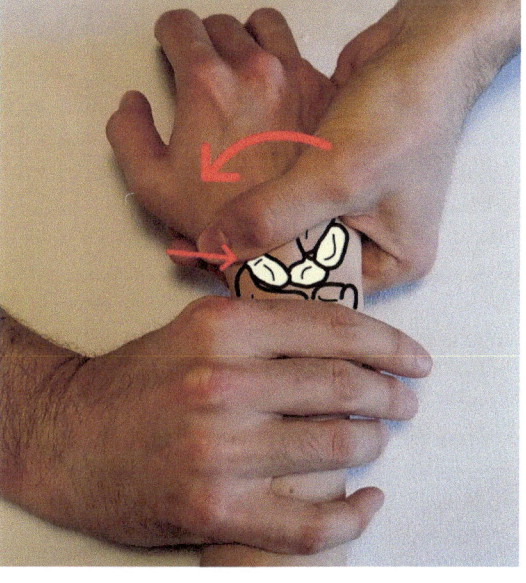

Fig. 5.14 Mobilization of the radiocarpal joint in radial deviation and ulnar translation

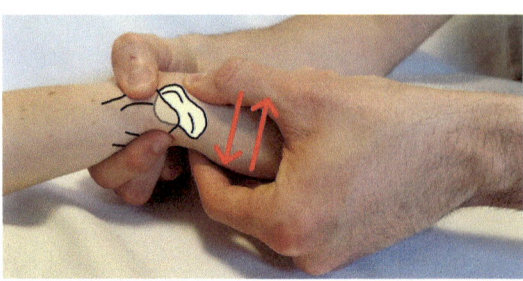

Fig. 5.15 Anteroposterior translations of the radioscaphoid joint

plexity of interactions between the eight carpal bones that make up the carpus and the numerous amounts of intrinsic and extrinsic ligaments, functional kinematics of the wrist is not yet well understood and is the subject of studies. Nevertheless, even though the way the wrist works remain in a theory and hypothesis stage, the carpus's role is well known. It facilitates the mobility of the wrist and transmits loads from the hand to the forearm. Any disturbance will lead to carpal instability with changes in local biomechanisms and changes load transmission, which will turn into pain and a loss of function [16].

For many years, two theories tried to explain wrist kinematics. The first one is the row theory which considers the carpus as a proximal and distal row [17]. The second one is the column theory which describes the carpal bones as three columns (radial, central, and ulnar) [18].

The row theory seems to be more adapted to described pathologies of the wrist, especially carpal instability dissociative. This theory describes a balanced mechanism of the lunate between the flexion moment applied by the scaphoid through the scapholunate ligament and the extension moment applied by the triquetrum through the lunotriquetral ligament [19]. In this theory, the bones of the proximal row are mobile in relation to each other whereas the bones of the distal row form a monolithic block with negligible intercarpal motion [20]. Therefore, and in practice, mobilizations within the distal row are not considered.

Nevertheless, there is no consensus among carpal motion theories allowing to understand all clinical observations. Moreover, with new tech-

nologies, new theories are emerging, as for example, the stable central column theory [21] in which the carpus functions around a stable central column composed of the lunate and the entire distal row. The scaphoid stabilizes the two rows, and the triquetrum restrains ulnar translation and controls lunate flexion. Finally, innovative imaging technologies, such as 4D-CT, allow making dynamic 3D representation of the wrist. These technologies will allow to improve and pursue studies of carpal kinematics [22].

While studying the midcarpal joint, the therapist should keep in mind his functional link with the radiocarpal joint in the motion of the wrist. As a matter of fact, in the sagittal plane, the central column divides the flexion for half in the radiocarpal joint and for the other half in the midcarpal joint. Likewise, for wrist extension, the central column divides the movement for 52% in the radiocarpal joint and for 48% in the midcarpal joint. However, the radial column shows a great difference in the separation between the radiocarpal joint part of the movement and the midcarpal joint part. This difference is greatly in favor of the radiocarpal joint or more precisely in favor of the radioscaphoid joint. The mobility of this joint represents 75% of the flexion mobility of the wrist and up to 92% of the extension mobility [23].

Therefore, in practice, midcarpal joint mobilizations need to be pair with radiocarpal joint mobilizations, described in the previous section.

Midcarpal joint mobilizations correspond to motions between proximal and distal row. Midcarpal joint is made of several plane joints. Therefore, the mobility of this anatomical area relies on accessory motions such as translations, rotations, and gapping [24].

Studies reveal the distal row motion in relation to the radius according to wrist's movements [25] (Table 5.4). By comparing the motion of the proximal and distal row in relation to the radius, we can draw conclusions on the motion between the two rows, which is the midcarpal joint mobility. Thus, we can notice that it exists synergetic and antagonistic motions between the two rows, according to wrist's movements (Table 5.5). In the frontal plane, the two rows always share synergetic motion. However, in the sagittal and transverse planes, the two rows can either have synergetic motions or antagonistic motions, depending on the overall wrist's motion.

Techniques of midcarpal joint mobilizations rely mainly on flexion-extension motion, pronation-supination motion, anteroposterior

Table 5.4 Summary of associated motions of the distal carpal row in relation to the radius according to wrist's movements

	Sagittal plane	Frontal plane	Tranverse plane
Wrist's flexion	Flexion	Slight ulnar deviation	Slight supination
Wrist's extension	Extension	Slight radial deviation	Slight pronation
Wrist's ulnar deviation	Slight flexion	Ulnar deviation	Slight pronation
Wrist's radial deviation	Slight extension	Radial deviation	Slight supination

Table 5.5 Summary of synergetic and antagonistic motions between the two carpal rows in relation to wrist's movements

	Sagittal plane	Frontal plane	Tranverse plane
Wrist's flexion	Synergetic motions	Synergetic motions	Scaphoid and triquetrum: antagonistic motions
			Lunate: synergetic motions
Wrist's extension	Synergetic motions	Synergetic motions	Scaphoid and triquetrum: antagonistic motions
			Lunate: synergetic motions
Wrist's ulnar deviation	Antagonistic motions	Synergetic motions	Scaphoid and lunate: synergetic motions
			Triquetrum: antagonistic motions
Wrist's radial deviation	Antagonistic motions	Synergetic motions	Synergetic motions

translations, and a specific mobilization according to the dart thrower's motion.

Mobilization Techniques

- **Flexion-extension mobilization**: The therapist holds the patient's wrist in neutral position. From one hand, he immobilizes the proximal carpal row. From the other hand, he holds on to the distal carpal row and mobilizes it with gapping motions toward flexion and extension (Fig. 5.16).
- **Pronation-supination mobilization**: These techniques imitate the rotation motions of the distal row compared to the proximal row. The therapist's hands are placed as for midcarpal joint flexion-extension mobilizations. The proximal hand holds the proximal row in place whereas the distal hand does rotation motions in the transversal plane. A medial rotation produces a pronation of the distal row. A lateral rotation produces a supination of the distal row (Fig. 5.17).
- **Anteroposterior translations**: The therapist uses the same hand position as before. The distal hand mobilizes the distal row doing anteroposterior tractions and thrusts (Fig. 5.18).
- **The Dart Thrower's Motion (DTM)**: DTM, defined by the International Federation of Societies for Surgery of the Hand as a motion from radial extension to ulnar flexion, is the

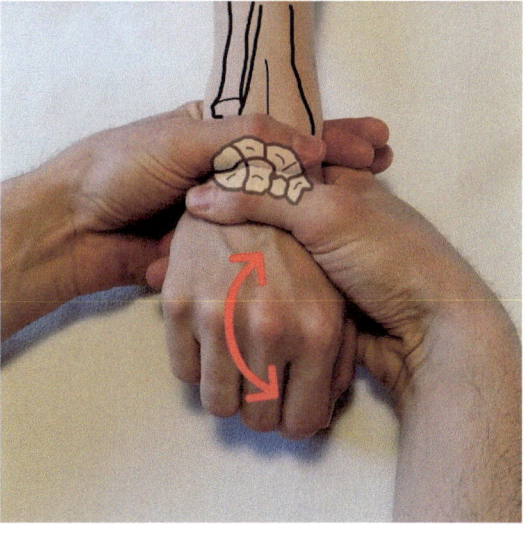

Fig. 5.16 Mobilization of the midcarpal joint in gapping motions in the sagittal plane

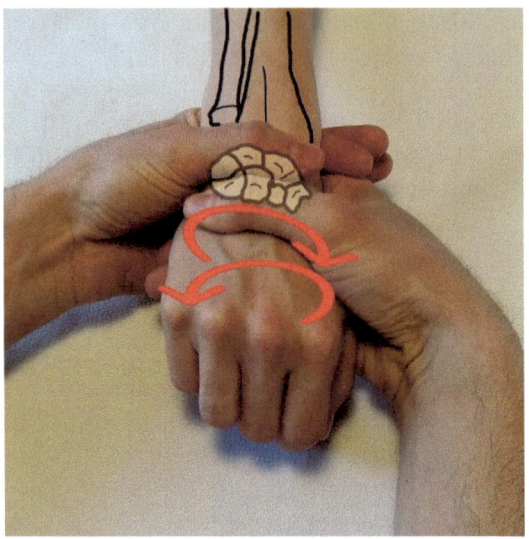

Fig. 5.17 Mobilization of the midcarpal joint in intracarpal pronation and supination

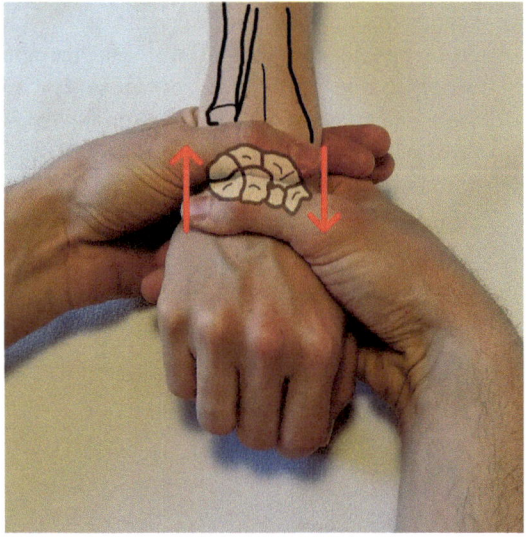

Fig. 5.18 Anteroposterior translations of the midcarpal joint

wrist's motion most involved in daily activities [14]. The plane of this motion is in a 45° in between the sagittal and frontal planes. This motion almost exclusively occurs in the midcarpal joint without participation of the radiocarpal joint. In practice, mobilizations in the plane of the DTM could allow to maintain a functional mobility of the wrist while restrict-ing radiocarpal motions and motions within the proximal carpal row. From a therapeutic point of view, this plane of motion could limit the stress upon the scapholunate ligament. Nevertheless, in the case of a complete scapholunate ligament rupture, DTM's dynamics is disrupted and the scaphoid acts as a bone of the distal carpal row. To realize this mobilization, the patient puts his elbow on the table with the forearm in a neutral pronation-supination position. The proximal hand of the therapist immobilizes the lower end of the forearm. His distal hand holds the distal carpal row and mobilizes the wrist between the radial extension and the ulnar flexion (Fig. 5.19).

5.2.4.3 Scapholunate and Lunotriquetral Joints

Within the proximal row of carpal bones, these two joints have compulsory mobilities for harmonious biomechanics of the wrist.

Scapholunate Joint Mobilization

The mobilization between the scaphoid and lunate resembles a scapholunate shear test [26]. Forearm in supination puts the scapholunate ligament in tension [27]. Therefore, for a well-executed mobilization, the patient's forearm is maintained in pronation to avoid this prejudicial tension.

The therapist holds, between his thumb and index finger, the scaphoid through its tubercle and dorsal surface. From his other hand, the therapist holds the dorsal and volar surface of the lunate between his thumb and index finger. The lunate is held in place whereas the scaphoid realizes translations between the two articular surfaces (Fig. 5.20).

Lunotriquetral Joint Mobilization

The therapist grasps the triquetrum through its volar (via the pisiform) and dorsal surface [28]. From his other hand, the therapist holds, as in scapholunate joint mobilization, the dorsal and volar surface of the lunate. The lunate is the fixed point of the mobilization, and the triquetrum is mobilized to achieve articular surfaces gliding (Fig. 5.21).

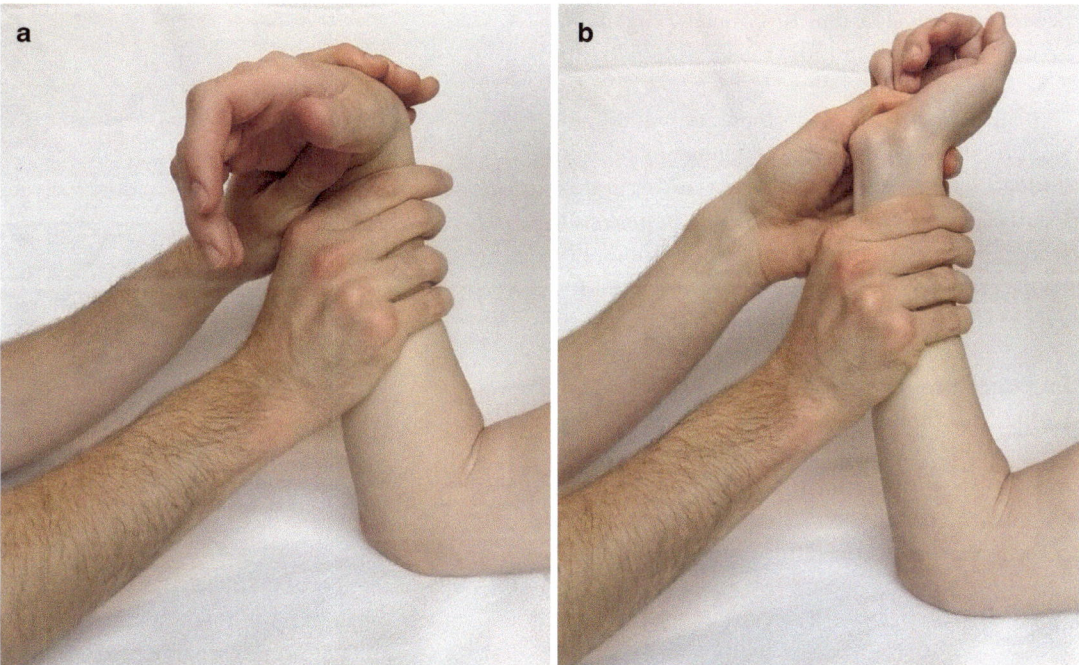

Fig. 5.19 The dart thrower's motion is a motion in an oblique plane from radial extension (in **a**) to ulnar flexion (in **b**)

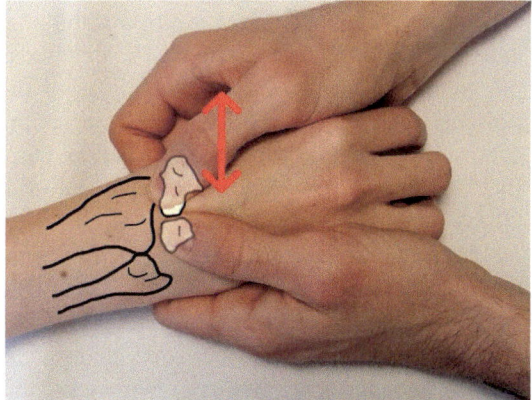

Fig. 5.20 Anteroposterior translations of the scapholunate joint

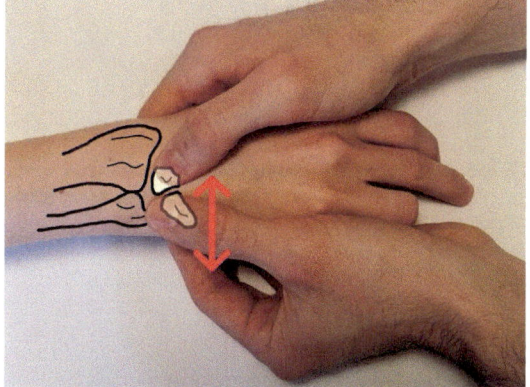

Fig. 5.21 Anteroposterior translations of the lunotriquetral joint

5.2.5 Finger Joints Mobilizations

5.2.5.1 Anatomical and Biomechanical Reminder

Metacarpophalangeal Joint

This joint unites the metacarpal head to the base of the proximal phalanx. It is a condyloid joint type with a two-degree-of-freedom kinematics.

In a sagittal plane, the metacarpophalangeal joint allows a flexion-extension motion along with an accessory translation according to the concavity rule [29].

In a frontal plane, the metacarpophalangeal joint allows an abduction-adduction motion. However, the lateral deviation of the joint only occurs in extension due to collateral ligaments laxity in this position [30] (Figs. 5.22, 5.23, and 5.24; Table 5.6).

In a transverse plane, there are automatic axial rotations of the metacarpophalangeal joint during flexion-extension motion. During a flexion, the index finger slightly moves in pronation while the rest of fingers moves in supination with a growing range of motion toward ulnar fingers [31].

Proximal Interphalangeal Joint

Unlike the biomechanical assumption that the proximal interphalangeal joint would act like a hinge type mechanism, the reality shows more complex biomechanics. The proximal interphalangeal joint is a nonconforming joint between

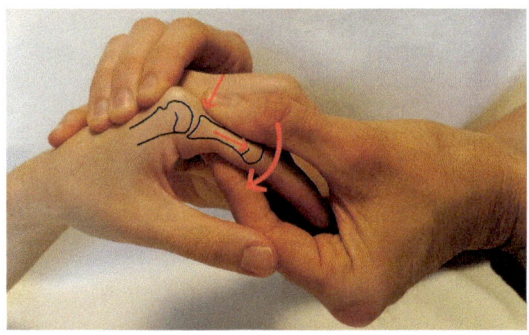

Fig. 5.22 Mobilization of the metacarpophalangeal joint in flexion combined with joint distraction and anterior translation

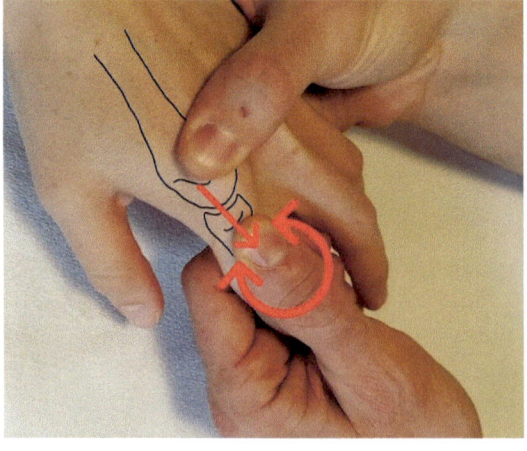

Fig. 5.23 Mobilization of the metacarpophalangeal joint in axial rotation combined with joint distraction

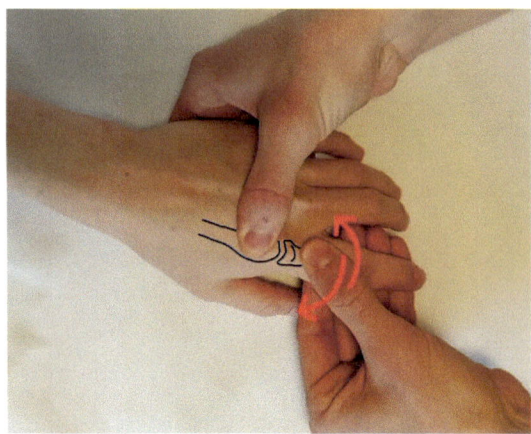

Fig. 5.24 Mobilization of the metacarpophalangeal joint in abduction and adduction, finger in extension

the head of the proximal phalanx and the base of the middle phalanx. Both articulating surfaces have two contact areas which means a four-degree-of-freedom kinematics [32]. Two of them can be observed in a sagittal plane, another in a frontal plane and the last one in a transverse plane.

In a sagittal plane, there are two simultaneous rotations around two centers. The first one is the center of curvature of the condyles of the proximal phalanx head. The second one is the center of curvature of the middle phalanx base. In practice, the proximal interphalangeal joint allows a flexion-extension motion with an instantaneous rotational center that shift during the movement according to the concavity rule (Figs. 5.25 and 5.26).

In a frontal plane, the joint allows an abduction-adduction motion. However, this motion is limited by collateral ligaments which confer stability from full flexion to full extension, with a maximal stability in extension [33].

In a transverse plane, just like in metacarpophalangeal joints, there are automatic axial rotations allowing the contact between the thumb and the fingers in prehension activity. These rotations show the same progression as for metacarpophalangeal joints. During a flexion, the index finger moves in pronation while the other of fingers move in supination [31].

Table 5.6 Summary of associated motions in relation to metacarpophalangeal joint mobilization

	Mobilization in flexion	Mobilization in extension
Frontal plane	–	Abduction/adduction
Transverse plane	Index finger: slight pronation	Index finger: slight supination
	Other fingers: supination	Other fingers: pronation
Translations	Anterior	Posterior

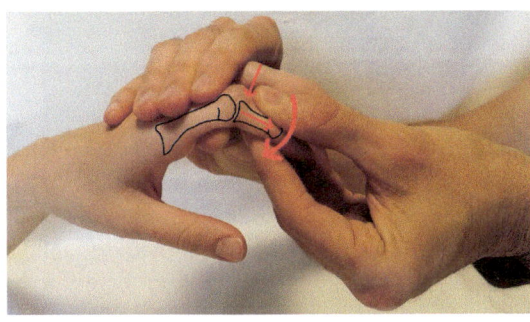

Fig. 5.25 Mobilization of the proximal interphalangeal joint in flexion combined with joint distraction and anterior translation

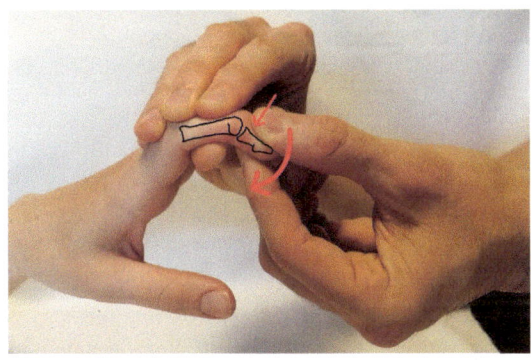

Fig. 5.27 Mobilization of the distal interphalangeal joint in flexion combined with a slight anterior translation

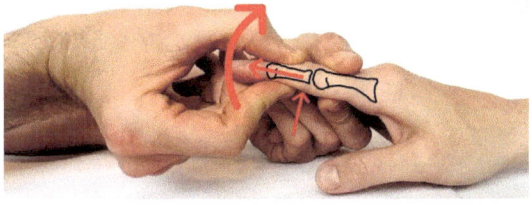

Fig. 5.26 Mobilization of the proximal interphalangeal joint in extension combined with joint distraction and posterior translation

Table 5.7 Summary of associated motions in relation to proximal interphalangeal joint mobilization

	Mobilization in flexion	Mobilization in extension
Transverse plane	Index finger: slight pronation	Index finger: slight supination
	Other fingers: supination	Other fingers: pronation
Translations	Anterior	Posterior

Thereby, proximal interphalangeal joint kinematics allows a flexion-extension motion along with an accessory translation according to the concavity rule and an axial rotation (Table 5.7).

Distal Interphalangeal Joint

There are few studies that described the distal interphalangeal joint. It is a nonconforming joint due to an asymmetry between the condyles of the middle phalanx head and the grooves of the distal phalanx base.

In a sagittal plane, distal interphalangeal joint kinematics allows a flexion-extension motion along with an accessory translation according to the concavity rule [34].

In a transverse plane, there are automatic axial rotations with a small range of motion. During a flexion, the index finger and middle finger slightly move in pronation while the two ulnar fingers slightly move in supination [31] (Fig. 5.27; Table 5.8).

5.2.5.2 Mobilization Techniques

All three finger joints have similar kinematics combining flexion-extension motion along with anteroposterior sliding and axial rotation motions. The main difference is based on the ability of the metacarpophalangeal joint to allow abduction-adduction motions in extension.

Table 5.8 Summary of associated motions in relation to distal interphalangeal joint mobilization

	Mobilization in flexion	Mobilization in extension
Transverse plane	Index and middle fingers: slight pronation	Index and middle fingers: slight supination
	Ring and small fingers: slight supination	Ring and small fingers: slight pronation
Translations	Anterior	Posterior

Table 5.9 Summary of analytical and accessory motions of the thumb carpometacarpal joint

	Analytical mobilizations	Accessory motions
Transverse axis	Flexion/extension	Radial/ulnar
Sagittal axis	Abduction/adduction	Dorsal/volar
Frontal axis	Medial rotation/lateral rotation	Axial distraction

To execute finger joint mobilizations, the proximal hand of the therapist immobilizes the head of the proximal bone and with his distal hand, he holds the base of the distal bone. Then, he pairs accessory motions with joint distraction to reduce pressure upon articulating surfaces, in all positions in the range of flexion-extension motion.

5.2.6 Thumb Joints Mobilizations

5.2.6.1 Thumb Carpometacarpal Joint

Anatomical Reminder

The ability to perform the thumb opposition movement is allowed by the saddle-shaped thumb carpometacarpal joint [35]. However, the great mobility of the carpometacarpal joint goes along with a mechanical disadvantage due to a reduced stability. Moreover, this joint is put to a great amount of compression loads, up to 12 times higher than the loads applied at the thumb fingertip [36].

There is a specific coordinate system used to describe the thumb carpometacarpal kinematics [37]. In this coordinate system, the joint can perform flexion/extension, adduction/abduction, internal rotation/external rotation as well as joint translations.

The thumb carpometacarpal joint allows a great mobility as well as a great motion complexity (Table 5.9). For example, a key pinch motion implies a flexion, an internal rotation, and a volar translation of the carpometacarpal joint. As for a cylinder grasping motion implies an external rotation, an abduction and three (ulnar, distal, and volar) translations in the carpometacarpal joint [38].

Mobilization Techniques

Mobilization techniques need to take oscillatory as well as accessory motions into account. The proximal hand of the therapist immobilizes the patient thumb base, composed of the scaphoid, trapezium, and trapezoid bones, between his thumb and index finger. The distal hand of the therapist takes hold of the thumb metacarpal base. Then, the therapist performs oscillatory movements of the joint along the distinct axis of the carpometacarpal joint coordinate system (Fig. 5.28). To facilitate the joint manipulation, a slight joint distraction can be combined. Concerning carpometacarpal accessory motions, dorsal-volar slides, ulnar-radial slides distractions and compressions can be realized. A circumduction motion slide can be used to work the overall accessory motions (Fig. 5.29).

5.2.6.2 Thumb Metacarpophalangeal Joint

Anatomical Reminder

The thumb metacarpophalangeal joint is a condyloid joint type that connects the thumb metacarpal head to the base of the proximal phalanx. The joint allows flexion/extension and abduction/adduction movements [39]. However, metacarpophalangeal mobility in abduction/adduction plane is limited by strong collateral ligaments. The proper collateral ligaments stabilize the joint in flexion and accessory collateral ligaments stabilize the joint in extension. Moreover, the metacarpophalangeal joint allows an axial rotation motion, which is essential for thumb positioning for opposition to the fingertips for prehension. Thereby, the flexion of the proximal phalanx promotes its pronation. On the contrary, the extension of the proximal pha-

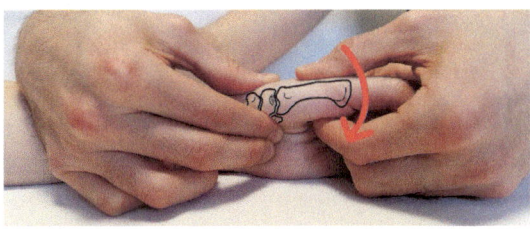

Fig. 5.28 Mobilization of the thumb carpometacarpal joint in flexion

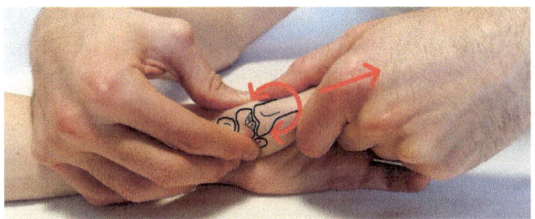

Fig. 5.29 Mobilization of the thumb carpometacarpal joint with joint distraction and circumduction motion

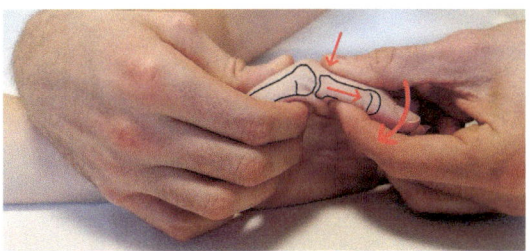

Fig. 5.30 Mobilization of the thumb metacarpophalangeal joint in flexion combined with joint distraction and anterior translation

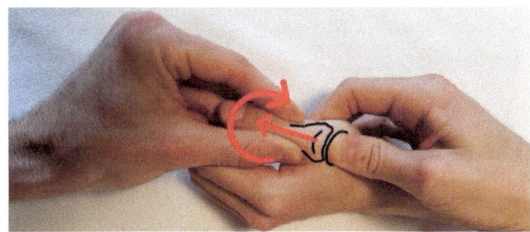

Fig. 5.31 Mobilization of the thumb metacarpophalangeal joint in pronation combined with joint distraction in flexed position

Table 5.10 Summary of associated motions in relation to thumb metacarpophalangeal joint mobilization

	Mobilization in flexion	Mobilization in extension
Anteroposterior translations	Anterior	Posterior
Axial rotations	Pronation	Supination

Table 5.11 Summary of thumb interphalangeal joint motions, according to the concavity rule

	Mobilization in flexion	Mobilization in extension
Anteroposterior translations	Anterior	Posterior

lanx promotes its supination. Furthermore, the thumb metacarpophalangeal joint responds to the concavity rule (Table 5.10).

Mobilization Techniques

The proximal hand of the therapist immobilizes the patient thumb metacarpal head between his thumb and index finger. The distal hand of the therapist takes hold of the base of the proximal phalanx. He produces flexion and extension motions combining with accessory slides. As always, a slight joint distraction can be used to facilitate the joint manipulation (Figs. 5.30 and 5.31).

5.2.6.3 Thumb Interphalangeal Joint

Anatomical Reminder

In the same way as for the fingers' distal interphalangeal joints, the thumb interphalangeal joint is a nonconforming articular joint connecting the two condyles of the thumb proximal phalanx head to the two grooves of the thumb distal phalanx base. Therefore, the joint allows flexion and extension motions as well as accessory slides according to the concavity rule (Table 5.11).

Mobilization Technique

From one hand, the therapist immobilizes the proximal phalanx head and from his second hand, the therapist seizes the thumb distal phalanx. With the help of a slight joint distraction, the therapist makes a flexion or extension joint motions along with a slight slide according to the concavity rule (Fig. 5.32).

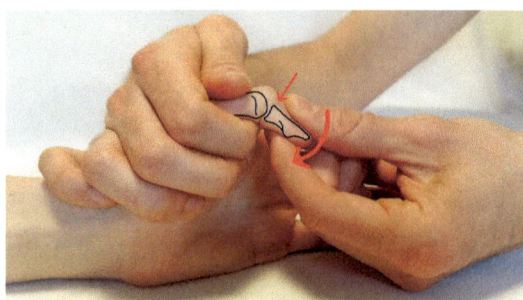

Fig. 5.32 Mobilization of the thumb interphalangeal joint in flexion combined with a slight anterior translation

References

1. Heiser R, O'Brien VH, Schwartz DA. The use of joint mobilization to improve clinical outcomes in hand therapy: a systematic review of the literature. J Hand Ther. 2013;26(4):297–311.
2. Glasgow C, Tooth LR, Fleming J. Mobilizing the stiff hand: combining theory and evidence to improve clinical outcomes. J Hand Ther. 2010;23(4):392–400.
3. Brody LT. Effective therapeutic exercise prescription: the right exercise at the right dose. J Hand Ther. 2012;25(2):220–31.
4. Flowers KR, LaStayo P. Effect of total end range time on improving passive range of motion. J Hand Ther. 1994;7(3):150–7.
5. Kaltenborn F. Manual mobilization of the extremity joints. 4th ed. Oslo, Norway: Olaf Norlis Bokhandel; 1989.
6. Maitland GD. Peripheral manipulation. 3rd ed. Boston: Butterworth-Heinemann; 1991.
7. Hing WA, Bigelow R, Bremner T. Mulligan's mobilisation with movement: a review of the tenets and prescription of MWMs. N Z J Physiother. 2008;36(3):144–64.
8. Stathopoulos N, Dimitriadis Z, Koumantakis GA. Effectiveness of Mulligan's mobilization with movement techniques on pain and disability of peripheral joints: a systematic review with meta-analysis between 2008-2017. Physiotherapy. 2019;105(1):1–9.
9. Ghossoub P, Dufour X, Barette G, Montigny J-P. Mobilisations spécifiques. EMC - Kinésithérapie - Médecine Phys - Réadapt. 2009;5(2):1–20.
10. Weiss AP, Hastings H. The anatomy of the proximal radioulnar joint. J Shoulder Elb Surg. 1992;1(4):193–9.
11. Dufour M, Neumayer M, Pillu M. Recherche de mobilités en glissements sagittaux dans l'articulation radioulnaire supérieure. Kinésithér Rev. 2008;5(37):35–40.
12. Nakamura T, Yabe Y, Horiuchi Y, Yamazaki N. In vivo motion analysis of forearm rotation utilizing magnetic resonance imaging. Clin Biomech (Bristol Avon). 1999;14(5):315–20.
13. Kaufmann R, Pfaeffle J, Blankenhorn B, Stabile K, Robertson D, Goitz R. Kinematics of the midcarpal and radiocarpal joints in radioulnar deviation: an in vitro study. J Hand Surg Am. 2005;30(5):937–42.
14. Crisco JJ, Coburn JC, Moore DC, Akelman E, Weiss A-PC, Wolfe SW. In vivo radiocarpal kinematics and the dart thrower's motion. J Bone Joint Surg Am. 2005;87(12):2729–40.
15. Atzei A, Luchetti R, Sgarbossa A, Carità E, Llusà M. Installation, voies d'abord et exploration normale en arthroscopie du poignet. Chir Main. 2006;25(Suppl 1):131–44.
16. Rainbow MJ, Wolff AL, Crisco JJ, Wolfe SW. Functional kinematics of the wrist. J Hand Surg Eur Vol. 2016;41(1):7–21.
17. Bryce TH. Certain points in the anatomy and mechanism of the wrist-joint reviewed in the light of a series of Röntgen ray photographs of the living hand. J Anat Physiol. 1896;31(Pt 1):59–79.
18. Navarro A. Luxaciones del carpo. Anal Fac Med. 1921;6:113–41.
19. Garcia-Elias M. Kinetic analysis of carpal stability during grip. Hand Clin. 1997;13(1):151–8.
20. Kamal RN, Starr A, Akelman E. Carpal kinematics and kinetics. J Hand Surg Am. 2016;41(10):1011–8.
21. Sandow MJ, Fisher TJ, Howard CQ, Papas S. Unifying model of carpal mechanics based on computationally derived isometric constraints and rules-based motion - the stable central column theory. J Hand Surg Eur Vol. 2014;39(4):353–63.
22. White J, Couzens G, Jeffery C. The use of 4D-CT in assessing wrist kinematics and pathology: a narrative view. Bone Joint J. 2019;101-B(11):1325–30.
23. Kaufmann RA, Pfaeffle HJ, Blankenhorn BD, Stabile K, Robertson D, Goitz R. Kinematics of the midcarpal and radiocarpal joint in flexion and extension: an in vitro study. J Hand Surg Am. 2006;31(7):1142–8.
24. Hamill J, Knutzen KM. Biomechanical basis of human movement. Philadelphia: Lippincott Williams & Wilkins; 2006. 486 p.
25. Camus EJ, Millot F, Lariviere J, Raoult S, Rtaimate M. Kinematics of the wrist using 2D and 3D analysis: biomechanical and clinical deductions. Surg Radiol Anat. 2004;26(5):399–410.
26. Stanley JK, Hodgson SP, Royle SG. An approach to the diagnosis of chronic wrist pain. Ann Chir Main Memb Super. 1994;13(3):202–5.
27. Esplugas M, Salvà-Coll G, Garcia-Elias M, Lluch-Bergadà A, Llusá-Pérez M. The scapholunate gap increases with forearm supination. A laboratory study. In: The XXIII FESSH Congress, Copenhagen, Denmark; 14 Jun 2018.
28. Tixa S. Atlas d'anatomie palpatoire. Tome 1: Cou, tronc, membre supérieur. 3ème. Paris: Elsevier Masson; 2012.
29. Pagowski S, Piekarski K. Biomechanics of metacarpophalangeal joint. J Biomech. 1977;10(3):205–9.
30. Sun YC, Sheng XM, Chen J, Qian ZW. In vivo metacarpophalanageal joint collateral ligament

length changes during flexion. J Hand Surg Eur Vol. 2017;42(6):610–5.

31. Degeorges R, Laporte S, Pessis E, Mitton D, Goubier JN, Lavaste F. Rotations of three-joint fingers: a radiological study. Surg Radiol Anat. 2004;26(5):392–8.

32. Dumont C, Albus G, Kubein-Meesenburg D, Fanghänel J, Stürmer KM, Nägerl H. Morphology of the interphalangeal joint surface and its functional relevance. J Hand Surg Am. 2008;33(1):9–18.

33. Pang EQ, Yao J. Anatomy and biomechanics of the finger proximal interphalangeal joint. Hand Clin. 2018;34(2):121–6.

34. Graham KS, Goitz RJ, Kaufmann RA. Curvatures of the DIP joints of the hand. Hand N Y. 2014;9(4):522–8.

35. Halilaj E, Moore DC, Patel TK, Laidlaw DH, Ladd AL, Weiss A-PC, et al. Thumb carpometacarpal joint congruence during functional tasks and thumb range-of-motion activities. In: Conf Proc Annu Int Conf IEEE Eng Med Biol Soc IEEE Eng Med Biol Soc Annu Conf. 2014; 2014. p. 4354–7.

36. Cooney WP, Chao EY. Biomechanical analysis of static forces in the thumb during hand function. J Bone Joint Surg Am. 1977;59(1):27–36.

37. Wu G, van der Helm FCT, Veeger HEJD, Makhsous M, Van Roy P, Anglin C, et al. ISB recommendation on definitions of joint coordinate systems of various joints for the reporting of human joint motion-- Part II: shoulder, elbow, wrist and hand. J Biomech. 2005;38(5):981–92.

38. Halilaj E, Rainbow MJ, Got C, Schwartz JB, Moore DC, Weiss A-PC, et al. In vivo kinematics of the thumb carpometacarpal joint during three isometric functional tasks. Clin Orthop. 2014;472(4):1114–22.

39. Leversedge FJ. Anatomy and pathomechanics of the thumb. Hand Clin. 2008;24(3):219–29.

Neurodynamic Mobilizations

6

Coline Geoffroy and Xabi Ezpeleta

6.1 General Notions

The nervous system is a continuous system. In fact, Littré [1] talks about a "dynamic interdependency" between its mechanics and its physiology: a mechanical alteration affects the physiology, which can then cause inflammation, peripheral sensitization, and mechano-sensitivity [2].

An impairment of this system usually leads to neuropathic pain, or even lack of mobility in most advanced cases [3].

6.1.1 Neuro-Mechanics

The nervous system's mechanical characteristics make it a mobile and viscoelastic system: the peripheral nerve trunks glide with movement, interacting with nearby structures and adapting to mechanical changes.

Therefore, they are under mechanical stress such as compression, gliding, displacement, tensioning, angulation and/or torsion, and vibration [4].

The nervous system has several mechanisms for decreasing nerve tension and/or elongation [5]. It adapts to tension, thanks to its internal structure made of "ripples" and its ability to glide at an intraneural and extraneural level [6]. As a matter of fact, a gliding movement is possible between the endoneurium and the perineurium, as well as between the paraneurium and the epineurium [7].

6.1.2 Neurophysiology

The physiological characteristics of the peripheral nervous system (PNS) make it sensitive to mechanical changes, with motor and sensorial functions. Its main role is to transfer information between the organs and the central nervous system (CNS).

Unlike the CNS, the PNS is protected neither by the skull and the spine, nor by the blood–brain barrier that isolates the CNS. This lack of defense leaves the PNS exposed to mechanical injuries and toxins.

To ensure axonal transport, the PNS has an intrinsic vascularization system (vasa vasorum) and an intrinsic innervation system (nervi nervorum) that are closely linked. The PNS represents 2–3% of the body weight but requires 20% of the blood flow [4].

Under normal conditions, when the nerve is excessively stimulated, it stimulates nociceptors and decreases blood flow and therefore axonal transports [4].

So, according to Sir Henry Head: "pain is the nerve screaming, deprived of its blood supply."

C. Geoffroy (✉) · X. Ezpeleta
Institut Sud Aquitain de la Main et du Membre Supérieur, Biarritz, France

© The Author(s), under exclusive license to Springer Nature Switzerland AG 2022
G. Mesplié (ed.), *Hand and Wrist Therapy*, https://doi.org/10.1007/978-3-030-94942-6_6

6.1.3 Patho-Neurodynamics

As long as the mechanical stress stays within the physiological limits, there are no symptoms: elongation and longitudinal gliding avoid over-tension, and transversal gliding prevents compression [4].

According to Kwan et al., a prolonged stress can affect the nerve's functional properties [8]: in case of undue stress, the nerve pressure gradient increases, and the intrinsic vascularization is altered, thus creating an inflammation of the nerve tissues and increasing its mechano-sensitivity: an edema can occur [9–11].

According to Lundborg and Rydevik [12], a tension of 5–10% applied on the nerve tissue is enough to make the first signs of changes in the blood supply appear in the epineurium and peri-neurium vessels. Moreover, an altered pressure (artery, capillary, venous return) can modify the circulation of the axoplasmic flow through the nerve [11, 13].

If this situation is maintained, fibrosis appears, and impedes the nerve's adapting capacities, thus leading to neurological symptoms [1, 14] (Fig. 6.1).

This intraneural or extraneural fibrosis prevents the nerve from gliding and lengthening, thus going against its adaptation to tension [6, 9, 15]. This way, there is less nerve tissue available when a joint moves, and the tension applied to the nerve tissue is more important [16]. This adaptation of the nervous system is expressed by a structural shortening causing a lack of mobility. Furthermore, according to Wall et al. [17], the damage caused on the nerve can be irreversible, even if the response to a prolonged nerve stretching does not occur immediately.

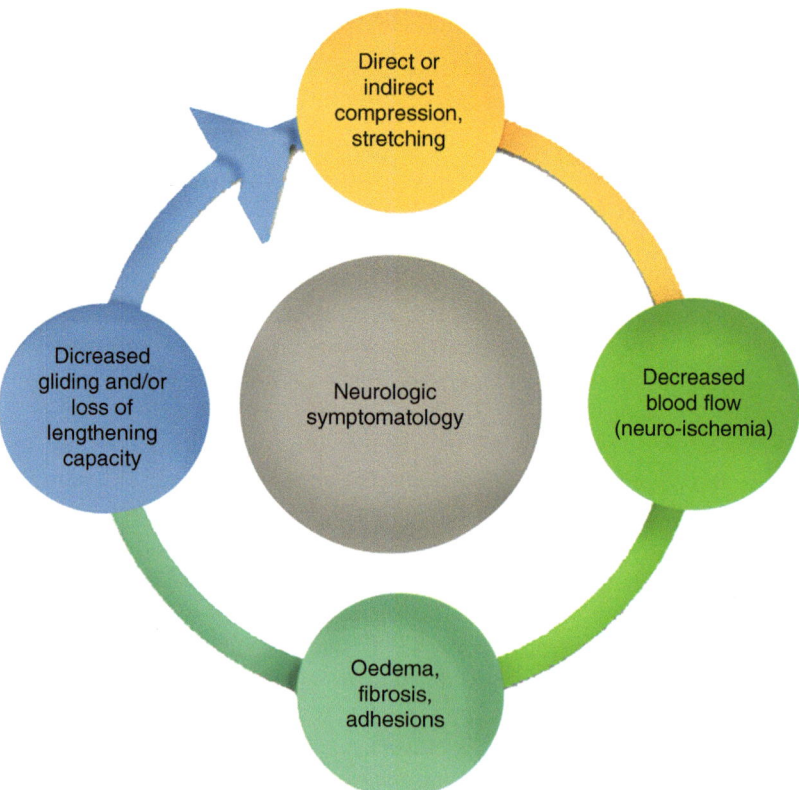

Fig. 6.1 Vicious circle of nerve degradation, according to B. Littré and J. de Laere

6.2   Neurodynamic Principles

To be as efficient in assessing as in rehabilitating, it is essential to integrate both the mechanics and physiology of the nervous system, as they both play an important role at a functional level [18].

Neurodynamic techniques are based on the nervous system's characteristics, and particularly on the close link between its mechanics and its physiology, as well as its relationship to the adjacent tissues. Therefore, the potential damage should be assessed and treated by mobilizing the nerve tissue as well as the adjacent tissues [1].

From an anatomical point of view, the techniques for assessing and treating the nervous system involve the mobilizations of joints that are along the peripheral nerve pathway. These mobilizations modify the nerves' tension and gliding [19–23].

6.2.1   Assessment

At first, neurodynamics were considered an evaluation method based only on nerve tension. However, this tension can cause symptoms and painful reactions that are too important to consider it a standard treatment [14]. According to Watanabe et al. [24], the elongation applied on the nerve must be under 4–6% of its resting length in order not to cause symptoms and/or injuries.

So, the mobilizations described by Butler et al. [25] in the Upper Limb Tension Tests (ULTT) will be used as a diagnostic tool and not as a therapeutic tool, as they stretch the nerves.

The pathological manifestations of a neurological dysfunction are symptoms like paresthesia, neuropathic pain, and lack of mobility of one or several segments of the concerned limb [26, 27] that can depend on the mobility of the spine or not. According to several studies [28–30], there can also be a "protecting" muscle contraction in the affected area.

However, one can wonder if using neurodynamic mobilizations such as ULTT is useful in a differential diagnosis. As these mobilizations include non-neural structures, how can we identify the structure causing the patient's pain? According to Coppieters et al. [31], using ULTT as a diagnostic tool is appropriate as it provokes important paresthesia in case of nerve damage, thus distinguishing it from a non-neural damage.

Walsh [3] suggests an assessment inspired by McClure's upper quadrant assessment [32], with several elements to look for in case of symptoms with a presumed neurodynamic origin.

The assessment starts with an anamnesis, to know the patient's history and symptoms. Neuropathic pain is a major component in case of neural dysfunction [3]. However, its differential diagnosis is complicated: the feeling and expression of pain are subjective variables. There are several scales that can help us make such a diagnosis, like the NP4, the Neuropathic Pain Scale [33], or the Neuropathic Pain Symptom Inventory [34].

A physical examination completes this first step, to study the patient's posture, with possible asymmetries and muscle atrophies. It can also be interesting to check tendon reflexes (biceps, brachioradialis, and triceps).

Furthermore, it is essential to know the anatomy of the nervous system as well as the innervation areas for each nerve, to direct the diagnosis towards one nerve or the other depending on the localization of the patient's symptoms (Figs. 6.2 and 6.3).

A sensitivity assessment can also be needed (see Chap. 7—"Physiology and Rehabilitation of Sensorial and Motor Disorders").

According to Walsh [3], five elements must be evaluated during the assessment, as they can confirm a neurodynamic dysfunction: a local dysfunction at the cervical level, an active dysfunction, pain when palpating the concerned nerve path, and sensitive points when palpating the tissues innervated by the concerned nerve (Fig. 6.4).

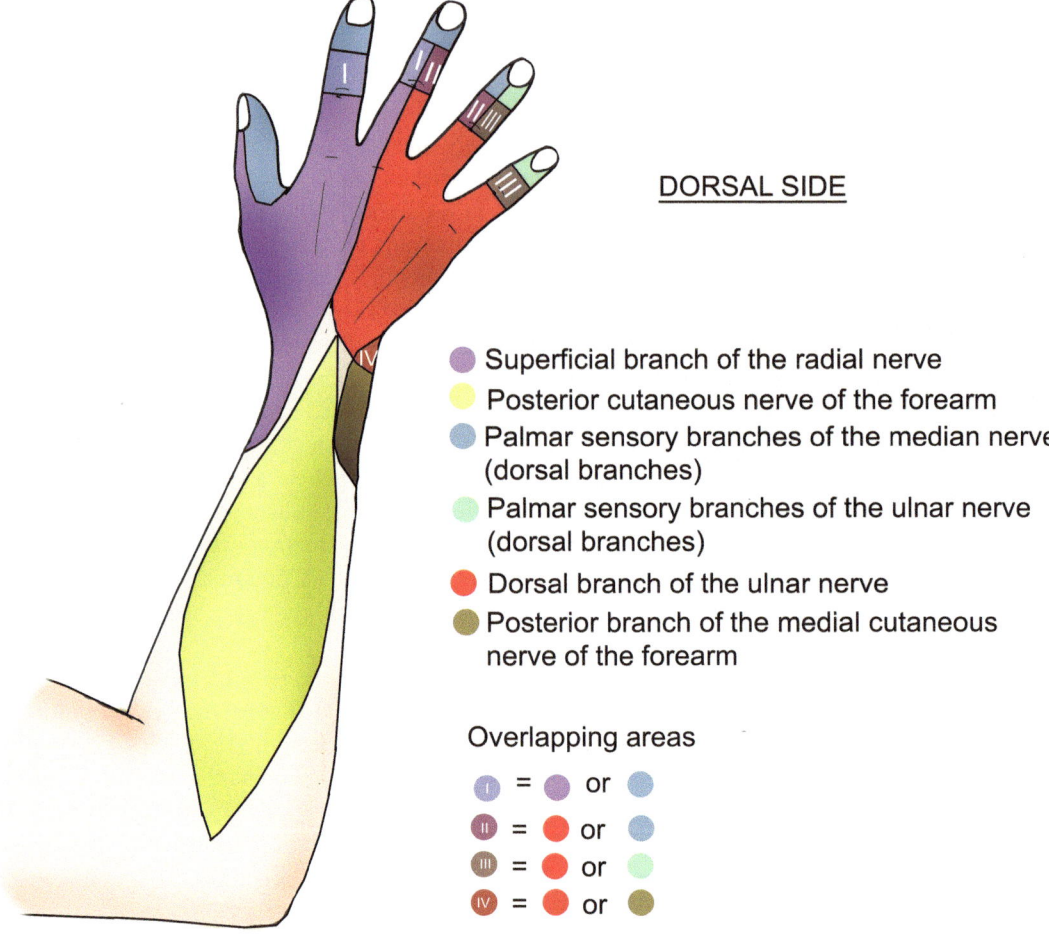

DORSAL SIDE

● Superficial branch of the radial nerve
○ Posterior cutaneous nerve of the forearm
● Palmar sensory branches of the median nerve
   (dorsal branches)
● Palmar sensory branches of the ulnar nerve
   (dorsal branches)
● Dorsal branch of the ulnar nerve
● Posterior branch of the medial cutaneous
   nerve of the forearm

Overlapping areas

ⅰ = ● or ●
ⅱ = ● or ●
ⅲ = ● or ●
ⅳ = ● or ●

Fig. 6.2 Innervation areas on the dorsal side of the hand, wrist, and forearm

The assessment will be considered positive if it reproduces the patient's symptoms and/or highlights lack of mobility caused by the neurodynamic dysfunction. It will have to be adapted to the patient's symptoms, especially in acute cases, in order not to worsen them: the therapist must pay attention to the patient's level of neuro-irritability (intensity and speed of his reactions), especially during the ULTT.

Regarding this, Walsh [3] also suggests a differential diagnosis based on decreasing the symptoms, rather than provoking them. By placing the tissues and joints that are far from the supposed compression/tension site in a position that decreases this mechanical stimulus, we can examine the patient without increasing the stress applied on a nerve that is possibly already mechanosensitive.

6.2.2 Treatment

A neurodynamic treatment is based on biomechanical components such as working on the lack of gliding and the excess of tension and/or compression. It is also based on physiological components that are

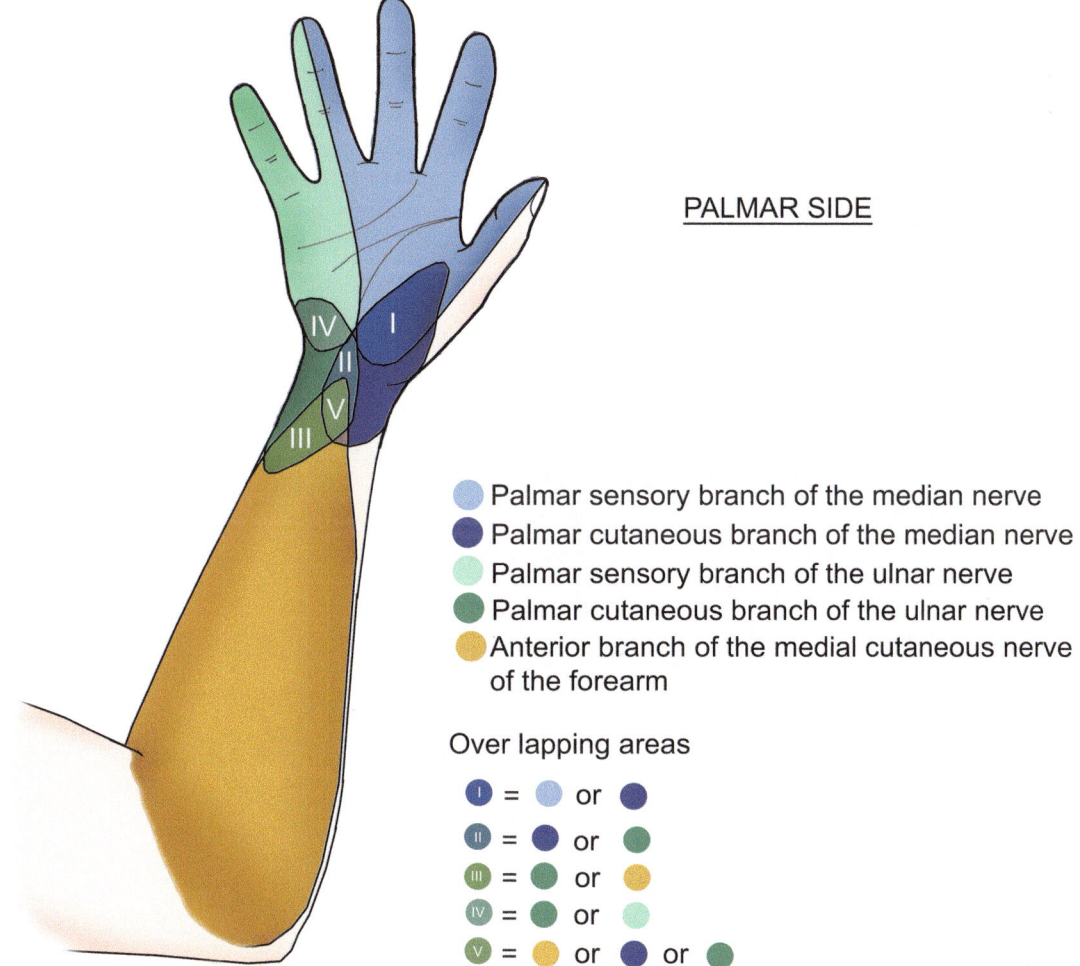

PALMAR SIDE

● Palmar sensory branch of the median nerve
● Palmar cutaneous branch of the median nerve
● Palmar sensory branch of the ulnar nerve
● Palmar cutaneous branch of the ulnar nerve
● Anterior branch of the medial cutaneous nerve
    of the forearm

Over lapping areas

I = ● or ●
II = ● or ●
III = ● or ●
IV = ● or ●
V = ● or ● or ●

Fig. 6.3 Innervation areas on the palmar side of the hand, wrist, and forearm

working on mechano-sensitivity and problems with nerve and blood circulation [25].

According to Wolny et al. [35], the efficacy of the neurodynamic treatment at the level of the carpal tunnel might come from the fact that it improves the nerve's viscoelasticity. The nerve ischemia changes its viscoelasticity, and therefore causes malfunctions in vascularization and peripheral innervation. Neuro-gliding mobiliza-

tions increase the efficacy of physiological processes within the nerve for a neuro-mechanical improvement [36].

Several studies [37–39] also conclude that a treatment including neurodynamic mobilization (especially neuro-gliding) seem more effective in decreasing the loss of function and the pain than a treatment without these mobilizations (manual therapy, orthosis, self-rehabilitation).

	Cervical dysfunction ?	Cervical tests (distraction, Spurling …) **Active mobility** **Passive mobility**	Tenderness to palpation of the segment related to the concerned peripheral nerve. Pain with active and/or passive movement. Hypo-mobility in segments related to the concerned peripheral nerve.
Anamnesis (history, symptoms, pain)			
Inspection (posture, asymmetry, muscle atrophy)	Active dysfunction ?	**Active mobility** of the joints in the upper limb **Myotomes** : C2-C4 (shrug of the shoulder) C5 (shoulder abduction, elbow fexion) C6 (elbow flexion, wrist extension) C7 (elbox extension, wrist flexion) C8 (thumb abduction) T1 (fingers abduction/adduction)	Restriction and/or pain. Motor weakness. Possible compensations and adaptations in motor patterns.
	Passive dysfunction ?	**Passive mobility** of the joints in the upper limb **Upper Limb Tension Tests** : median nerve (ULTT 1 and ULTT 2a) ulnar nerve (ULTT 3) radial nerve (ULTT 2b)	Restriction and/or pain. Muscle contraction (protective reflex).
Deep tendon reflexes (biceps, brachioradialis, triceps)		**Palpation** along the nerves and in areas where we most frequently find nerve compressions : brachial plexus : supraclavicular area, axilla median nerve : along the medial side of the humerus, along the medial side of the biceps, pronator teres, carpal tunnel ulnar nerve : along the medial side of the humerus, ulnar tunnel, proximal insertion of the flexor carpi ulnaris, Guyon's canal radial nerve : along the torsion channel of the humerus, anterior to the radial head, radial tunnel.	Pain and/or paresthesia
Sensitivity (innervation areas)	Neural sensitivity ?	**Palpation** of the surrounding tissues and/or the tissues innervated by the concerned peripheral nerve and/or cervical segment.	Tenderness and/or pain

Fig. 6.4 Neurodynamic assessment according to M.T. Walsh and P. McClure

6.3 Neurodynamic Mobilization Techniques

A systematic review by Littré [1] concludes that nerve mobilizations have an interesting efficiency in compressive neuropathies, but these techniques must be adapted to the type of neuropathy.

There are several techniques for neurodynamic treatment: nerve tension, nerve gliding, self-mobilization, tissue interface liberation.

As a rule, neurodynamic mobilizations (tension and gliding) must not reproduce or provoke the patient's symptoms [40], nevertheless several studies [31, 41] describe important reactions in asymptomatic patients when realizing ULTT (sensation of stretching, pain, paresthesia, etc.).

Moreover, in case of neurodynamic dysfunction, the patients mostly seek a consultation because of pain or paresthesia. If there is a lack of mobility, it is mostly due to the patient's protection position as he tries to avoid pain and/or paresthesia. In view of this, "stretching" a nerve with neuro-tension mobilizations seems to be of little interest to us.

Besides, according to Coppieters and Butler [42], neuro-gliding mobilizations are less harsh on the nerve and are therefore more suited in acute phases or after a surgery. This study shows that the tension on the median nerve is significantly smaller when performing nerve gliding than when applying tension on it. Nerve tension mobilizations apply a tension of more than 4% on the nerve, while the maximal tension applied should be under 4–6% in order not to cause symptoms and/or injuries, as mentioned earlier [24].

As the exact percentage of tension applied on the nerve is difficult for the therapist to evaluate, if not impossible, it seems more appropriate to use neuro-gliding mobilizations throughout the treatment, to avoid injuring the nerve more [3].

These techniques will be applied paying attention to the patient's feedback so that we do not reproduce or provoke his symptoms [3].

Another advantage of neuro-gliding techniques is that they produce a bigger nerve excursion than neuro-tension techniques. For example, Coppieters and Butler measured an excursion of 12.6 mm for the median nerve in the wrist and 8.3 mm for the ulnar nerve in the elbow with neuro-gliding techniques, while they measured excursions of 6.1 and 3.8 mm, respectively, with neuro-tension techniques [42].

Regarding the speed of execution, several studies [8, 43, 44] concluded that a slow application lets the nerve tissues adapt better to the nerve movements.

To sum up, we suggest applying neuro-gliding mobilizations, slowly, and respecting the patient's feedback to stay beneath the neurological symptoms triggering threshold.

In relation to the treatment of tissues adjacent to or innervated by the concerned nerve, Walsh [3] suggests two different approaches depending on whether we are dealing with intraneural or extraneural fibrosis. In case of intraneural fibrosis, he recommends treating the tissues far from the site of the supposed injury. In case of extraneural fibrosis, he recommends treating the tissues having a contact with the nerve at the level of the supposed injury.

6.3.1 Median Nerve

The carpal tunnel syndrome is the peripheral neuropathy with the highest incidence [42, 45].

According to Wolny et al. [35], neurodynamic mobilizations and passive techniques like ultrasounds and laser both improve the symptoms of a carpal tunnel syndrome. However, the patients treated with neurodynamic techniques improved better. The surgical treatment seems to be more effective than the conservative treatment but given that it is only proposed in advanced cases, neurodynamic mobilizations are interesting for moderate cases.

They can also be used if the nerve is compressed at a more proximal level: under the lacertus fibrosus, between the two fascicles of the pronator teres muscle, or under the arcade of the flexor digitorum superficialis muscle (Fig. 6.5).

6.3.1.1 Nerve Tension

These mobilizations, described by Butler, will be mostly used as a diagnostic tool. For the median nerve, they are the ULTT 1 and the ULTT 2a [25].

The ULTT 1 includes the following steps (Fig. 6.6):

- 90° of shoulder abduction (110° for the roots between C5 and C7)
- Slight shoulder depression
- Wrist and fingers supination and extension, elbow flexion
- 90° shoulder external rotation
- Elbow extension
- Contralateral head inclination

The ULTT 2a is based on the combination of shoulder traction/external rotation (Fig. 6.7):

- Position with a "triple grip" (therapist's pelvis and two hands)
- Strong shoulder depression
- Elbow extension
- Shoulder supination and external rotation

Fig. 6.5 Most common
compression sites for the
median nerve, other than
the carpal tunnel:
lacertus fibrosus
syndrome, pronator teres
syndrome, and anterior
interosseous nerve
syndrome

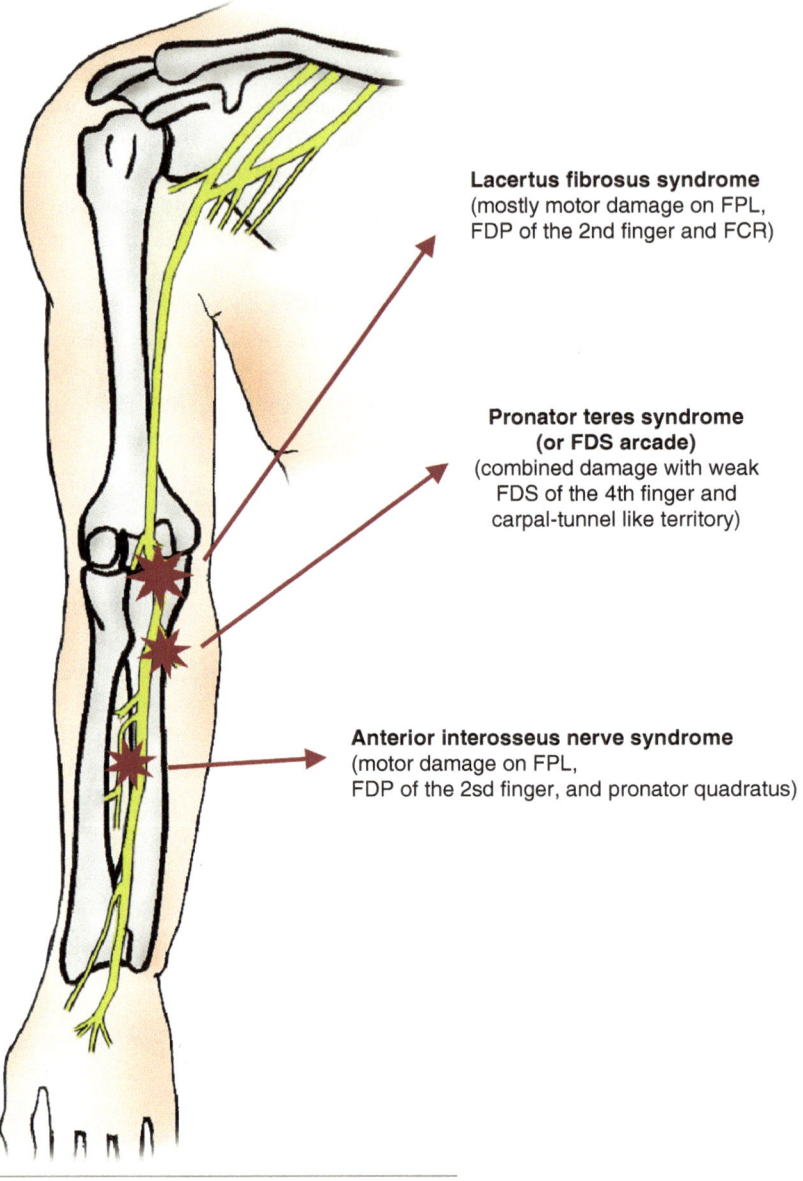

Lacertus fibrosus syndrome
(mostly motor damage on FPL,
FDP of the 2nd finger and FCR)

**Pronator teres syndrome
(or FDS arcade)**
(combined damage with weak
FDS of the 4th finger and
carpal-tunnel like territory)

Anterior interosseus nerve syndrome
(motor damage on FPL,
FDP of the 2sd finger, and pronator quadratus)

- Wrist and fingers extension
- Shoulder abduction until 30°

6.3.1.2 Nerve Gliding

According to Coppieters and Butler [42], to achieve nerve gliding without applying tension on it, the adjacent joints must be placed to alternatively increase and decrease the length of the nerve's path.

The median nerve is mostly shortened with an elbow extension and supination and a wrist and

fingers extension. The opposite position (elbow flexion and pronation and wrist and fingers flexion) relaxes it.

Based on biomechanics, we suggest the following mobilization (Fig. 6.8):

- Elbow extension and supination, wrist and fingers flexion.
- Elbow flexion and pronation, wrist and fingers extension.

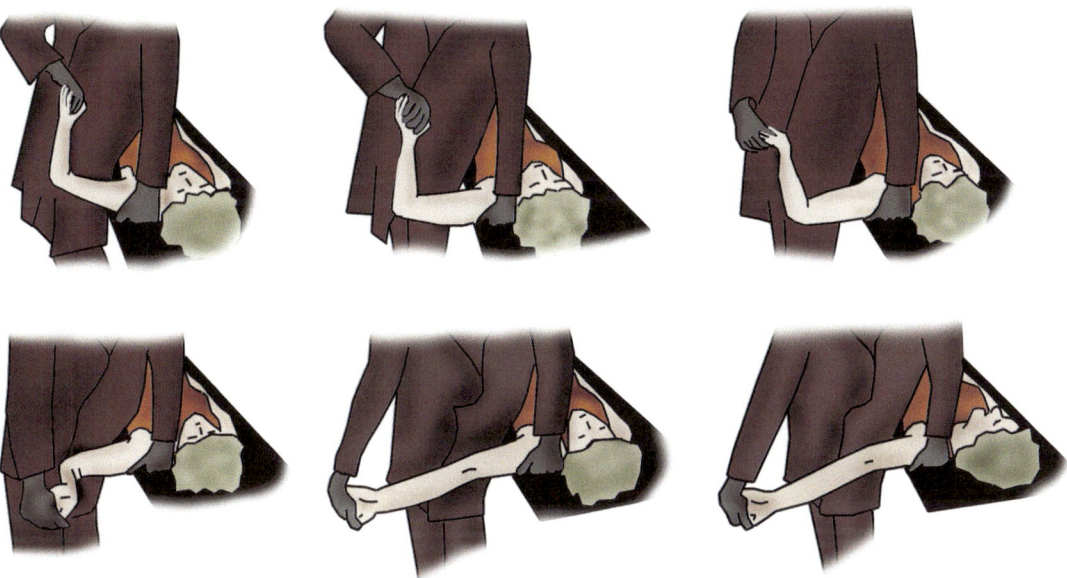

Fig. 6.6 Mobilization of the median nerve (ULTT 1). • 90° of shoulder abduction (110° for the roots between C5 and C7), • Slight shoulder depression, • Wrist and fingers supination and extension, elbow flexion, • 90° shoulder external rotation, • Elbow extension, • Contralateral head inclination

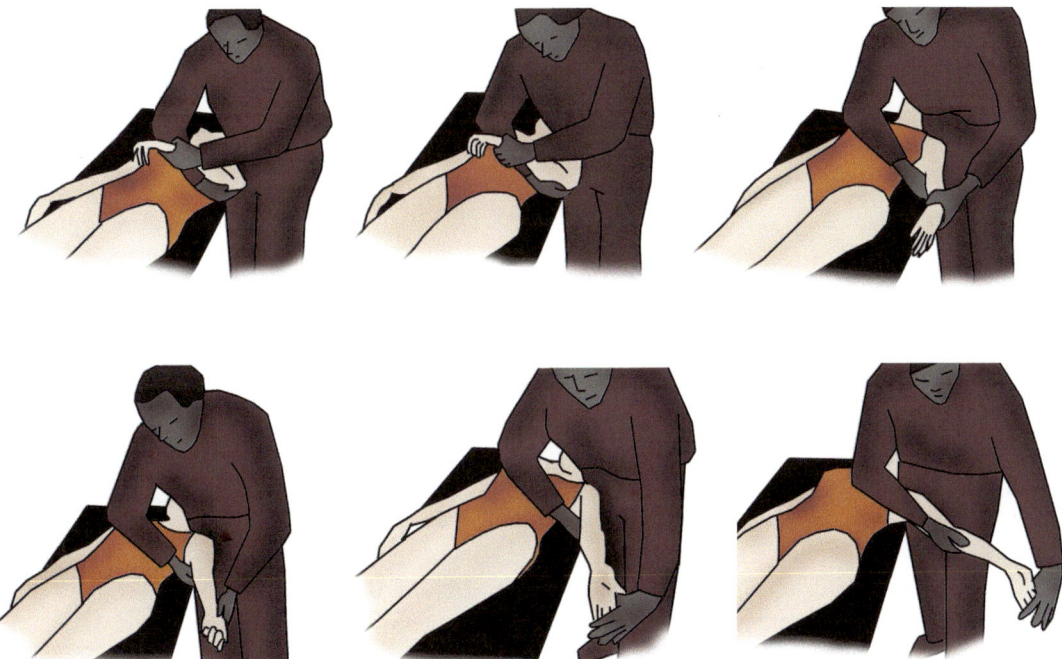

Fig. 6.7 Mobilization of the median nerve (ULTT 2a). • Position with a "triple grip" (therapist's pelvis and two hands), • Strong shoulder depression, • Elbow exten-sion, • Shoulder supination and external rotation, • Wrist and fingers extension, • Shoulder abduction until 30°

Fig. 6.8 Gliding without tension of the median nerve. • Elbow extension and supination, wrist and fingers flexion.
• Elbow flexion and pronation, wrist and fingers extension

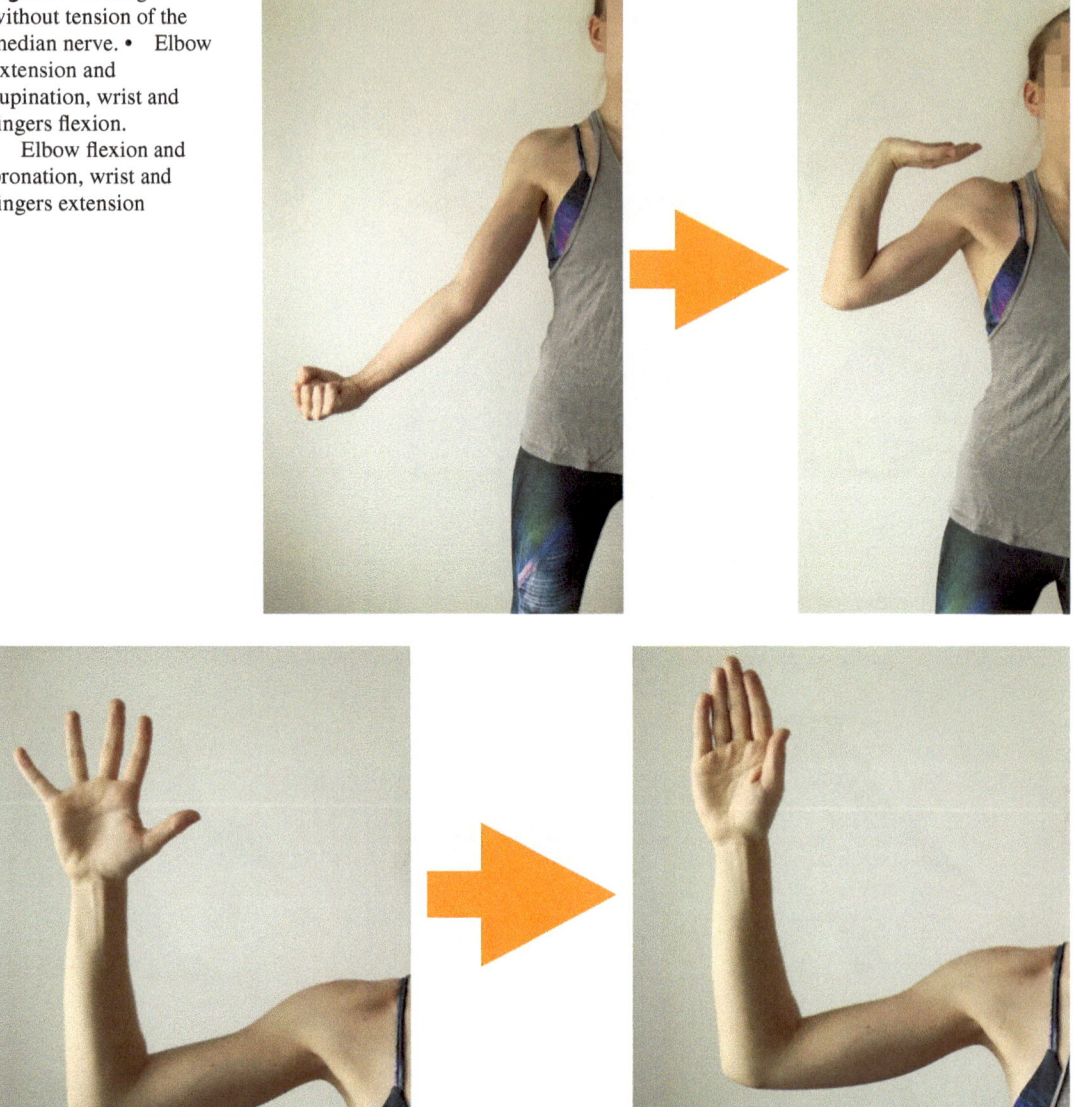

Fig. 6.9 Mobilization of the median nerve in the carpal tunnel according to Meng et al. • Shoulder abduction, • 90° of elbow flexion, • Neutral wrist position, • Fingers abduction/adduction

However, according to a recent study [45], these mobilizations do not result in the most important longitudinal gliding of the median nerve inside the carpal tunnel. This study suggests another mobilization to achieve that maximal gliding in the carpal tunnel (Fig. 6.9):

• Shoulder abduction
• 90° of elbow flexion

• Neutral wrist position
• Fingers abduction/adduction

6.3.1.3 Self-Mobilizations

They include the neuro-gliding mobilizations described earlier (Figs. 6.8 and 6.9).

Moreover, in less acute cases, the patient can realize a self-mobilization including the proximal part of the nerve, and working on the general

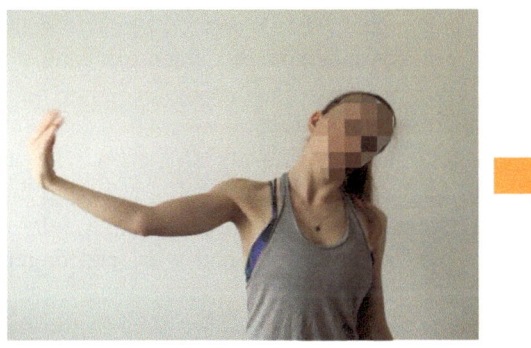

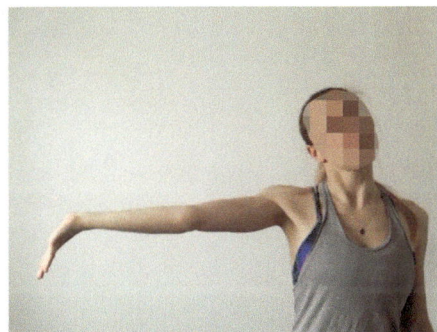

Fig. 6.10 Self-mobilization of the median nerve from proximal to distal. • Lowering the shoulder, • Shoulder abduction and external rotation, • Forearm supination,

• Wrist flexion and contralateral head inclination,
• Wrist extension and homolateral head inclination

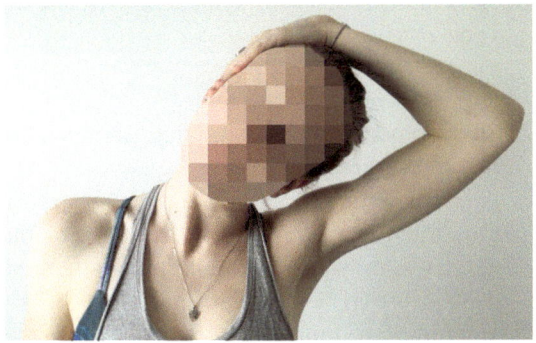

Fig. 6.11 Self-stretching of the superior fibers of the trapezius muscle. • The patient is sited, the homolateral hand holds the chair to lower the shoulder. • The contralateral hand brings the head in flexion, contralateral inclination, and homolateral rotation of the cervical spine

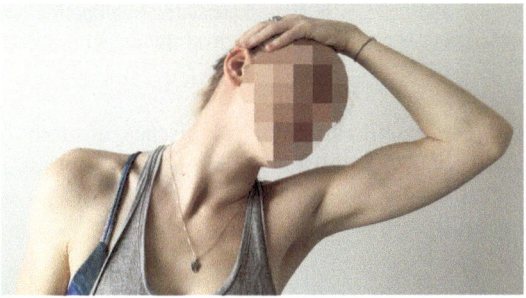

Fig. 6.12 Self-stretching of the superior fibers of scalene muscles. • The patient is sited, the homolateral hand holds the chair to lower the shoulder. • The contralateral hand brings the head in extension, contralateral inclination, and contralateral rotation of the cervical spine

gliding between the cervical spine and the distal extremity of the limb (Fig. 6.10):

- Lowering the shoulder
- Shoulder abduction and external rotation
- Forearm supination
- Wrist flexion and contralateral head inclination
- Wrist extension and homolateral head inclination

It is also interesting to add cervical spine self-mobilizations and to stretch the muscles that can be involved in a compression and/or a lack of gliding of the nerve:

- Superior fibers of the trapezius muscle (Fig. 6.11): passive flexion, contralateral incli-

nation, and homolateral rotation of the cervical spine.
- Superior fibers of scalene muscles (Fig. 6.12): passive extension, contralateral inclination, and contralateral rotation of the cervical spine.
- Levator scapulae muscle (Fig. 6.13): passive flexion, contralateral inclination, and contralateral rotation of the cervical spine.

6.3.1.4 Working on Adjacent Tissues
Alternating contraction-relaxation stretching of the adjacent muscles creates a peri-neural pumping that improves local trophicity and maintains inter-tissue gliding.

For example, when there is a total excursion of the fingers flexors tendons, the lumbrical muscles influence the pressure inside the carpal tunnel and should therefore be solicited [46].

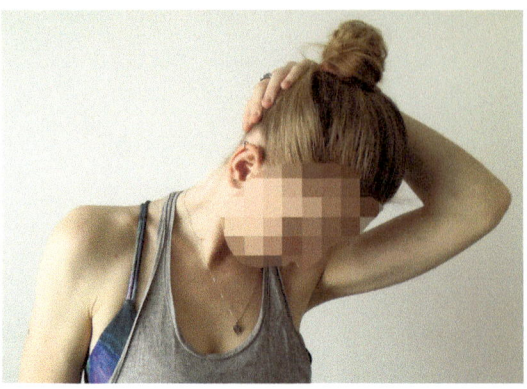

Fig. 6.13 Self-stretching of the levator scapulae muscle. • The patient is sited, the homolateral hand holds the chair to lower the shoulder. • The contralateral hand brings the head in flexion, contralateral inclination, and contralateral rotation of the cervical spine

The mobilization of the tissues around the nerve can be realized alternating movements in the wrist and fingers, allowing a dissociative contraction of the muscles adjacent to the median nerve.

Massages against fibrosis (dot-shaped, glided pressures, and kneading) can be realized along the median nerve, on the anterior part of the forearm, at the level of the flexor retinaculum and the thenar muscles. They improve local trophicity, fight against peri-neural fibrosis, and relax the muscles adjacent to the nerve [14].

6.3.2 Ulnar Nerve

6.3.2.1 Nerve Tension

For the ulnar nerve, the mobilization is based on the ULTT 3 and has several steps [25] (Fig. 6.14):

- 90° of shoulder abduction that can be combined with a slight shoulder depression
- Wrist extension and supination
- Blocking the shoulder to avoid anteflexion and external rotation
- Arm abduction with the palm of the hand touching the ear without losing the previous components
- Contralateral inclination of the head

Just as the ULTT 1 and ULTT 2a for the median nerve, it is more of a diagnostic tool.

6.3.2.2 Nerve Gliding

The ulnar nerve is mostly shortened with an elbow flexion and pronation and a wrist and fingers extension. The opposite position (elbow extension and supination and wrist and fingers flexion) relaxes it.

Based on biomechanics, we suggest the following mobilization (Fig. 6.15):

- Elbow flexion and pronation, wrist and fingers flexion.
- Elbow extension and supination, wrist and fingers extension.

6.3.2.3 Self-Mobilizations

They include the neuro-gliding mobilization described earlier (Fig. 6.15).

Moreover, in less acute cases, the patient can realize a self-mobilization including the proximal part of the nerve, and working on the general gliding between the cervical spine and the distal extremity of the limb (Fig. 6.16):

- Lowering the shoulder
- Shoulder abduction
- Forearm pronation
- Wrist extension and homolateral head inclination
- Wrist flexion and contralateral head inclination

It is also interesting to add cervical spine self-mobilizations and to stretch the muscles that can be involved in a compression and/or a lack of gliding of the nerve (Figs. 6.11, 6.12, and 6.13).

6.3.2.4 Working on Adjacent Tissues

Alternating contraction-relaxation stretching of the adjacent muscles creates a peri-neural pumping that improves local trophicity and maintains inter-tissue gliding. These mobilizations are realized preferentially on the flexor carpi ulnaris for proximal compressions and on the hypothenar muscles for distal compressions.

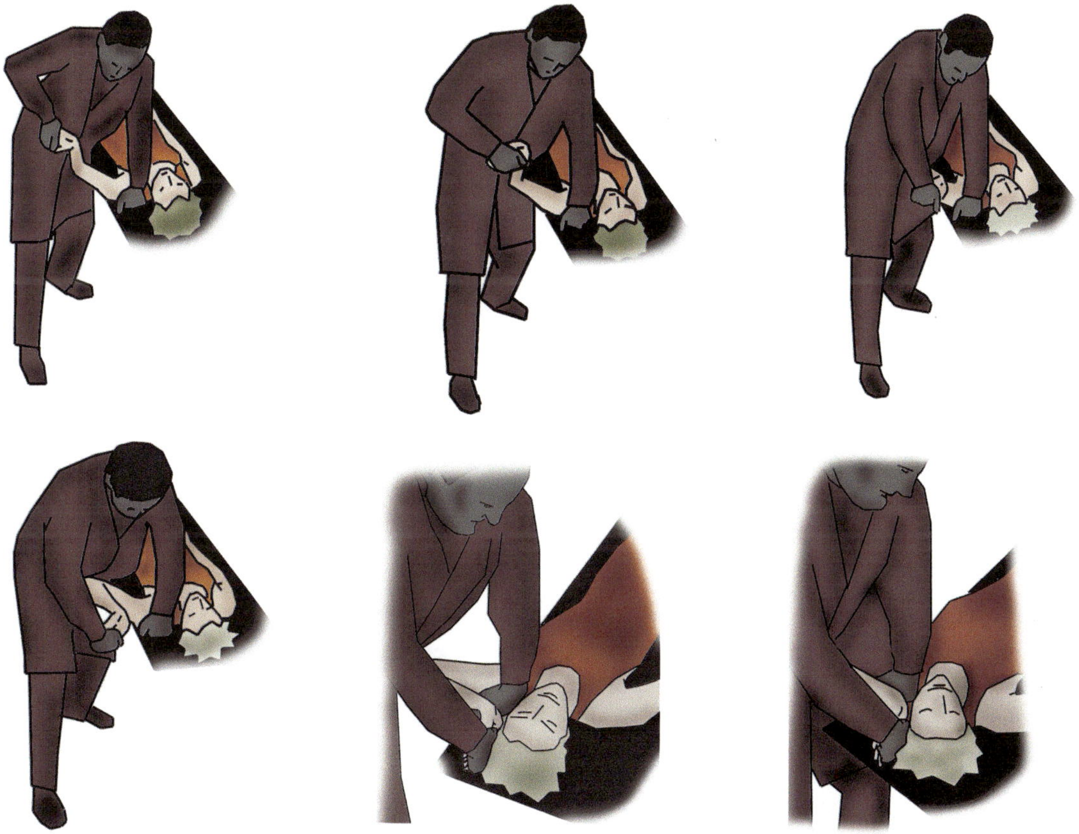

Fig. 6.14 Mobilization of the ulnar nerve (ULTT 3). • 90° of shoulder abduction that can be combined with a slight shoulder depression, • Wrist extension and supination, • Blocking the shoulder to avoid anteflexion and external rotation, • Arm abduction with the palm of the hand touching the ear without losing the previous components, • Contralateral inclination of the head

Fig. 6.15 Gliding without tension of the ulnar nerve. • Elbow flexion and pronation, wrist and fingers flexion. • Elbow extension and supination, wrist and fingers extension

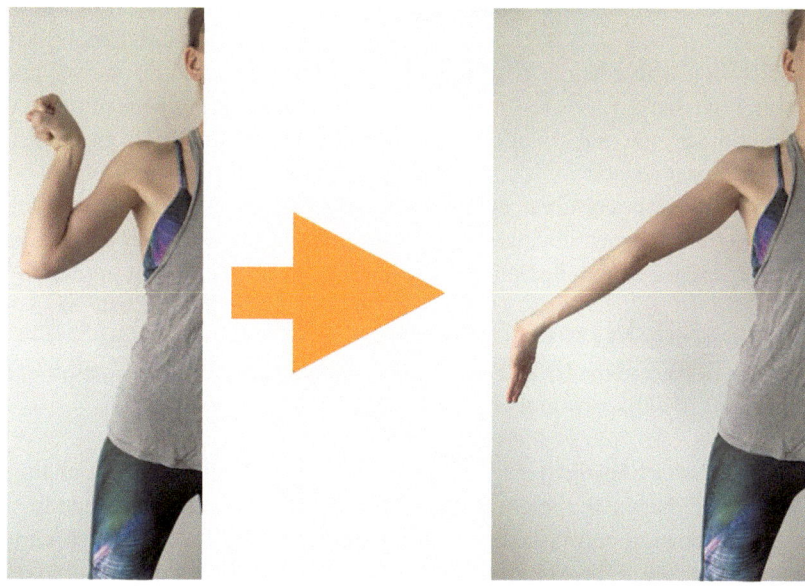

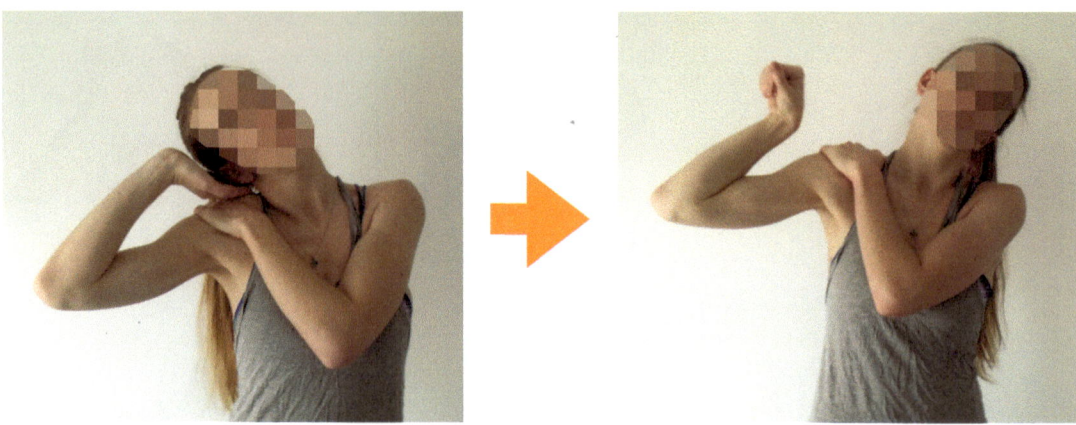

Fig. 6.16 Self-mobilization of the ulnar nerve from proximal to distal. • Lowering the shoulder, • Shoulder abduction, • Forearm pronation, • Wrist extension and homolateral head inclination, • Wrist flexion and contralateral head inclination

Massages against fibrosis (dot-shaped, glided pressures, and kneading) can be realized along the ulnar nerve, on the internal side of the forearm, around the pisiform, and on the hypothenar muscles. They improve local trophicity, fight against peri-neural fibrosis, and relax the muscles adjacent to the nerve [14].

6.3.3 Radial Nerve

6.3.3.1 Nerve Tension
For the radial nerve, the mobilization is based on the ULTT 2b and has several steps [25] (Fig. 6.17):

- Position with a "triple grip" (therapist's pelvis and two hands)
- Shoulder internal rotation, pronation, and strong depression
- Wrist flexion and ulnar inclination to put the superficial branch in tension
- Fingers and thumb flexion

Just as the ULTT 1 and ULTT 2a for the median nerve and the ULTT 3 for the ulnar nerve, it is more of a diagnostic tool.

6.3.3.2 Nerve Gliding
The radial nerve is mostly shortened with an elbow extension and pronation and a wrist and fingers flexion. The opposite position (elbow flexion and supination and wrist and fingers extension) relaxes it.

Based on biomechanics, we suggest the following mobilization (Fig. 6.18):

- Elbow flexion and supination, wrist and fingers flexion.
- Elbow extension and pronation, wrist and fingers extension.

6.3.3.3 Self-Mobilizations
They include the neuro-gliding mobilization described earlier (Fig. 6.18).

Moreover, in less acute cases, the patient can realize a self-mobilization including the proximal part of the nerve, and working on the general gliding between the cervical spine and the distal extremity of the limb (Fig. 6.19):

- Lowering the shoulder
- Shoulder abduction and internal rotation
- Forearm pronation
- Wrist extension and contralateral head inclination
- Wrist flexion and homolateral head inclination

It is also interesting to add cervical spine self-mobilizations and to stretch the muscles that can be involved in a compression and/or a lack of gliding of the nerve (Figs. 6.11, 6.12, and 6.13).

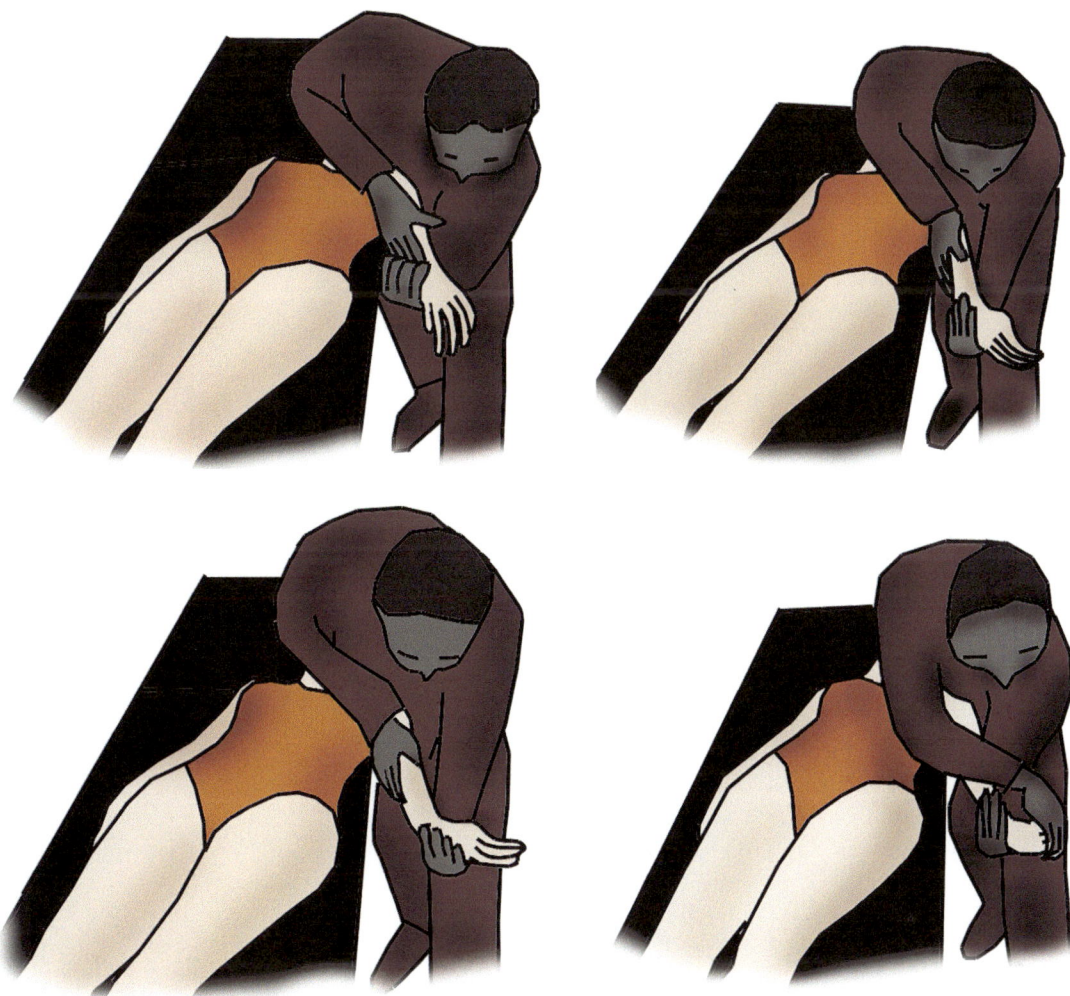

Fig. 6.17 Mobilization of the radial nerve (ULTT 2b). • Position with a "triple grip" (therapist's pelvis and two hands), • Shoulder internal rotation, pronation, and strong depression, • Wrist flexion and ulnar inclination to put the superficial branch in tension, • Fingers and thumb flexion

6.3.3.4 Working on Adjacent Tissues

Alternating contraction-relaxation stretching of the adjacent muscles creates a peri-neural pumping that improves local trophicity and maintains inter-tissue gliding.

These mobilizations are realized preferentially on the supinator muscle in posterior interosseous nerve syndromes, on the brachialis and brachioradialis in radial tunnel syndromes, and on the brachioradialis in Wartenberg's syndromes.

Massages against fibrosis (dot-shaped, glided pressures, and kneading) can be realized along the radial nerve, on the posterior and lateral sides of the forearm and hand. They improve local trophicity, fight against peri-neural fibrosis, and relax the muscles adjacent to the nerve [14].

Fig. 6.18 Gliding without tension of the radial nerve. • Elbow flexion and supination, wrist and fingers flexion. • Elbow extension and pronation, wrist and fingers extension

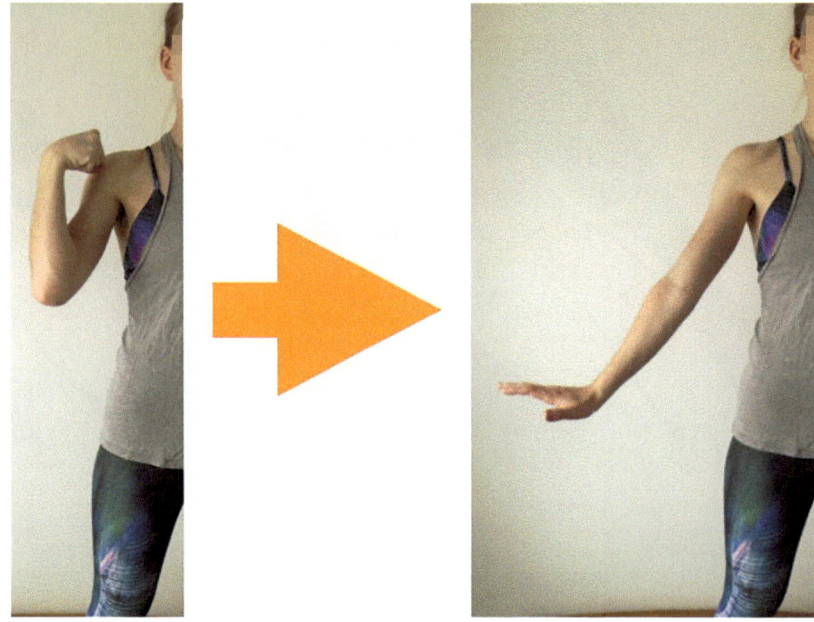

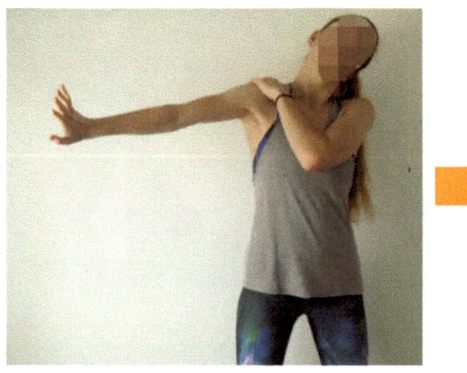  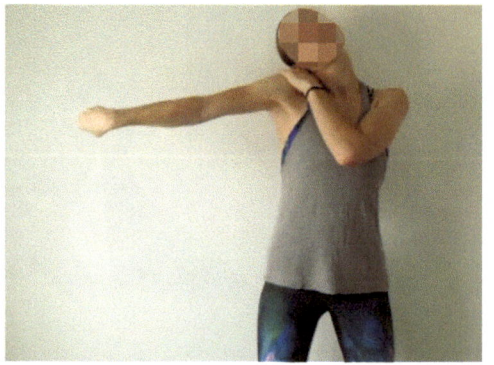

Fig. 6.19 Self-mobilization of the radial nerve from proximal to distal. • Lowering the shoulder, • Shoulder abduction and internal rotation, • Forearm pronation, • Wrist extension and contralateral head inclination, • Wrist flexion and homolateral head inclination

References

1. Littré B. Neurodynamique et neuropathie compressive du membre supérieur: revue systématique. Kinesither Rev. 2018;18(195):10–22.
2. Shacklock M. Biomechanics of the nervous system. Breig revisited. Adelaide, Australia: Neurodynamic Solutions; 2007.
3. Walsh MT. Neurodynamic treatment, examination, and intervention with nerve gliding. In: Skirven TM, Osterman AL, Fedorczyk JM, Amadio PC, Feldscher SB, Shin EK, editors. Rehabilitation of the hand and upper extremity. Philadelphia: Elsevier; 2021. p. 1433–50.
4. de Laere J. Thérapie manuelle neurodynamique: du bilan diagnostique au traitement manuel, 1ère partie. Prof Kinésithér. 2010;25:28–33.
5. Dilley A, et al. Quantitative in vivo studies of median nerve sliding in response to wrist, elbow, shoulder and neck movements. Clin Biomech. 2003;18:899–907.
6. Sunderland S. Nerve and nerve injuries. London: Churchill and Livingston; 1978.
7. Millesi H, Zoch G, Reihsner R. Mechanical properties of peripheral nerves. Clin Orthop Relat Res. 1995;314:76–83.

8. Kwan M, et al. Strain, stress, and stretch of peripheral nerve: rabbit experiments in vitro and in vivo. Acta Orthop Scand. 1992;63:267–72.

9. Butler D. The sensitive nervous system. Adelaide, Australia: Noigroup Publications; 2000.

10. Lundborg G. Intraneural microcirculation. Orthop Clin North Am. 1988;19:1–12.

11. Mackinnon S, Dellon A. Experimental study of chronic nerve compression clinical implications. Hand Clin. 1986;2:639–50.

12. Lundborg G, Rydevik B. Effects of stretching the tibial nerve of the rabbit. A preliminary study of the intraneural circulation and the barrier function of the perineurium. J Bone Joint Surg. 1973;55B:390–401.

13. Upton A, McComas A. The double crush in nerve entrapment syndrome. Lancet. 1973;2:359–62.

14. Walsh MT. Upper limb neural tension testing and mobilization. Fact, fiction, and a practical approach. J Hand Ther. 2005;18:241–58.

15. Lundborg G, Dahlin L. The pathophysiology of nerve compression. Hand Clin. 1992;8:215–27.

16. Zoech G, et al. Stress strain in peripheral nerves. Neuro Orthop. 1991;10:73–82.

17. Wall E, et al. Experimental stretch neuropathy: changes in nerve conduction under tension. J Bone Joint Surg. 1992;74B:126–9.

18. Ellis RF, Hing WA. Neural mobilization: a systematic review of randomized controlled trials with an analysis of therapeutic efficacy. J Man Manip Ther. 2008;16(1):8–22.

19. Wright T, Cowin D, Wheeler D. Radial nerve excursion and strain at the elbow and wrist associated with upper-extremity motion. J Hand Surg Am. 2005;30A:990–6.

20. Wright T, et al. Ulnar nerve excursion and strain at the elbow and wrist associated with upper extremity motion. J Hand Surg Am. 2001;26A:655–62.

21. Wright T, et al. Excursion and strain of the median nerve. J Bone Joint Surg. 1996;78A:1897–903.

22. Kleinrensink G, et al. Upper limb tension tests as tools in the diagnosis of nerve and plexus lesions. Clin Biomech. 2000;15(1):9–14.

23. Lewis J, Ramot R, Green A. Changes in mechanical tension in the median nerve: possible implications for the upper limb tension test. Physiotherapy. 1998;84:254–61.

24. Watanabe M, et al. The implication of repeated versus continuous strain on nerve function in a rat forelimb model. J Hand Surg Am. 2001;26A:663–9.

25. Butler D, et al. Mobilization of the nervous system. Melbourne, Australia: Churchill Livingstone; 1991.

26. Shacklock M. Improving application of neurodynamic (neural tension) testing and treatments: a message to researchers and clinicians. Man Ther. 2005;10(3):175–9.

27. Shacklock M. Clinical neurodynamics: a new system of musculoskeletal treatment, vol. 1. 1st ed. Philadelphia: Elsevier Butterworth Heinemann; 2005. p. 251.

28. Elvey R. Physical evaluation of the peripheral nervous system in disorders of pain and dysfunction. J Hand Ther. 1997;10:122–9.

29. Balster S, Jull G. Upper trapezius muscle activity during the brachial plexus tension test in asymptomatic subjects. Man Ther. 1997;2:144–9.

30. van der Heide B, Allison G, Zusman M. Pain and muscular responses to a neural tissue provocation test in the upper limb. Man Ther. 2001;6:154–62.

31. Coppieters M, et al. Addition of test components during neurodynamic testing: effect on range of motion and sensory responses. J Orthop Sports Phys Ther. 2001;31(5):226–37.

32. McClure P. Upper-quarter screen. In: Skirven TM, Osterman AL, Fedorczyk JM, Amadio PC, Feldscher SB, Shin EK, editors. Rehabilitation of the hand and upper extremity. Philadelphia: Elsevier; 2021. p. 117–24.

33. Galer B, Jensen M. Development and preliminary validation of a pain measure specific to neuropathic pain: the neuropathic pain scale. Neurology. 1997;48:332–8.

34. Bouhassira D, et al. Development and validation of the neuropathic pain symptom inventory. Pain. 2004;108:248–57.

35. Wolny T, et al. Effect of manual therapy and neurodynamic techniques vs ultrasound and laser on 2PD patients with CTS: a randomized controlled trial. J Hand Ther. 2016;29:235–45.

36. Shacklock M. Clinical neurodynamics. A new system of musculoskeletal treatment. Toronto, Canada: Elsevier; 2005.

37. Nee R, et al. Neural tissue management provides immediate clinically relevant benefits without harmful effects for patients with nerve-related neck and arm pain: a randomized trial. J Physiother. 2012;58:23–31.

38. Day J, et al. Outcomes following the conservative management of patients with non-radicular peripheral neuropathic pain. J Hand Ther. 2014;27(3):192–200.

39. Pinar L, et al. Can we use nerve gliding exercises in women with carpal tunnel syndrome. Adv Ther. 2005;22:467–75.

40. Nee R, Butler D. Management of peripheral neuropathic pain: integrating neurobiology, neurodynamics, and clinical evidence. Phys Ther Sport. 2006;7:36–49.

41. Lohkamp M, Small K. Normal response to upper limb neurodynamic Test 1 and 2A. Man Ther. 2011;16:125–30.

42. Coppieters MW, Butler DS. Do 'sliders' slide and 'tensioners' tension? An analysis of neurodynamic techniques and considerations regarding their application. Man Ther. 2008;13:213–21.

43. Haftek J. Stretch injury of peripheral nerve: acute effects of stretching on rabbit nerve. J Bone Joint Surg. 1970;52B:354–65.

44. Rydevik B, et al. An in vitro mechanical and histological study of acute stretching on rabbit tibial nerve. J Orthop Res. 1990;8(5):694–701.

45. Meng S, et al. Longitudinal gliding of the median nerve in the carpal tunnel: ultrasound cadaveric evaluation of conventional and novel concepts of nerve mobilization. Arch Phys Med Rehabil. 2015;96:2207–13.

46. Cobb TK, An KN, Cooney WP. Effect of lumbrical muscle incursion within the carpal tunnel on carpal tunnel pressure: a cadaveric study. J Hand Surg Am. 1995;20(2):186–92.

Physiology and Rehabilitation of Sensorial and Motor Disorders

Grégory Mesplié

7.1 Nerve Physiology [1]

A peripheral nerve [2] is made of fascicles surrounded by connective tissue (the endoneurium) and contained in the perineurium. These fascicles are gathered in another tissue, the epineurium, which ensures the fixation and gliding of the nerve respective to the adjacent structures.

These fascicules describe a wavy path and absorb the stretching stress before they are transmitted to the proper fibers.

The peripheral nerves have a double vascularization:

- Extrinsic, from the adjacent vascular systems.
- Intrinsic, via a longitudinal web that anastomoses to create a link between the vessels of the epineurium and the perineurium.

The low energetic needs of the nerve, the wavy path of the fascicles, and the double vascularization allow supporting a nerve elongation until a certain point. Beyond that point, the diameter of the fascicle decreases, and the intra-fascicular pressure increases. This can compromise the vascularization and have irreversible side-effects.

The importance of the stress imposed on the nerve depends on the applied strength, its speed, and duration.

G. Mesplié (✉)
Institut Sud Aquitain de la Main et du Membre Supérieur, Biarritz, France

7.2 Functional Classification of Nervous Injuries

Seddon first made this classification in 1943 and includes three types of nervous injuries: neurapraxia, axonotmesis, and neurotmesis. Sunderland then added two other stages [3] (Fig. 7.1):

1. **Neurapraxia or Sunderland's first stage**: Damage of the myelin but preservation of the axonal continuity. There is usually a full recovery in 3–12 weeks.
2. **Axonotmesis or Sunderland's second stage**: Damage of the fascicle, but conservation of the endoneural tubes. Therefore, there is usually a full recovery except if the denervation lasts too long and causes irreversible damages in the motor plate or the sensorial receptors. The motor plate stays functional during approximately a year while the sensorial receptors can survive several years. An axonal regrowth can happen, thanks to the preservation of the internal histological structures of the nerve. The regeneration speed is hard to assess with precision, but according to some authors it is of 8.5 mm a day in the arm, 2 mm a day in the wrist, and 0.5 mm a day in the fingers—not 1 mm a day everywhere as we can usually hear [4]. For other authors, the regeneration speed is approximately of 1 mm a day in the hand but can go up to 3 mm a day for more proximal injuries [5].

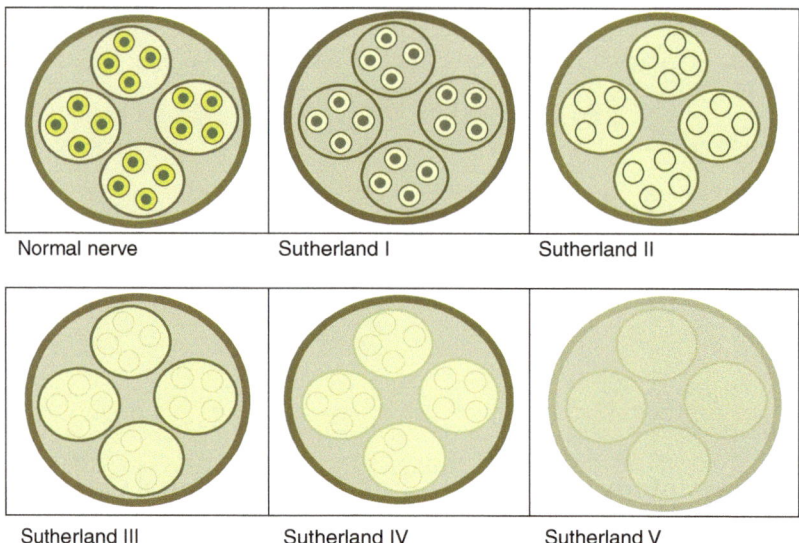

Normal nerve　　　　　Sutherland I　　　　　Sutherland II

Sutherland III　　　　　Sutherland IV　　　　　Sutherland V

Sutherland	Axon	Endoneurium	Perinerium	Epineurium	Seddon	Clinical correspondence
Stage 1					Neurapraxia	Quick spontaneous recovery when the compression stops
Stage 2					Axonotmesis	Spontaneous recovery: the axon grows back
Stage 3						A spontaneous recovery is possible but always partial
Stage 4						No spontaneous recovery, nerve reparation with a suture or a graft
Stage 5					Neurotmesis	No spontaneous recovery, nerve reparation with a suture or a graft

Fig. 7.1 Functional classification of nervous injuries and synthesis (according to Liverneaux and Nonnenmacher [3])

3. **Stage 3 with damage of the endoneural tubes but preservation of the perineurium**: The axon is damaged and the prognosis uncertain.
4. **Stage 4 with damage of the perineurium but preservation of the epineurium**: The continuity of the nerve is only due to the epineurium. Surgery is necessary for any hope of recovery.
5. **Neurotmesis or Sunderland's fifth stage**: Total rupture of the nerve, there is no continuity anymore and surgery is needed.

7.3　Chronology of Re-Afferentation [6–8]

At a peripheral level, there are no new sensorial receptors produced after an injury. However, the denervated sensorial receptors reconnect with each other through regenerating axons from the injured nerve and axons from the healthy adjacent nerves (collateral sprouting).

The free nerve endings (nociceptors and thermoreceptors) responsible for pain and thermal sensitivity are the first ones to recover. At the beginning of regeneration, there is an imbalance between myelinated and unmyelinated fibers: there are more unmyelinated fibers (linked to free nerve endings) than myelinated fibers (linked to mechanoreceptors) [9].

The mechanoreceptors do not all act the same after a peripheral nerve injury. Merkel cells degenerate faster than Meissner corpuscles [10]. Ruffini corpuscles seem relatively stable even with a deteriorated morphology, and the evolution of Ruffini corpuscles is not well known.

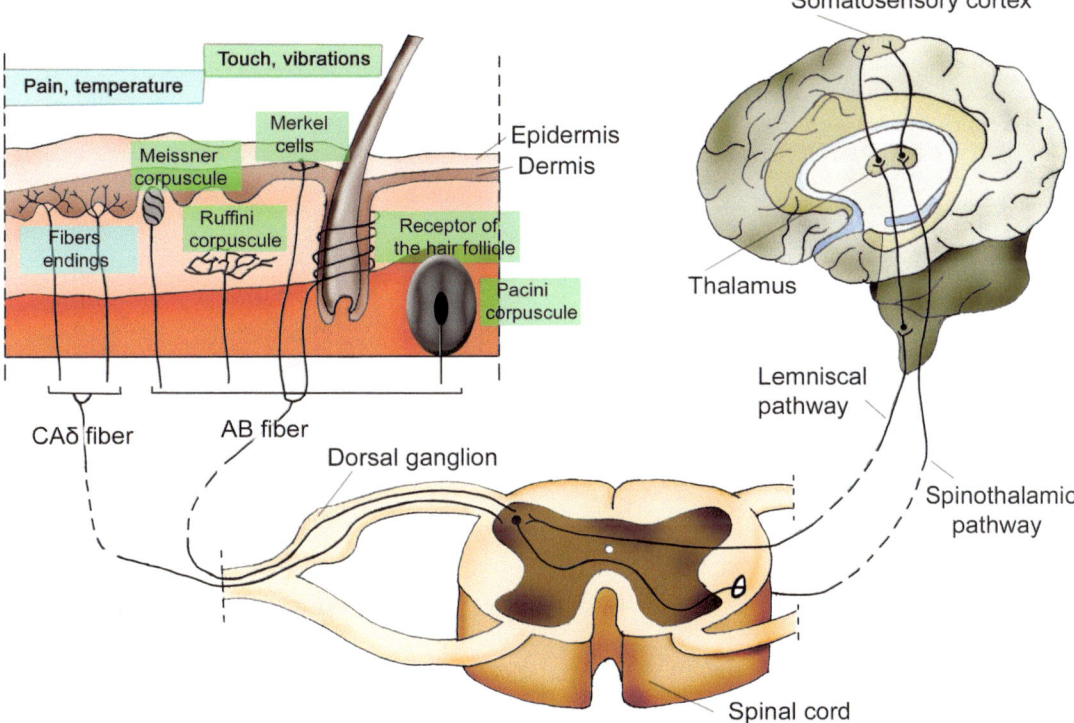

Fig. 7.2 Elements participating in the hand's sensitivity (according to Bonnafond and Schwebel)

Recovering the ability to detect a stimulus moving on the skin (Meissner corpuscle) comes before recovering the ability to detect a static stimulus (Merkel cells). This explains why the two-point mobile test is often passed before the two-point static test.

Finally, the perception of low-frequency vibrations is recovered before the perception of high-frequency vibrations [9].

7.4   Sensorial Physiology

The sensitivity of the hand and wrist allows transmitting to the cortex any information that brings an adapted motor answer. The skin mechanoreceptors of the palm of the hand are the most precise and transform the mechanical stimulus in nerve impulse, which travels towards the somesthetic cortex through diverse types of nerve fibers corresponding to distinct types of sensitivities (Fig. 7.2).

The proprioceptive sensitivity combined with the skin sensitivity allow precise motor responses, needed for complex prehensions.

7.4.1   Receptors for Skin Sensitivity (Table 7.1) [8]

The hand has approximately 17,000 tactile unities, which gives it important precision allowing very precise prehensions. The discriminative sensitivity can be lower than 2 mm between the thumb and the radial index.

There are two big categories of receptors that work differently and do not react the same when receiving a stimulus. The main difference is that the fast-adapting receptors (FA) react to the stimulus with only one pulse whereas the slow-adapting receptors (SA) modify the frequency of their pulses.

Hairless skin presents several types of receptors that react to mechanical, thermic, or painful stimuli.

Table 7.1 Hand's cutaneous receptors (modified according to Roudaut et al. [8])

Receptor	Fast adapting receptors		Slow adapting receptors		
	Meissner corpuscle	Pacini corpuscle	Ruffini corpuscle	Merkel cell (complex neurite cell)	Free nerve ending
Sensory function	Skin movement taking an object	Vibration when grasping an object	Skin stretching, movement direction, hand shape, finger position	Fine tactile discrimination, perception of shapes, and textures	Pain, nociception
Skin stimulus	Dynamic deformation	Vibration	Skin stretching	Deep stimulations	Painful stimulations
Location	Dermal papilla	Deep dermis	Dermis	Basal layer of the epidermis	Epidermis/ dermis
Associated fiber	Aβ	Aβ	Aβ	Aβ	Aδ C-HTMR
Conduction speed	35–70 m/s	35–70 m/s	35–70 m/s	35–70 m/s	5–30 m/s 0.5–2 m/s
Receptive field	22 mm²	Finger, hand	60 mm²	9 mm²	1–3 mm²

7.4.1.1 Mechanoreceptors

Their location changes a lot in the skin (Fig. 7.3), and their functional capacities are complementary, to perceive a wide array of stimuli.

- **Meissner corpuscles**: Localized in the papillary groove between the epidermis and the dermis. They are fast-adapting receptors and are sensitive to low frequencies (1–300 Hz) and to exploratory touch.
- **Pacini corpuscles**: Localized in the deep dermis and the subcutaneous tissue. They are fast-adapting receptors, sensitive to frequencies between 5 and 1000 Hz.
- **Merkel cells**: Localized at the level of the junction between the epidermis and the dermis. They are slow-adapting receptors, and they can modulate their pulses, which favors the touch and pressure evaluation. Cold temperatures increase their excitability while hot temperatures inhibit them.
- **Ruffini corpuscles**: Localized in the dermis. They are slow-adapting receptors, sensitive to pressure, and play a role in detecting movements and positions. They are more sensitive to skin stretching than to vertical pressures and are excited by cold temperatures and inhibited by hot temperatures.

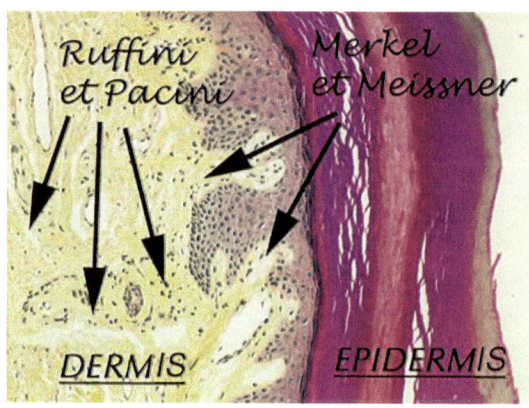

Fig. 7.3 Location of the mechanoreceptors in the hand (modified according to a picture form Pr Casoli's anatomical laboratory—Bordeaux)

7.4.1.2 Thermoreceptors (Fig. 7.4)

- **Hot receptors** are point-located, which explains why the thermo-sensitivity works by "stains" of approximately 1 mm. They are active from 30 °C to liberate a pulse peak between 38 and 43 °C. They stop emitting this pulse below 32 °C or above 48 °C (then the nociceptive fibers are the ones that are active).
- **Cold receptors** are also point-located, with a reception field of 1 mm. They are active from approximately 10 °C to liberate a pulse peak between 20 and 30 °C. They stop emitting this

Frequency of the action potentials (by s.)

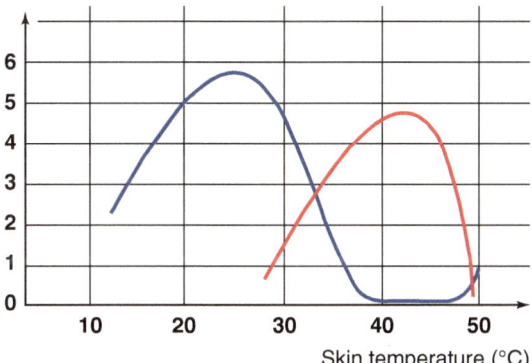

Fig. 7.4 Thermo-receptors' activity depending on the cutaneous temperature (hot receptors—red line and cold receptors—blue line)

pulse below 10 °C and between 38 and 48 °C. Between 48 and 50 °C, they react paradoxically, creating a cold feeling.

When we put the hand in cold water, the thermoreceptors' activity is important at first, but then it decreases. This can explain the fact that water seems less cold after a short time. The same phenomenon exists with hot temperatures.

7.4.1.3 Nociceptors

They are activated by stimulations which excitement threshold is higher than for other types of receptors. They allow defining risky stimulations that can be potentially damaging. There are three types of receptors (mechano-nociceptors, thermo-nociceptors, and polymodal), related to fibers with different diameters. This allows transmitting a well-localized acute pain followed by a delayed burning pain, less localized but lasting longer.

7.4.2   Receptors for Muscles, Tendons, and Joints

They play an important part in collective proprioceptive information that will be transmitted to the cortex. This information will help maintaining the joint homeostasis and realizing precise motor control.

7.4.2.1 Musculo-Tendinous Captors
- **Golgi tendon receptors** that give information about the tendon tension via Aβ fibers and has an inhibitory role on motoneurons during tendon stretching (inverse stretch reflex).
- **Neuromuscular bundle**, made up of two types of receptors: Nuclear chain fibers reacting to continuous stretching and nuclear bag fibers reacting to short stretching. It activates motoneurons and the two polar parts are innervated by motor γ fibers. When these motor fibers contract, they stretch the sensorial equatorial zone, which increases its sensitivity. On the other hand, the muscle contraction inhibits the bundle's activity. Thanks to this complex system, the neuromuscular bundle plays a "starter" role for voluntary movements and participates in regulating the motor control by transmitting information about the instant length and stretching speed of the muscle. The number of fibers in the bundle is particularly important in the hand for precise movements.

7.4.2.2 Joint Captors (Table 7.2)
They give information about the joint position, its moving speed, its acceleration, and its tissue tension [11].

7.4.3   Protopathic Sensitivity (Thermo-Algesia or "Protective Sensitivity")

7.4.3.1 Nociceptive Sensitivity: Types of Pain
Pain is defined by the International Association for the Study of Pain (IASP) as "an unpleasant sensory and emotional experience associated with, or resembling that associated with, actual or potential tissue damage."

This definition highlights the multifactorial aspect of pain [12] (Fig. 7.5) and the fact that its intensity is not always related to the severity of the tissue injury.

This paragraph is about peripheral pain and does not cover central pain, which is usually treated in specialized centers. However, it is important to know how to detect it to refer the patient to an adapted center.

Table 7.2 Joint receptors (according to Hagert [11])

Name	Neurophysiological characteristics	Role on the joint's function
Ruffini	Slow adaptation, low threshold	Joint position, modification of the speed/amplitude
Pacini	Fast adaptation, low threshold	Acceleration/deceleration
Golgi	Fast adaptation, high threshold	Extreme amplitudes
Free nerve endings	Fast Aδ fibers, slow C fibers	Pain, inflammation, harmful situation
Unclassifiable	Unknown	Unknown

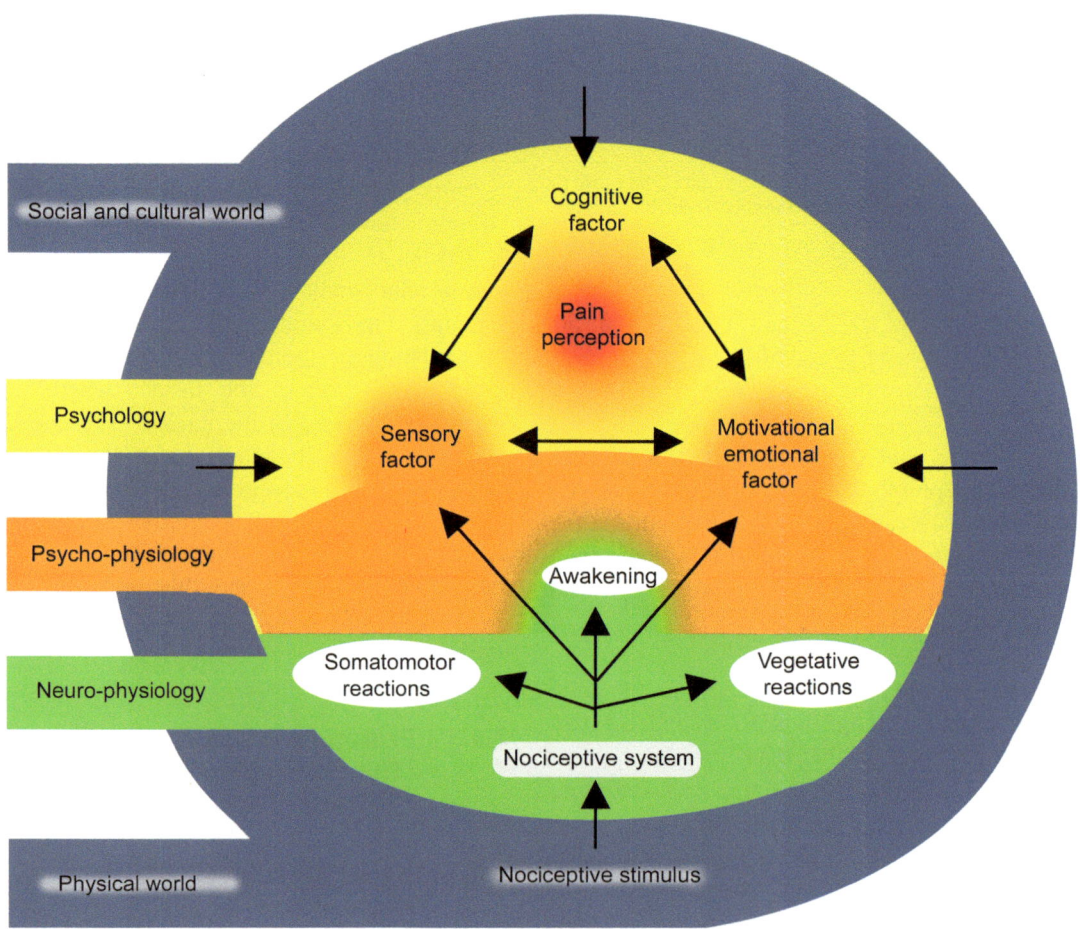

Fig. 7.5 Multifactorial aspect of pain (according to Le Bars and Plaghki [12])

- **Nociceptive pain**: It is a sharp pain related to a tissue injury. In these cases, the injury causing the painful message should be at the center of the treatment. The therapeutic orientation will depend on the other elements of the clinical assessment.

  The therapist should try to define as precisely as possible what the patient feels regarding the type of pain, its rhythm, location, and intensity, and what eases the pain. If the assessment is realized while the patient is taking an analgesic treatment, it should be stated to avoid a possible bias when comparing with the following assessments.

It should be noted than we can be dealing with referred pain, so the origin of the pain is in a different area than the painful one…

The rhythm can be mechanical (after an effort) or inflammatory (during the night, with morning stiffness). The pain can be sharp, stabbing, burning, electrical, associated with a sensation of compression.

The therapist must identify precisely the movements causing pain, and therefore assess the different structures in the painful area with techniques such as palpation and tissue tensioning. For example, if the pain is triggered by an active mobilization and not by a passive one, then pain probably comes from a muscular or tendinous structure.

The location can be widespread or precise. Using a print of a hand or upper limb drawing during the assessment can facilitate communication between the members of the caring team.

The pain intensity is assessed with the Visual Analog Scale described earlier (see Chap. 1). The therapist should always assess the pain at the moment of the assessment, as well as the highest and lowest levels of pain felt during the last 15 days.

Knowing what eases the patient's pain can be useful to pinpoint what causes pain and to choose the techniques we are going to use.

- **Neuropathic pain**: It is a chronic pain, where the tissues are no longer the main cause of the problem: the tissue nociception—granted it still exists—is only participating in the clinical picture. Trying to decrease it usually has little positive impact on the patient [13].

The NP4 can be used to determine if the pain we are dealing with is neuropathic or not (sensitivity 80% and specificity 92%) [14]. We can also add other criteria to differentiate a neuropathic pain and a non-neuropathic central sensitization (Table 7.3).

A neuropathic pain can be associated with a mechanical allodynia.

7.4.3.2 Nociceptive Sensitivity: Transmission of the Nociceptive Message

The nociceptors are either Aδ receptors responding to mechanical and hot stimulations, or C

Table 7.3 Factors participating in differentiating neuropathic pain and central sensitization

Neuropathic pain	Non-neuropathic central sensitization
The patient's history and the related medical diagnoses (stroke, diabetes, cancer, herpes zoster etc.) suggest an injury or a disease affecting the somatosensory system	The patient's history and the related medical diagnoses don't suggest a pathology affecting the somatosensory system
There is evidence (clinical/laboratory/imagery) confirming an injury or a disease affecting the somatosensory system	There is no evidence confirming an injury or a disease affecting the somatosensory system
Pain is logical, from a neuro-anatomical point of view	The location of the pain does not match a peripheral nerve territory or the body schema in the central nervous system
The pain is typically described as burning, throbbing, and tingling	The pain is mostly described as dull and diffuse
Sensory dysfunctions (hypoesthesia, allodynia) are found in the symptomatic area	Sensory dysfunctions are found outside and far away from the symptomatic area

nociceptors responding to intense mechanical, thermal, or chemical stimuli.

They convey the pain message towards the spine through Aδ fibers poorly myelinated (localized and sharp pain) or C fibers unmyelinated (delayed and widespread pain). These fibers have a moderate diameter and a conduction speed inferior to one of the Aβ and Aα fibers conveying sensitivity for fine touch (Fig. 7.6).

These fibers enter the dorsal horn of the spinal cord where there is a medullary relay with two types of neurons:

- Specific nociceptive neurons that only convey pain messages.
- Polymodal neurons that convey any kind of information, whether it is nociceptive or not, coming from the skin, the guts, or the muscles. The convergence of information at the cortical level can lead to a processing "error" that can cause referred pain, where we find a cutaneous metameric pain when the origin is visceral, articular, or muscular.

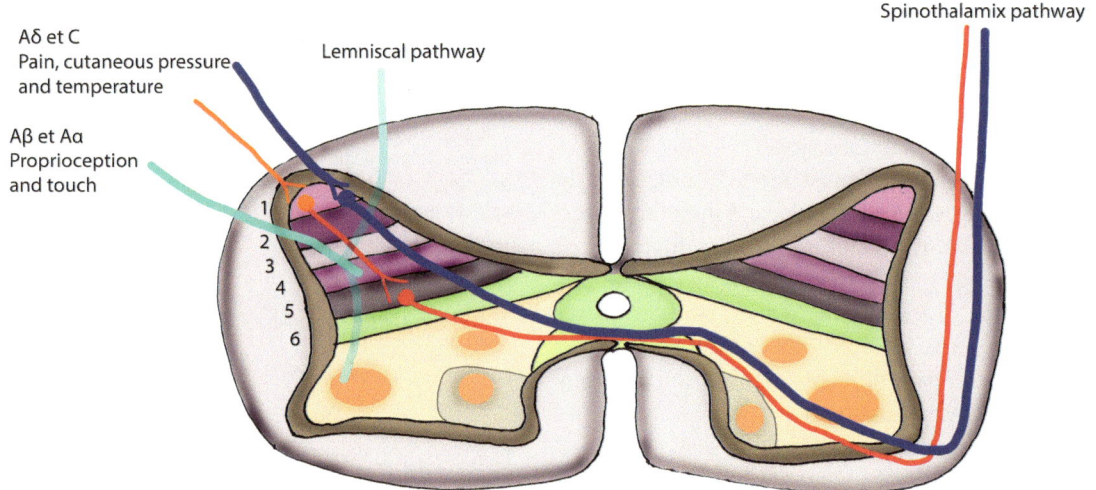

Fig. 7.6 Afferent messages at a spinal level. Protopathic messages are conveyed by Aδ and C fibers until the layers 1–2 of the spinal cord, and then to the brain through the spinothalamic pathway. Epicritic and proprioceptive mes-sages are conveyed by Aβ and Aα fibers until the layers 3–4 of the spinal cord, and then to the brain through the lemniscal pathway

On its way towards the brain, the pain message is modulated by several factors that can amplify or inhibit it [1]:

- **Nociceptor sensitivity**: The substances released around the damaged tissues can increase the inflammatory phenomena, lowering the excitability threshold and causing allodynia.
- **Pain memory**: The pain message lasts too long, the hormonal and chemical phenomena involved in the message transmission can "soak up" the nerve cells that "remember" this pain signal. Any other signal is then transcripted as if it were nociceptive.
- **Axon reflex**: In the dorsal horn, the affluence of nociceptive messages can create a neurogenic inflammation that can maintain pain.
- **Gate-control** or Mailsack and Wall theory: Large fibers have an inhibitory action on the nociceptive message conveyed by Aδ fibers and C fibers with antidromic conduction.
- **The opioid system**: The opioid receptors of the nervous system are present at the level of the central and peripheral system and oppose nociceptive messages.

Finally, there is an integration of pain in the brain where there is also a modulation of the pain message that depends on the circumstances of the injury, and the individual's culture and background.

7.4.3.3 Protopathic Sensitivity Other than Nociceptive

Aside from the nociceptive message, Aδ and C fibers convey information about temperature and cutaneous pressure.

The thermoreceptors react after 45 °C and under 10 °C and can convey a pain message in case of important stimulus.

The information arrives in the dorsal horn of the spinal cord at the level of convergent cells that receive nociceptive information and other sensorial messages.

7.4.4 Epicritic Sensitivity

7.4.4.1 Vibrotactile Sensitivity

The vibrotactile sensitivity conveys information of fine and discriminative movements, pressure, or vibration through Aβ fibers. Two types of mechanoreceptors that collect mechanical information and change it in nervous impulses are as follows:

- Type 1 receptors are small and cover a small skin surface.
- Type 2 receptors cover a wider surface and do not have precise limits.

Each of these receptor types can have a slow adaptation (and send the message during the whole stimulation) or a fast adaptation (and send the message at the beginning and at the end of the stimulation).

There are many cutaneous territories in the hand, and they all have distinct roles. Therefore, the hand can perceive several stimuli with a great precision, especially regarding the discriminative sensitivity (Fig. 7.7).

In the hand, the cutaneous territory concerned by one receptor is small, which explains the important sensorial precision at this level.

The sensorial message coming from these receptors is conveyed by Aβ fibers that are large, myelinated fibers with important conduction speeds.

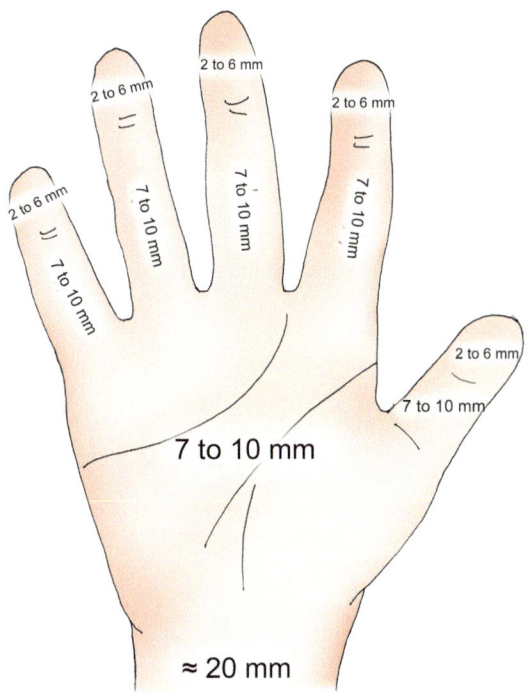

Fig. 7.7 Normal values of the discriminative sensitivity in the palmar side of the hand

7.4.4.2 Proprioceptive Sensitivity

It conveys information concerning the limbs' position and movements through Aα fibers. This information is essential for the cortex to regulate the muscular tensions and adapt to every situation.

The proprioceptive sensitivity relies on several mechanoreceptors at a muscular, tendinous, and articular level, to which we must add cutaneous receptors that also participate in the formation of the proprioceptive message.

7.4.5   Autonomic System

The autonomic system concerns the innervation of the guts and the endocrine and exocrine glands, as well as the vasomotor activity. On a sensorial level, it conveys the visceral sensitivity.

The autonomic system consists of the following two antagonist but complementary systems:

- The parasympathetic system whose role is to reduce the use of energy (tropho-tropism).
- The sympathetic system that produces energy (ergo-tropism).

Any disturbance in the balance between them can lead to important autonomic disorders, like the ones we can find in Complex Regional Pain Syndrome where the predominance of the sympathetic system causes vasomotor, pilomotor, and sweating disorders, as well as pain exacerbation by axon reflex.

7.5   Rehabilitation of Sensorial Disorders

7.5.1   Rehabilitation of Hyposensitivity

It is based on the brain's neuroplasticity that allows the somesthetic cortex, which reacts to tactile stimulations, to reorganize [15–17] (Fig. 7.8).

The patient will only be able to decode this added information with training. The new message is the result of the summons of mechanore-

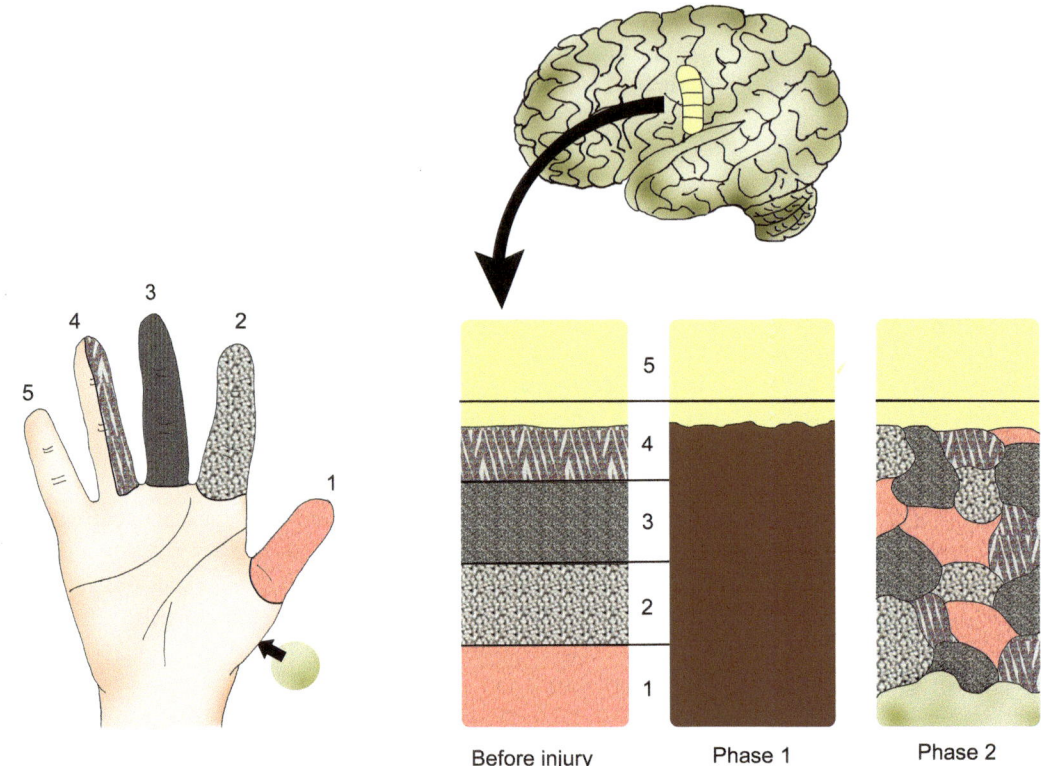

Fig. 7.8 The brain's neuroplasticity allows the somesthetic cortex (that reacts to tactile stimulation) to reorganize after an injury causing sensory disorders (according to Rosen et al. [17])

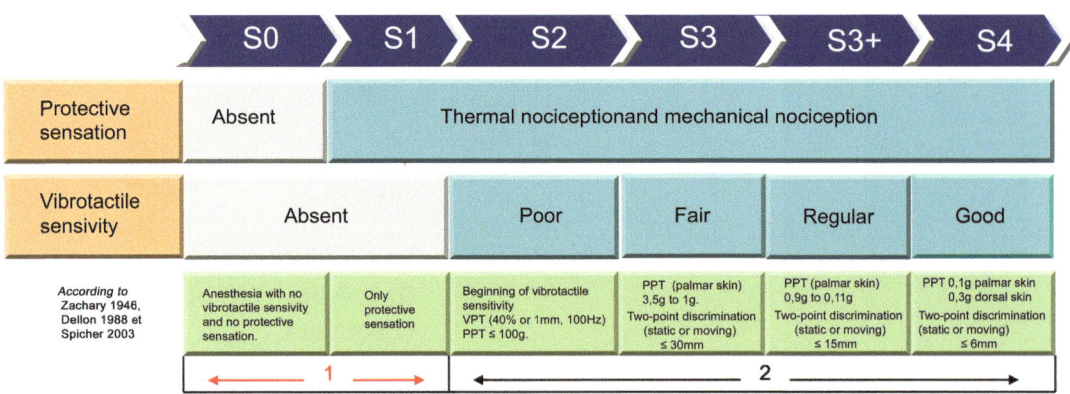

Fig. 7.9 The stages of recovery allow to define two rehabilitation phases. Phase 1 corresponds to the stages S0 to S1 where we must maintain the hand's cortical representation using the brain's dynamic capacities. Phase 2 corresponds to the stages S2 to S4 and its goal is to increase the stimulations to widen the corresponding cortical area, and to vary the stimulations to stimulate different types of sensitivity and promote an optimal functional recovery

ceptors whose number, variety, and locations are different from the previous conditions.

The rehabilitation goals will be adapted to the phase of recovery (Fig. 7.9) and are as follows:

- To maintain the cortical representation of the hand using the brain's dynamic abilities (phase 1).
- To improve the quantity of stimuli to expand the corresponding cortical area [15] and to

vary the stimulations to solicit several types of sensitivity. This will avoid the deterioration of the tensorial representation of the hand in the somatosensory cortex, which could lead to losing motor control [18] (phase 2).

7.5.1.1 Phase 1: Vibrotactile Anesthesia (S0 and S1)

The rehabilitation aims at protecting the patient from traumatisms to which he might be exposed and from which he is not protected in case of anesthesia (hot and cold burns, sharp or pointed objects, etc.) and to limit the risks of exclusion in and around the damaged area.

In these phases, we ask the patient to realize motor and sensorial actions and to imagine touching various kinds of textures and shapes. The motor actions get increasingly complex with time [19–21].

During this phase, using Motor Imagery can be extremely useful (see Chap. 9).

7.5.1.2 Phase 2: Vibrotactile Rehabilitation (S2 to S4)

We start with this phase when the patient can perceive a pressure of 100 g.

- **Location exercise**: It is the first type of exercise implemented in this phase. We use the thickest monofilament so that the exercise is not biased by a bad pressure perception. The pressure is applied perpendicularly to the area for 1.5 s, with the patient keeping his eyes closed. He must then draw on a picture where he felt the pressure (Fig. 7.10).
- **Touch exercise**: We realize these exercises when the level of hyposensitivity is low (PPT < 3.5 g). They consist in asking the patient to touch various kinds of objects and analyze the sensations he gets, comparing with the healthy side. First the exercises are realized with visual control, and then the eyes closed with everything accessible to the hand (trousers, jumper, blanket, face, etc.) (Fig. 7.11). The analysis gets more complex with

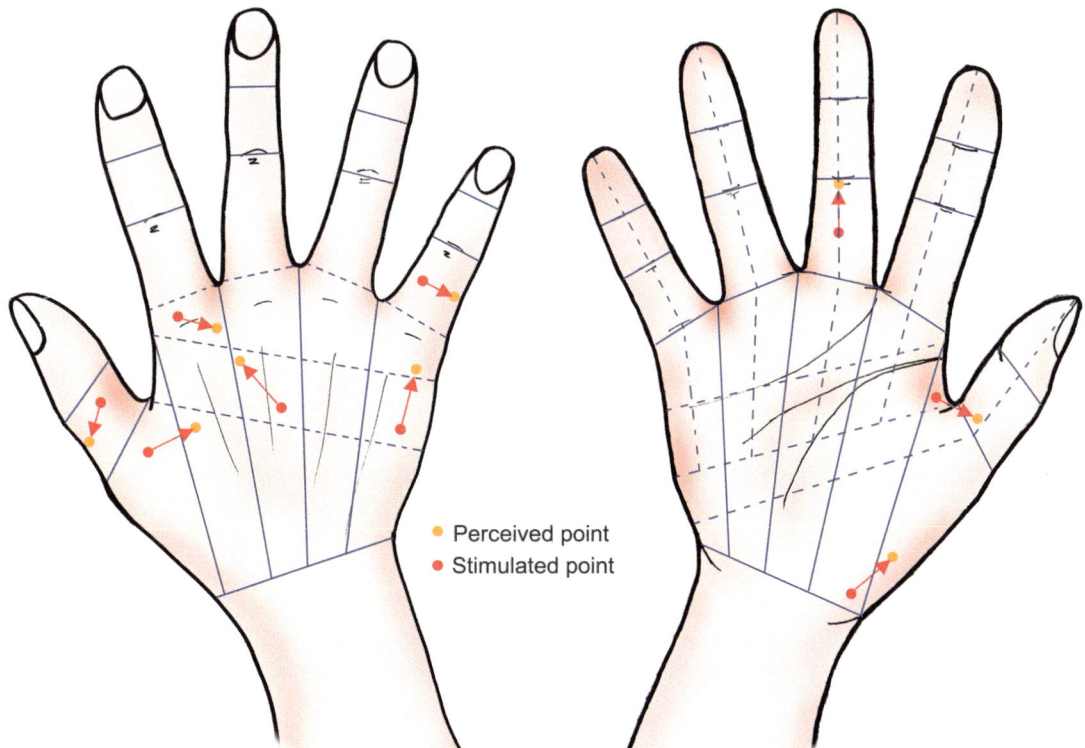

- Perceived point
- Stimulated point

Fig. 7.10 Hand diagram showing the touched areas and the perceived areas to evaluate location mistakes

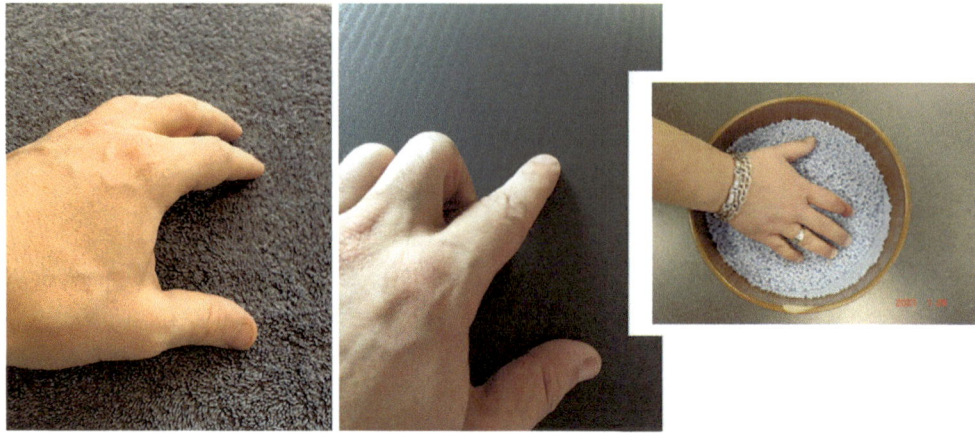

Fig. 7.11 Exercise for the touch: the patient is asked to touch different objects and to analyze the sensations by comparing them to the ones on the healthy side

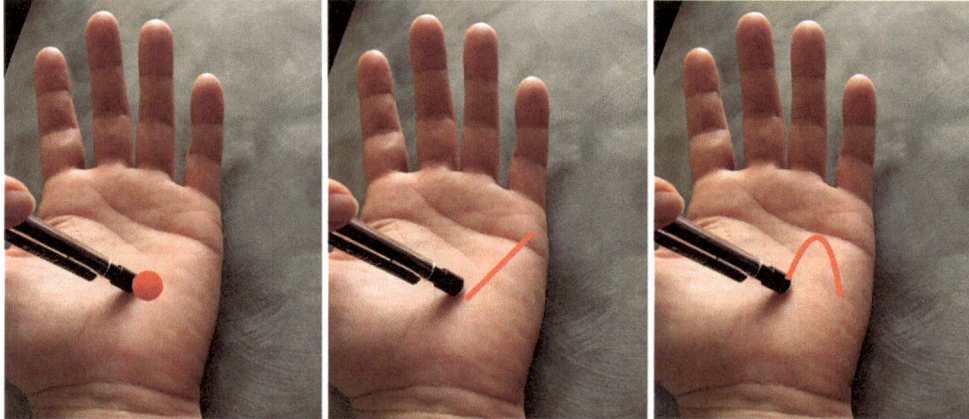

Fig. 7.12 With a rubber, the patient must differentiate a fixed point from a moving point and a straight line from a curve, by reproducing the pattern made by a third party

the patient's evolution and becomes multifactorial (shape and temperature, shape and texture, shape and weight, texture, and temperature, etc.). The exercises are realized four times a day for 5 min.

- **"Trace" rehabilitation**: We realize this rehabilitation when the level of hyposensitivity is important (PPT > 3.5 g). With a pencil rubber, the patient must differentiate a fixed point from a mobile point, then a straight line from a curved line. We can vary and increase the difficulty asking alternatively to locate and analyze the stimulus (Fig. 7.12). The exercises are realized five times a day for 5 min.
- **Transcutaneous vibratory stimulations**: They consist in stimulating the skin with a

vibration generator with a variable frequency and asking the patient to compare the perceived sensations with the healthy side. When there is no injury, the receptors on the fingertips can perceive mechanical waves up to a frequency of 1000 Hz (Fig. 7.13). After nerve suture, vibrations should be applied distally, with no direct contact for 3 weeks. Applying these waves must be completely pain-free and the nerve regrowth site should not be directly stimulated.

- **Complex activities**: Global exercises are used when the patient has recovered enough not to fail. They concern performances, sensorial functional exploration, fine prehensions, object and texture recognition (Fig. 7.14). The

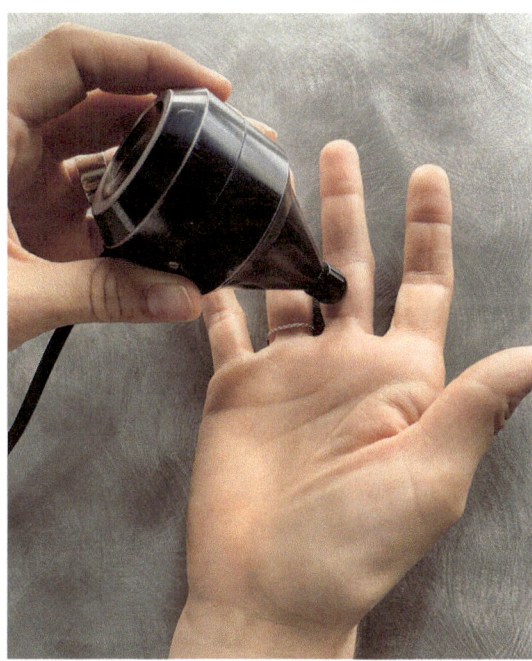

Fig. 7.13 Transcutaneous vibratory stimulations with different frequencies, asking the patient to compare his sensations with the healthy side

functional tests participate in this rehabilitation, in addition to assessing the patient's performances and progress (see Chap. 1).

7.5.2 Rehabilitation of Sensorial Disorders (Not Allodynia)

7.5.2.1 Terminology of the Concerned Disorders [22]

They are sensorial disorders, frequent in hand rehabilitation but with different origins (scar, neuroma, entrapment syndrome, etc.). They are a priority in sensorial rehabilitation and must be treated before going any further:

- **Hyperesthesia**: Increased sensitivity to a somesthetic stimulation (tactile, thermal, or painful), except for special senses. Hyperalgesia (increased reaction to a usually painful stimulation) and allodynia (pain produced by stimulations that usually cause no pain) are hyperesthesias, but allodynia is treated with distant vibrotactile counter-stimulation, not with the techniques described in this paragraph.

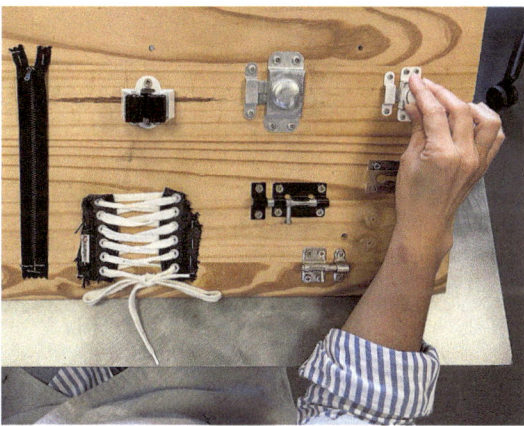

Fig. 7.14 Realizing more and more complex functional exercises

- **Paresthesia**: Abnormal spontaneous or provoked sensation.
- **Dysesthesia**: Abnormal and unpleasant spontaneous or provoked sensation.

These sensorial disorders are rehabilitated according to a specific protocol, but the therapist must treat hyposensitivity first, as these abnormal sensations often disappear when hyposensitivity is treated.

7.5.2.2 Rehabilitation of Sensorial Disorders (Not Allodynia)

These disorders are treated combining a desensitization protocol with electrotherapy and treating the hypoesthesia according to the modalities described previously.

- **Desensitization**: The goal is to stimulate the damaged area with painless contacts to short-circuit the painful interpretation of the brain [23]. Painful contacts must be avoided as it would maintain pain phenomena.

We use massages, transcutaneous vibratory stimulations, and any other element allowing a progressive contact on the damaged area.

At the beginning of the protocol, we use superficial massages on the area or far from it if it is painful, and contacts on the skin with soft elements.

Transcutaneous vibratory stimulations are applied on the area if they do not produce pain, making circular movements with high-frequency waves (>200 Hz if the generator can). The intensity should be low and adapted to the patient's pain threshold. The habituation effect allows the patient to tolerate more intense stimulations, with high intensities and low frequencies. The treatment lasts 20 min. This protocol seems to significantly decrease the perceived pain [24].

The other elements of the protocol evolve the same way: we realize deeper massages and less soft contacts as the patient progresses. If the applied contacts begin to feel painful again, we go back to less harsh techniques before following the progression.

It should be noted that these techniques are interesting for treating the symptoms described previously but must not be used on a healthy nerve regrowth site in order not to interfere with the process. Using a "tingling test" is important to differentiate the symptoms' origins (see Chap. 1).

- **Electrotherapy**: The nociceptive stimulus is transmitted by unmyelinated nervous fibers (small diameter) to the spinal cord, where a transmission control is realized in superior centers by inhibitory neurons. Stimulating large fibers activates these neurons, blocking the transmission of the nociceptive impulse towards the superior centers ("gate control").

Analgesia is immediate and lasts from 30 min to a few hours.

We use a high-frequency TENS current (see Chap. 3), with a 40–75 ms pulse width, and a wobble frequency between 25 and 150 Hz (a wobble frequency varies to limit habituation without increasing intensity). The currents we use are bipolar with a zero mean.

We place two electrodes around the painful area, or proximally to it, depending on the concerned nerve path.

The intensity must produce a "tingling" sensation in the concerned area, intense but comfortable. We apply the current for 30 min.

Stimulating large fibers can be done with other techniques like massage, active or passive mobilization, or any painless sensorimotor stimulation.

The treatment of hypoesthesia in the territory of the nerve is described in the paragraph (Sect. 7.5.1) if necessary.

7.5.3 Rehabilitation of Allodynia

Allodynia is pain caused by a stimulus that does not normally produce pain.

There are two types of allodynia: mechanical (pain produced by a static stimulus like pressure) and dynamic (pain produced by a mobile stimulus like water or air on the skin).

7.5.3.1 Distant Vibrotactile Counter-Stimulation (DVCS)

It is a technique that uses a tactile and vibratory therapeutic agent to allow the patient to perceive a non-nociceptive stimulus on an allodynic territory in a comfortable way, while stopping any contact with the concerned area [25].

This concept comes from the counter-stimulation of medullary neurostimulators, based on Melzack and Wall's gate-control theory.

This technique "consists, for the patient, in perceiving a non-nociceptive stimulus in a non-nociceptive way, first on a non-allodynic territory and then on a surface closer and closer to the allodynic territory, until the allodynic territory" [4].

The first crucial point is to explain to the patient that he must avoid any contact with the allodynic territory in order not to maintain the painful phenomenon. This step is essential in the protocol's success and supposes a significant involvement from the patient.

With very soft materials (rabbit skin, very soft brush, Alcantara, etc.), the patient must stimulate a precise area for 45 s (or less if it becomes unpleasant), eight times a day. This stimulation must never produce unpleasant sensations.

Vibrotactile stimulations can be localized in three areas as follows, preferring the one closest to the allodynic territory:

- **Area proximal to the allodynic territory**: Stimulations are realized proximally to the territory of the damaged nervous branch.
- **"Cousin" area**: We apply stimulations on a "cousin" nervous branch of the damaged branch. They are part of the same brachial plexus cord (lateral, posterior, or medial) [26] (Fig. 7.15). In this kind of area, we stimulate the "cousin" branches proximally to the

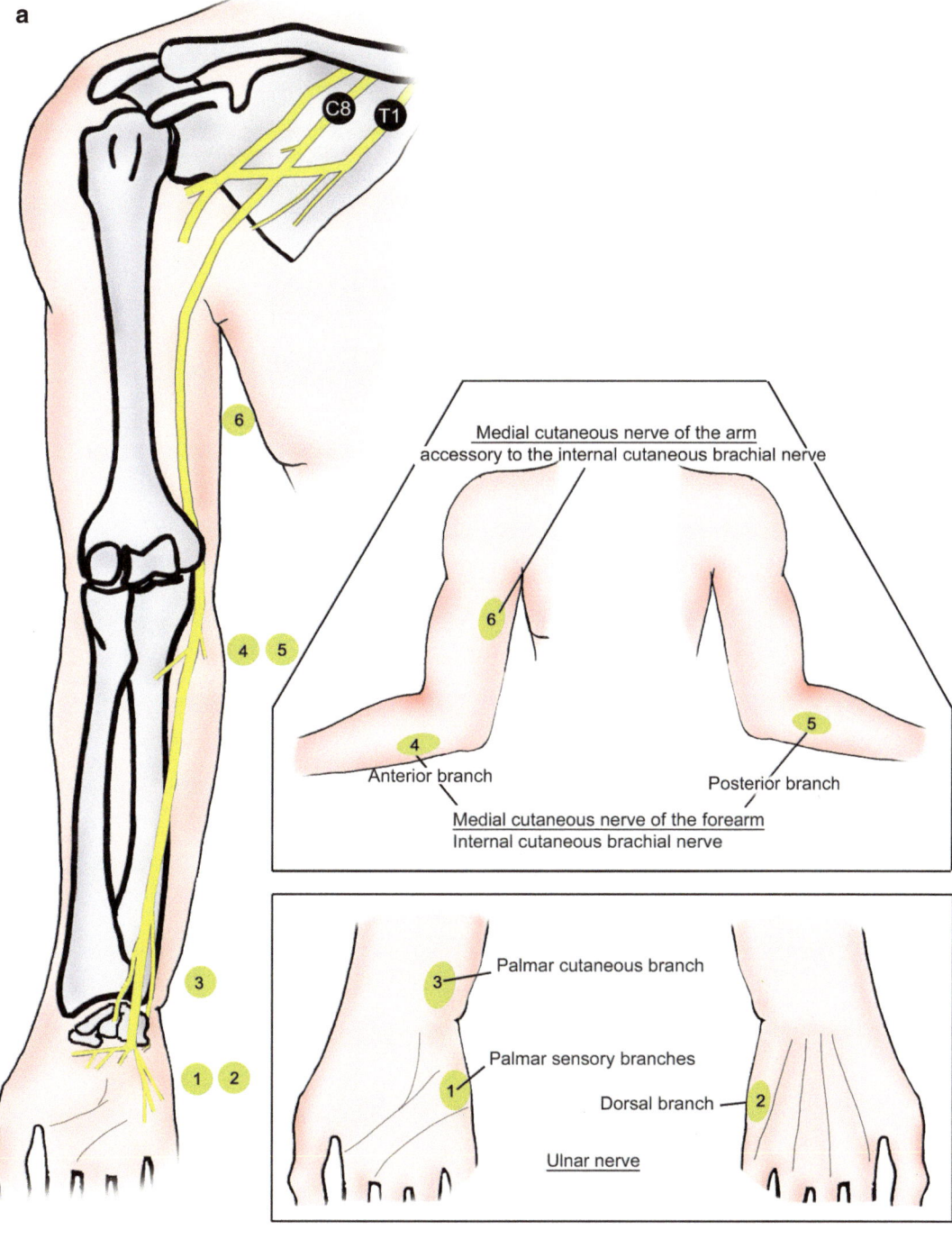

Fig. 7.15 "Cousin" areas corresponding to nerves from the same accessory trunk (modified from Spicher and Kohut [24]). Medial (**a**), lateral (**b**), and posterior (**c**) trunks

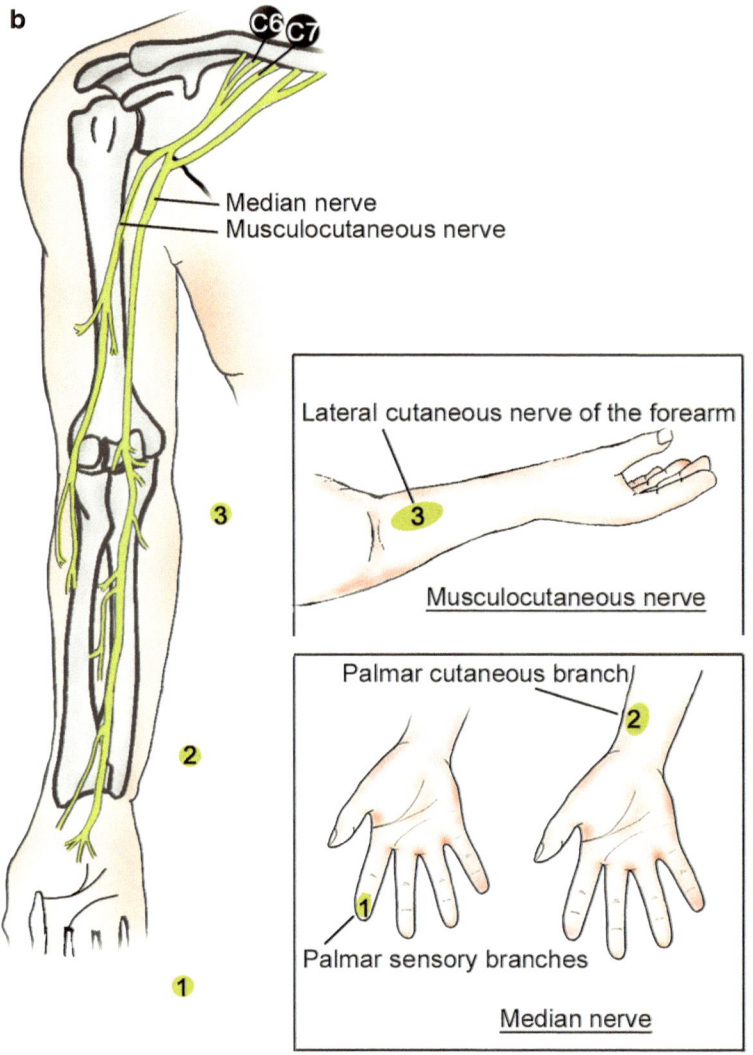

b

Median nerve
Musculocutaneous nerve

Lateral cutaneous nerve of the forearm

3

Musculocutaneous nerve

Palmar cutaneous branch

2

Palmar sensory branches

Median nerve

Lateral secondary branch of the brachial plexus (C6-C7)

Fig. 7.15 (continued)

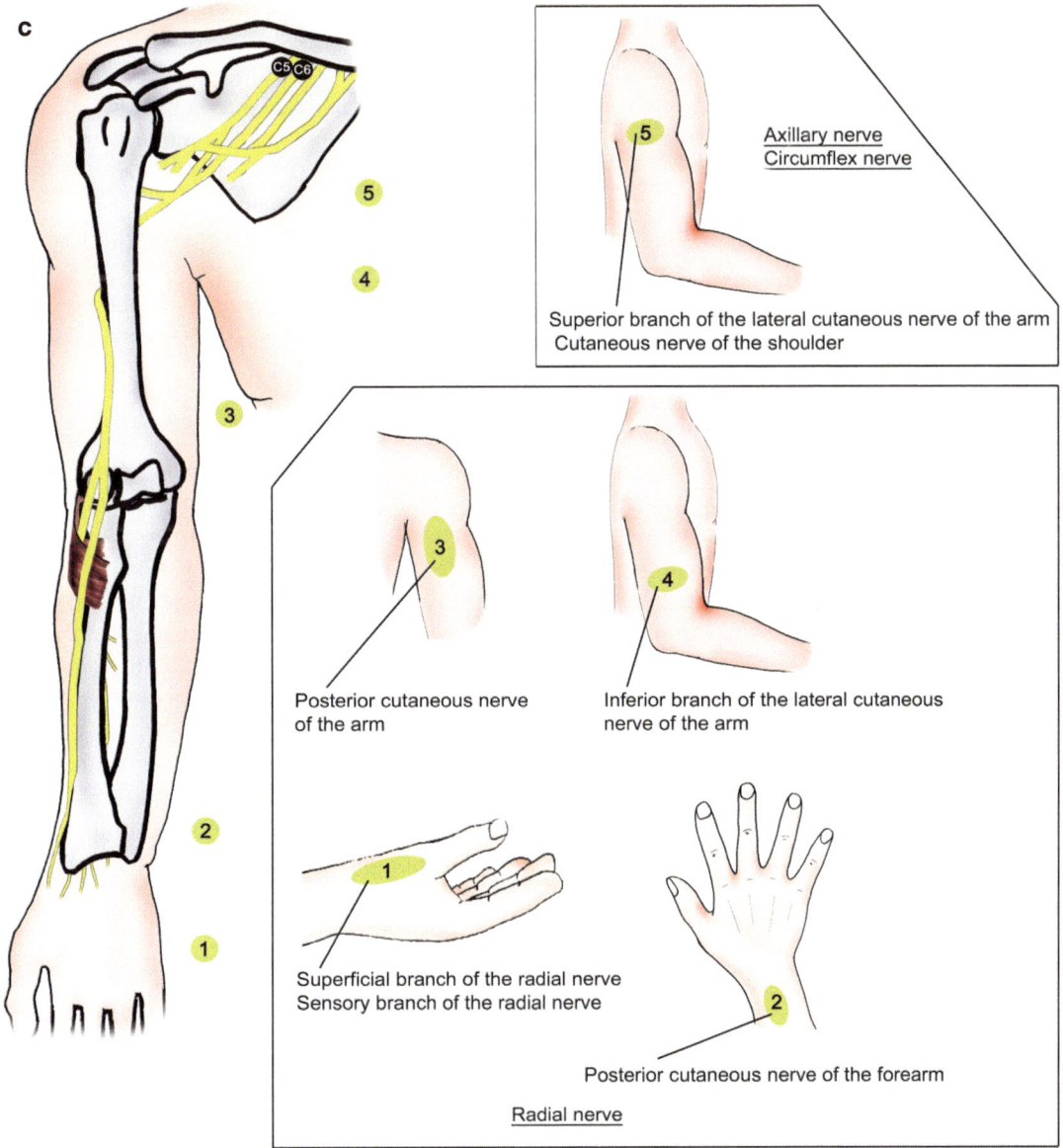

c

C5 C6

5

4

3

2

1

Axillary nerve
Circumflex nerve

Superior branch of the lateral cutaneous nerve of the arm
Cutaneous nerve of the shoulder

Posterior cutaneous nerve
of the arm

Inferior branch of the lateral cutaneous
nerve of the arm

Superficial branch of the radial nerve
Sensory branch of the radial nerve

Posterior cutaneous nerve of the forearm

Radial nerve

Posterior secondary branch of the brachial plexus (C5-C6)

Fig. 7.15 (continued)

damaged branch, if there are no unpleasant sensations.

- **Segmental area**: Stimulations are applied at the segmental level when "cousin" branches cannot be used (unpleasant sensations, pain, etc.). In the inferior limb, we stimulate the segmental level inferior to the damaged branch.

We can also realize a vibratory counter-stimulation on the territories previously described using precise parameters: 0.06 mm with the vibradol, 0.9 V and 300 Hz with the old vibralgic, 2% and 100 Hz with the new vibralgic.

Once treated, the former allodynic area stays hyposensitive. We assess and treat this hypoesthesia like hypoesthesia without allodynia, adapting the tests and rehabilitation in order not to trigger allodynia again. Therefore, the tests are shorter with less stimulations and touch rehabilitation starts with rabbit skin and stimulations of 15 s during the first week. It progressively evolves towards "normal" hyposensitivity rehabilitation if there are no complications.

7.5.3.2 Gradual Motor Imagery
See Chap. 9

7.6 Rehabilitation of Motor Disorders

The innervation of striated muscles is organized around $A\alpha$ and $A\gamma$ fibers, corresponding respectively to the muscle fibers and the muscle spindle.

Therefore, α motoneurons are responsible for the muscle contraction while γ and β motoneurons regulate the muscle tone through the γ loop.

Various muscular fibers depend on one motor neuron; together they form the motor unit.

Tonic muscles have a postural or stabilization function. They have many muscular fibers for one neuron. These muscles do not allow fine gestures as only one neuron has to "manage" a lot of muscular fibers.

On the contrary, phasic muscles have a very little number of fibers for one neuron. Therefore, they can realize very fine movements and are well represented in the hand.

7.6.1 Rehabilitation Depending on Stages

The exercises realized after a peripheral nervous injury require a lot of concentration and will from the patient. We must pay particular attention to the patient's tiredness and mood.

It is usually better to realize short sessions several times a day.

The techniques for peripheral motor disorders are directly related to the stages determined during the assessment:

7.6.1.1 Stages 0 and 1
The denervated muscle atrophies and the therapist's main goals are to fight against fibrosis and vicious attitudes.

We start working with analytical contractions of the concerned muscle as early as possible but avoid making the patient permanently face failure (little repetitions, learning the movement with the healthy side, active-assisted work so the patient feels the movement, etc.).

Massages against fibrosis are realized with glided pressures and kneading, avoiding areas of nerve regrowth that are usually painful.

Facilitation techniques based on percussions and stretching can be realized when there are signs of regrowth and the nervous suture (if there is one) is not very fragile, usually after 1 month and after surgical advice.

The psychological interest of these techniques is to trigger an ideo-muscular response related to the histological characteristics of the muscular fibers without fibrosis (percussions) and to trigger the tendon reflex (stretching). Therefore, we must at least be in stage 1 to realize this technique.

Using electrostimulation for denervated (stage 0) or partially innervated (stage 1) muscles can be done to maintain muscular trophicity and favor muscle regeneration (see Chap. 3—"Physical Agents").

7.6.1.2 Stage 2
The exercises are realized analytically, active without gravity or active-assisted against gravity.

Facilitation techniques like PNF (Proprioceptive Neuro Facilitation) are started in this stage, as they stimulate damaged muscles.

They use "trigger" muscles preserved from the nervous injury and "target" damaged muscles.

Irradiation is realized working against a dynamic or static resistance for the "trigger" muscles and working with active (without gravity) or active-assisted (against gravity) contractions for the "target" muscles.

We complete this protocol with electrotherapy for partially innervated muscles.

Using visual feedback can improve the contraction quality. We ask the patient to reach a pre-established threshold, and then to maintain the contraction during a certain time. The threshold can be increased from one session to the other depending on the patient's progress.

7.6.1.3 Stage 3

The exercises are analytical, active, or active-assisted against gravity.

Facilitation techniques like PNF are prolonged but the exercises for "target" muscles can be realized against gravity.

We complete this protocol with feedback systems and electrostimulation for partially innervated muscles.

7.6.1.4 Stages 4 and 5

The goal is to regain mechanical and physiological capacities in the damaged muscles.

We start a muscular reinforcement protocol adapted to the patient's capacities and needs, associated to proprioception exercises following the usual steps in proprioceptive rehabilitation (see Chap. 8—"Rehabilitation of Proprioception").

Facilitation techniques like PNF are realized, placing adaptive resistances on "trigger" and "target" muscles.

The functional reintegration of the hand, including occupational therapy [1], is essential in this stage to optimize the functional result and help the patient go back to his sports and work activities.

References

1. Valembois B, et al. Rééducation des troubles de la sensibilité de la main. In: EMC Kinésithérapie - Médecine physique - Réadaptation. Paris: Masson; 2006.
2. Antoine J. Anatomie et physiologie du nerf périphérique. In: EMC Appareil locomoteur, vol. 14005-A-10. Paris: Elsevier; 1999.
3. Liverneaux P, Nonnenmacher J. Lésions nerveuses et vasculaires du poignet et de la main. In: Dubert T, Masmejean E; C.d.e.d.l. SOFCOT, editor. Plaies de la main. Paris: Elsevier Masson; 2006. p. 109–22.
4. Spicher C. Manuel de rééducation sensitive du corps humain. Genève, Paris: Médecine et hygiène; 2003.
5. Menorca RM, Fussell TS, Elfar JC. Nerve physiology: mechanisms of injury and recovery. Hand Clin. 2013;29(3):317–30.
6. Basset N. Bilan et rééducation des troubles de la sensibilité de la main. In: EMC - Kinésithérapie - Médecine physique – Réadaptation, vol. 26-064-A-10. Paris: Masson; 2016. https://doi.org/10.1016/S1283-0887(16)60201-3.
7. Noel L, Liverneaux P. Prise en charge et rééducation des lésions nerveuses périphériques. In: EMC - Kinésithérapie - Médecine physique - Réadaptation. Paris: Masson; 2013. p. 9 (10).
8. Roudaut Y, et al. Touch sense: functional organization and molecular determinants of mechanosensitive receptors. Channels (Austin). 2012;6(4):234–45.
9. Mabin D. Bilan de la sensibilité: aspects anatomo-physiologiques. In: Séméiologie de la main et du poignet. Montpellier: Sauramps Medical; 2001. p. 87–96.
10. Mackel R. Human cutaneous mechanoreceptors during regeneration: Physiology and interpretation. Neurological Progress. First published: August 1985.
11. Hagert E. Proprioception of the wrist joint: a review of current concepts and possible implications on the rehabilitation of the wrist. J Hand Ther. 2010;23(1):2–16; quiz 17.
12. Le Bars D, Plaghki L. Douleurs: bases anatomiques, physiologiques et psychologiques. Douleurs aiguës, douleurs chroniques, soins palliatifs. Paris: éditins Med-line; 2001. p. 43–82.
13. Woolf C. What to call the amplification of nociceptive signals in the central nervous system that contribute to widespread pain? Pain. 2014;155(10):1911–2.
14. Spallone V, et al. Validation of DN4 as a screening tool for neuropathic pain in painful diabetic polyneuropathy. Diabet Med. 2012;2012(29):578–85.
15. Godde B, Spengler F, Dinse HR. Associative pairing of tactile stimulation induces somatosensory cortical reorganization in rats and humans. Neuroreport. 1996;8:281–5.
16. Westlake KP, Byl NN. Neural plasticity and implications for hand rehabilitation after neurological insult. J Hand Ther. 2013;26(2):87–92; quiz 93.

17. Rosen B, Björkman A, Lundborg G. Sensory relearning and the plastic brain. In: Rehabilitation of hand and upper extremity. Paris: Elsevier Masson; 2020. p. 597–607.

18. Byl N, Melnick M. The neural consequences of repetition: clinical implications of a learning hypothesis. J Hand Ther. 1997;10:160–74.

19. Rizzolatti G. The mirror neuron system and its function in humans. Anat Embryol (Berl). 2005;210(5–6):419–21.

20. Rizzolatti G, Sinigaglia C. The mirror mechanism: a basic principle of brain function. Nat Rev Neurosci. 2016;17(12):757–65.

21. Schmidt TT, Ostwald D, Blankenburg F. Imaging tactile imagery: changes in brain connectivity support perceptual grounding of mental images in primary sensory cortices. NeuroImage. 2014;98:216–24.

22. ANAES. Évaluation et suivi de la douleur chronique chez l'adulte en médecine ambulatoire. Service de recommandations et références professionnelles; 1999. p. 66–68. http://www.anaes.fr.

23. Lasserre R. La désensitization. Feuillet du GEMMSOR; 2003.

24. Spicher C, Kohut G. Rapid relief of a painful, long-standing posttraumatic digital neuroma treated by transcutaneous vibratory stimulation (TVS). J Hand Ther. 1996;9(1):47–51.

25. Packham TL, et al. Somatosensory rehabilitation for allodynia in complex regional pain syndrome of the upper limb: a retrospective cohort study. J Hand Ther. 2018;31(1):10–9.

26. Spicher C, et al. Atlas des territoires cutanés. 3e édition. Montpellier: Sauramps Médical; 2017.

Rehabilitation of Proprioception

Grégory Mesplié

Proprioception is the ability to feel and perceive oneself [1] and helps maintaining joint homeostasis. This homeostasis is defined as a dynamic process in which the organism maintains and controls its environment despite external perturbations [2]. This ability, combined with a realized movement projection system, is essential for an adapted motor control [3] (Fig. 8.1).

8.1 Sensory Perception

An external stimulus can be detected through several receptors: exteroceptive receptors, interoceptive receptors, and joint mechanoreceptors.

8.1.1 Exteroceptive Receptors

They gather the five senses of a human being: sight, smell, hearing, touch, and taste. They react to an external stimulation.

8.1.2 Interoceptive Receptors

They react to a stimulation coming from the organ itself. It corresponds to a very deep sensitivity of the body itself. The nerve impulses coming from this internal stimulation bring information to the central nervous system. This information can be conscious or unconscious. The pancreas' Pacini corpuscles can be cited as an example.

8.1.3 Joint Mechanoreceptors (Fig. 8.2)

These receptors, combined with the receptors in the muscles, tendons, and skin [4–7], deliver information about the position, movement speed, amplitude, acceleration, and tension of the concerned tissues (see Chap. 7).

G. Mesplié (✉)
Institut Sud Aquitain de la Main et du Membre
Supérieur, Biarritz, France

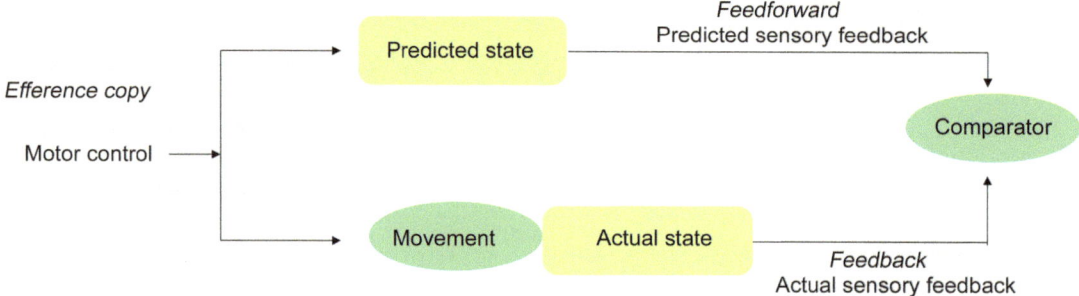

Fig. 8.1 Motor control model based on the efference copy theory [3]

Name	Neurophysiological characteristics	Role on the joint's function
Ruffini	Slow adaptation, low threshold	Joint position, Modification of the speed/amplitude
Pacini	Fast adaptation, low threshold	Acceleration/deceleration
Golgi	Fast adaptation, high threshold	Extreme amplitudes
Free nerve endings	Fast Aδ fibers, slow C fibers	Pain, inflammation, harmful situation
Unclassifiable	Unknow	Unknow

Fig. 8.2 Joint mechanoreceptors

8.2 Conscious and Unconscious Proprioception

8.2.1 Conscious Proprioception

It is part of the conscious sensitivity (somatosensorial) [1, 8] (Fig. 8.3). Thanks to it, we can picture the position of our different body parts in relation to each other and the position of the body at any moment [9]. Its pathways are projected on the primary somesthetic cortex. Goll's fasciculus and Burdach's bundle are made of long fibers of T-shaped cells, placed along the spinal cord until Goll's and Burdach's nuclei.

They carry messages from the sheaths, tendons, myo-fasciae, and joint capsules. These messages are responsible for conscious proprioceptive sensitivity.

Discriminative tactile sensitivity also travels through these pathways. Ruffini corpuscles give information about the speed and direction of the

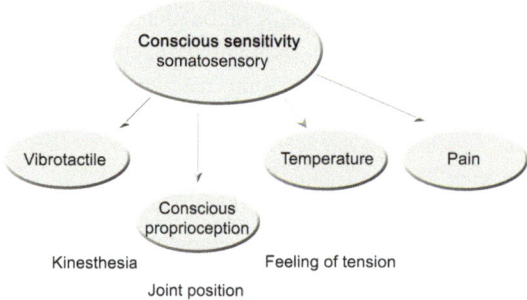

Fig. 8.3 Elements constituting the conscious sensitivity

movement, while Pacini corpuscles give information about acceleration and deceleration. They play an essential role in movement coordination.

8.2.2 Unconscious Proprioception

It allows controlling posture and joint stability and guarantees feedforward (Fig. 8.4). Its path-

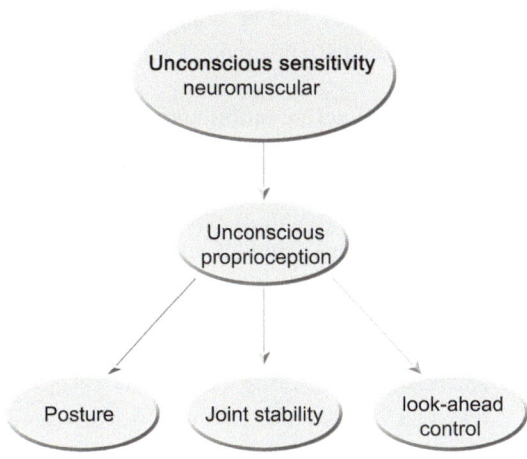

Fig. 8.4 Elements constituting the unconscious sensitivity

ways are projected on the nuclei of the cerebellum. Their afferences do not reach the cortex so they stay unconscious.

The direct and crossed bundles of the cerebellum carry impulses from the neuromuscular spindles (sensitive to length and speed), the Golgi neurotendinous organ (protecting against excessive stretching or contraction), and the vestibular system (sensitive to the head movement). All these systems produce unconscious sensations. The two bundles are projected at the level of the cerebellum and allow this organ playing a regulating role for the muscle tone, a coordinating role for automatic movements, and an equilibration role.

There are two main bundles:

- **The direct or posterior bundle** travels through the inferior pedicle of the cerebellum until it reaches the cerebellum. It conveys afferences from the trunk. The information from the right part of the trunk is projected on the right part of the cerebellum, and vice versa.
- **The crossed or anterior bundle** travels through the superior pedicle of the cerebellum until it reaches the cerebellum too. It conveys afferences from the limbs. The information from the right limbs is projected on the left part of the cerebellum, and vice versa.

8.2.2.1 Feedback and Feedforward
(Fig. 8.5)

Until recently, proprioception was considered a feedback mechanism only. Feedback is a reflex reaction to a stimulus, like a muscle contraction responding to a joint instability. To sum up, first the body moves (or is moved), then the information is sent to the brain, and then adjustments are made.

However, there is evidence showing that this feedback mechanism takes longer to appear than the duration of the injury mechanism. For example, for the knee (the most studied joint), the injury mechanism for a sprain takes 34 ms, while the protective feedback mechanism happens in 89 ms. This long latency time renders the reflexes' role limited, so there must be another way to protect the joint: it is the feedforward.

Feedforward must act to protect the joint in the time gap between the injury mechanism and the feedback. Its base is the central control. This model suggests that the subject also has centralized information about his body position before he reaches said position. Therefore, movement should be used to develop this ability. In the case of the wrist, it will be important to (re)learn movements so that the joint is in a good position when being solicited (pression, ball, fall). For that reason, we can talk about anticipation.

Rehabilitation can act on feedforward to (re) create motor patterns that are underdeveloped or impaired by a trauma. If we want both these controls to work correctly, all the proprioceptive receptors must work correctly as well, therefore stimulating these receptors is an important part of rehabilitation.

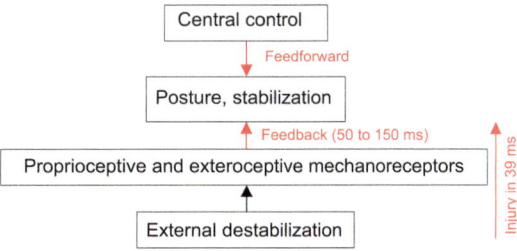

Fig. 8.5 Feedback and feedforward systems working in synergy to optimize the speed and quality of the proprioceptive response

8.3   Rehabilitation Steps (Fig. 8.6)

The rehabilitation program aiming at improving joint stability must consider the three levels of motor control—spinal reflexes, adjustments by the brain stem, and cognitive programming [10, 11]—by combining exercises for conscious and unconscious proprioception.

The first steps of this program correspond to a "classic" rehabilitation and will not be developed in this chapter.

8.3.1   First Stages Recovered: Conscious Proprioception

8.3.1.1 Proprioceptive Consciousness (Hagert's Second Stage)

This step corresponds to the elements that are available to us to maintain or stimulate proprioceptive consciousness during and right after the immobilization phase.

The techniques will be adapted to the tissue healing and the patient's pain. They can be:

- **Passive and active mobilizations**.
- **Self-mobilizations** controlling the stress applied on tissues with a closed kinetic chain, for example, using a medicine ball [12] (Fig. 8.7). This kind of exercise helps the patient perceive his joint better and anticipate risky situations better too, at a time when tissues are not strong yet.
- **Exercises stimulating cutaneous receptors** (exercises where the patient touches various materials for example).
- **Transcutaneous vibratory stimulations** with a frequency of 80 Hz applied on a tendon for 30 min [13].
- **Massages**.
- **Electric stimulations** (TENS) with high and low frequencies, or electrostimulations if the tissue healing allows it.

Rehabilitation steps for proprioception	Treatment plan	Goal	Techniques
1	Classic rehabilitation	Fight against pain, trophic disorders and mobility	Classic techniques
2	Proprioceptive consciousness	Improve conscious joint control	Graded motor imagery
3	Joint position sensitivity	Ability to reproduce a predefined joint position	Blind passive and active reproduction of a joint angle
4	Kinesthésia	Ability to feel a joint mobilization without visual or audible information	Detection of a movement with an arthro-motor
5	Conscious neuromuscular rehabilitation	Strength of specific muscles allowing to improve joint stability	Auxotonic contractions, co contraction
6	Unconscious neuromuscular rehabilitation	Muscle reactivation (speed and quality)	Destabilizing plyometric exercices

1 = Conscious proprioception (cortical interactions)
2 = Unconscious proprioception (spinal and cerebellar interactions)

Fig. 8.6 Rehabilitation steps according to Hagert

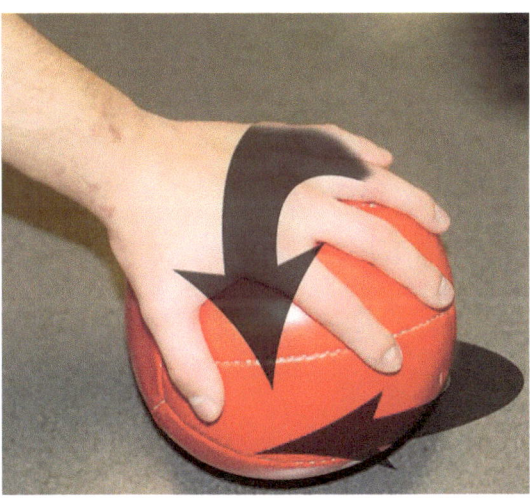

Fig. 8.7 Self-mobilizations in a closed chain, with controlled tissue stress, with a medicine ball

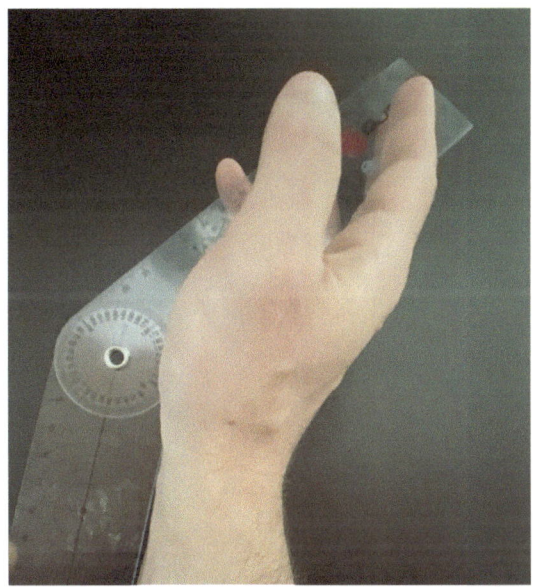

Fig. 8.8 Assessment of the joint position sense (statesthesia)

8.3.1.2 Joint Position Perception (Hagert's Third Stage)

It is defined as the ability to precisely reproduce a given joint angulation [1].

The rehabilitation of this perception is done in three steps. In the first step, the therapist places the patient's forearm in a defined joint position and controls the joint amplitude with a goniometer.

In the second step, the forearm is placed in another position, indifferently. In the third step, the patient must place his forearm in the first position [1, 14] (Fig. 8.8).

The exercise is realized with the patient's eyes closed to avoid any visual afference. An error margin of 4° is considered normal in adults (at the level of the wrists).

8.3.1.3 Kinesthesia (Hagert's Fourth Stage)

It is defined as the ability to detect a passive movement. The therapist realizes the movement while the patient keeps his eyes closed and tells him when he perceives the movement.

This exercise is easy to realize at the physiotherapy office or at home but does not allow a precise analysis regarding the patient's perception threshold.

Using an arthromotor device allows analyzing more precisely the movement speed and the studied angular sector.

A laser can also be a very helpful tool to improve conscious proprioceptive abilities. The patient must follow trajectories becoming increasingly complex, going faster and faster (Fig. 8.9).

8.3.2   Last Stages Recovered: Unconscious Proprioception

As shown in several studies on other joints [2, 10, 15], proprioceptive rehabilitation is essential for an optimal joint function: it decreases the latency period and the quality of the motor response when the joint's environment changes.

The two last steps of the protocol should be implemented only after the injured tissues are healed [8, 16].

8.3.2.1 Conscious Neuromuscular Rehabilitation (Hagert's Fifth Stage)

Several strengthening modes have been described to improve neuromuscular capacities. They help increasing the basic muscle tone and therefore the joint's dynamic stability [2].

Every contraction mode has its particularities and must be requested during rehabilitation to help the patients with all their functional needs.

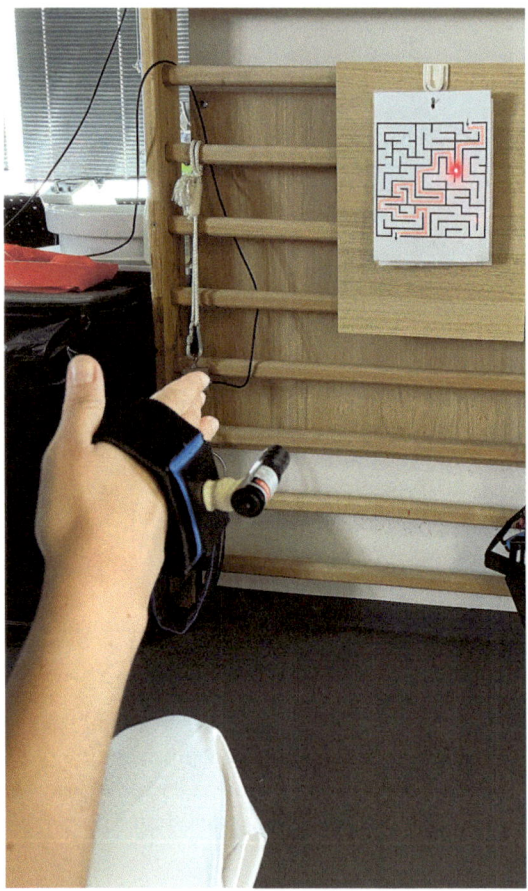

Fig. 8.9 Using a laser to improve conscious proprioceptive abilities

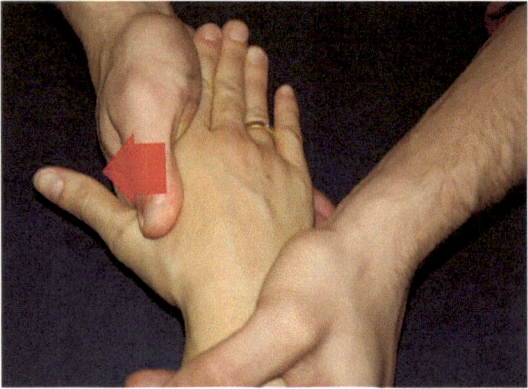

Fig. 8.10 Static contractions using target muscles and minimizing joint and muscle stress

Static Contractions

Static contractions have a resistance moment equal to their moment of muscular force. This corresponds to a contraction with a fixed joint angle [1]. This type of contraction is the least stressful for the involved joint and muscles.

During rehabilitation, it helps strengthening the targeted muscle by modifying the position of the unstable joint, from the stable position towards a more unstable position, always respecting the tissue healing time (Fig. 8.10).

Dynamic Contractions

They are defined by a difference between the resistance moment and the moment of muscular force [17].

If the moment of muscular force is greater than the resistance moment, the muscle insertions move closer to one another, and the muscle shortens: it is a concentric contraction. The movement is produced by the increase of the muscle tension.

On the contrary, if the moment of muscular force is lower than the resistance moment, the muscle insertions move apart from each other, and the muscle lengthens: it is an eccentric contraction. The movement is produced when the resistance is higher than the force produced by the muscle.

In most functional movements, there is a natural and permanent interaction between dynamic and static contractions, as the stress load and the speed vary. It is called auxotonic contraction.

These exercises can be easily realized with weighted sticks or other tools designed for this purpose.

Finally, an isokinetic contraction is defined as a muscle contraction with a constant angular speed. It is concentric when the resistance opposed to the muscle contraction adapts so that the speed is constant. It is eccentric when the device maintains a constant speed against which the patient must resist [18].

Using a 3D device like the "kinevolution" helps getting closer to a functional movement using proprioceptive neuromuscular facilitation (Fig. 8.11).

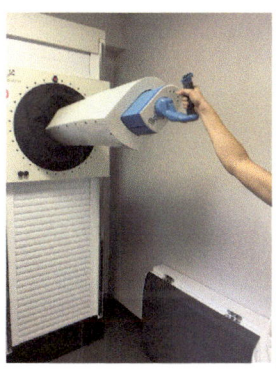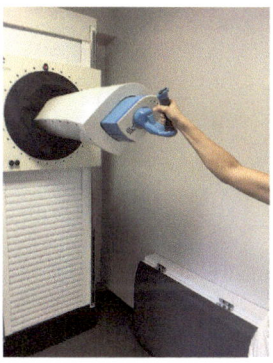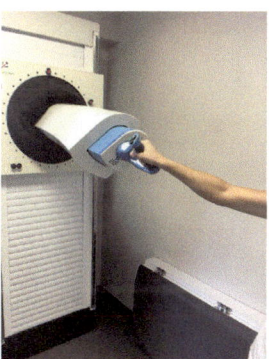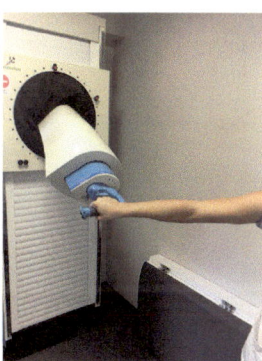

Fig. 8.11 Global exercise for the superior limb muscles (isokinetic mode)

There is a high level of evidence showing the interest of isokinetic exercises to improve strength, endurance, and all the joints' proprioceptive functions in athletes with knee, ankle, and shoulder instability. Unfortunately, this kind of device is expensive and therefore rarely available for therapists.

8.3.2.2 Unconscious Neuromuscular Rehabilitation or Reflex Muscle Activation (Hager's Sixth Stage)

Conscious neuromuscular rehabilitation intentionally targets the requested muscles. On the contrary, unconscious neuromuscular rehabilitation uses the reflexes that actively lock the joints, which can partially compensate a passive instability.

Reflex muscle activation can be disturbed in any joint with ligamentous injuries and its adapted rehabilitation helps getting back protective neuromuscular reflexes that exist in all normal joints [16].

The exercises can be done in open chain and in closed chain, from the stable position to the unstable position to get closer to the superior limb's global function, targeting the patient's functional needs.

To work on reflex neuromuscular control in a closed chain, the exercise can be, for example, using a medicine ball with the patient's hands on it (two hands then one hand), and the therapist destabilizing the ball in different directions.

When the patient knows the modalities of destabilization, we work on feedforward with an anticipated contraction happening before the sensorial detection of the destabilization.

We can also work on feedback when the patient has his eyes closed and does not know what the modalities of destabilization are going to be. This corresponds to a corrective contraction after the sensorial detection of the destabilization [19].

A similar exercise in semi-closed chain can be realized with a plastic tube half-full of water. The patient holds it in the palm of his hand and controls the oscillations in pronation and supination.

Other reflex muscle activation exercises can be done using a ball on a racket or an oscillating bar. Other more specific and complex devices can be interesting too, such as the "inimove"© and the "powerball"© (Fig. 8.12).

Plyometric exercises refer to an eccentric contraction immediately followed by a concentric contraction. They have shown their interest in improving the global stability of the inferior limb by bettering the muscle activation and creating adaptations in the sensorimotor system [20].

They can be realized asking the patient to "jump" against a wall or against the floor first, then against a Swiss ball (Fig. 8.13).

In proprioceptive rehabilitation, it is essential to respect a progression to optimize the functional recovery and reduce the risk of relapse. In fact, a settled proprioceptive deficit can be responsible for a decrease of neuromuscular control, overstressing the ligaments and resulting in a relapse [10, 21] (Fig. 8.14).

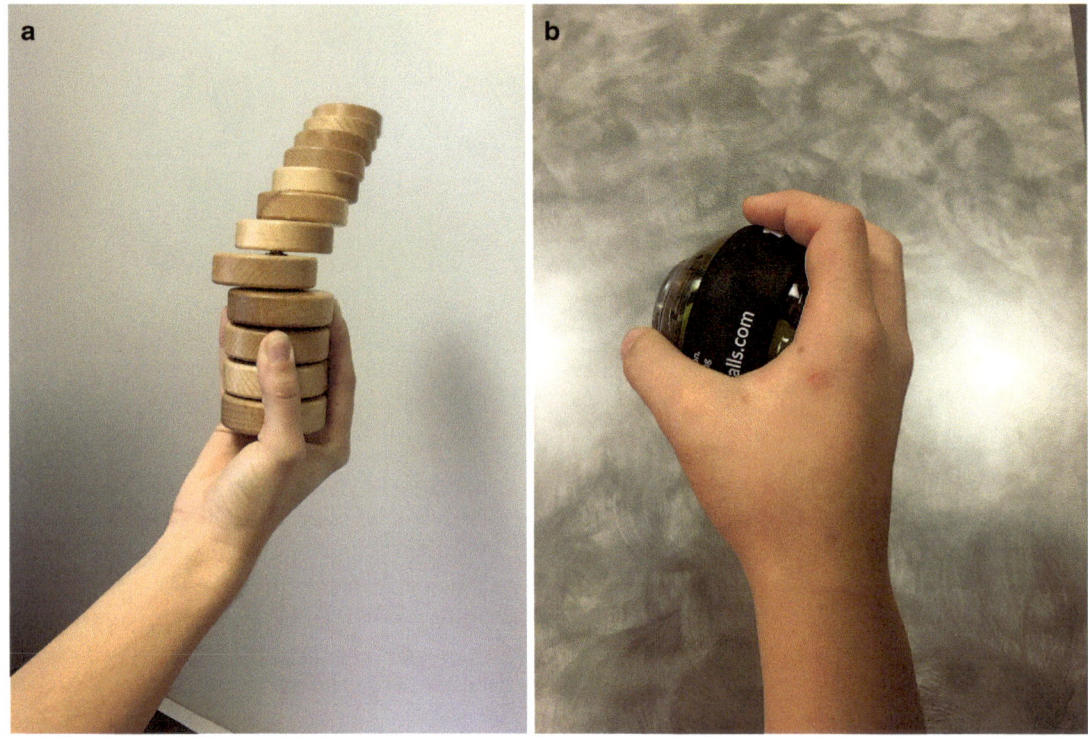

Fig. 8.12 Example of exercise allowing to stimulate reflex muscle activation abilities, aligning magnetic discs with the Inimove© (**a**) and rotating a full ball in a sphere with the Powerball© (**b**)

Fig. 8.13 Example of plyometric exercise with a Swiss ball

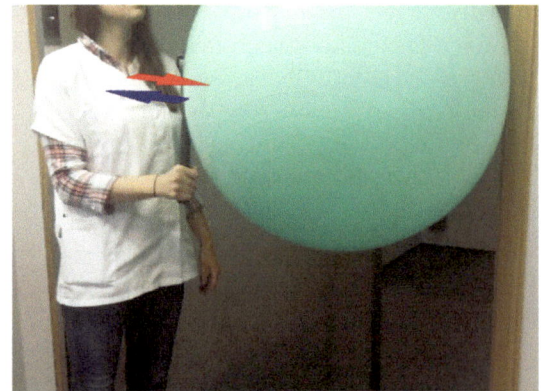

Fig. 8.14 Importance of proprioceptive rehabilitation to improve the patient's abilities and to reduce the risk of recurrence

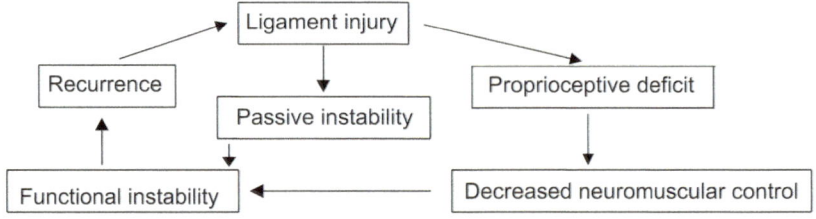

References

1. Hagert E. Proprioception of the wrist joint: a review of current concepts and possible implications on the rehabilitation of the wrist. J Hand Ther. 2010;23(1):2–16; quiz 17.

2. Riemann B, Lephart S. The sensorimotor system, part 1: the physiologic basis of functional joint stability. J Athl Train. 2002;37(1):71–9.

3. Blakemore S, Frith C, Wolpert D. Spatio-temporal prediction modulates the perception of self-produced stimuli. J Cogn Neurosci. 1999;11(5):551–9.

4. Hagert E, Ferreres A, Garcia-Elias M. Nerve-sparing dorsal and volar approaches to the radiocarpal joint. J Hand Surg Am. 2010;35(7):1070–4.

5. Hagert E, Forsgren S, Ljung BO. Differences in the presence of mechanoreceptors and nerve structures between wrist ligaments may imply differential roles in wrist stabilization. J Orthop Res. 2005;23(4):757–63.

6. Hagert E, et al. Immunohistochemical analysis of wrist ligament innervation in relation to their structural composition. J Hand Surg Am. 2007;32(1):30–6.

7. Hagert E, Lee J, Ladd AL. Innervation patterns of thumb trapeziometacarpal joint ligaments. J Hand Surg Am. 2012;37(4):706–14. e1.

8. Hagert E, Karagiannopoulos C, Rein S. Proprioception in hand rehabilitation. In: Rehabilitation of the hand and upper extremity. St. Louis: Elsevier; 2021.

9. Lamy J-C. Bases neurophysiologiques de la proprioception. Kinésithér Scient. 2006;472:15–23.

10. Lephart S, et al. The role of proprioception in the management and rehabilitation of athletic injuries. Am J Sports Med. 1997;25:130–7.

11. Lotters FJB, Schreuders TAR, Videler AJ. SMoC-Wrist: a sensorimotor control-based exercise program for patients with chronic wrist pain. J Hand Ther. 2020;33(4):607–15.

12. Carlson L, Watson K. Treatment of reflex sympathetic dystrophy using the stress-loading program. J Hand Ther. 1988;1:149–54.

13. Roll R, et al. Illusory movements prevent cortical disruption caused by immobilization. NeuroImage. 2012;62(1):510–9.

14. Karagiannopoulos C, et al. Responsiveness of the active wrist joint position sense test after distal radius fracture intervention. J Hand Ther. 2016;29(4):474–82.

15. Fitzgerald G, Axe M, Snyder-Mackler L. The efficacy of perturbation training in nonoperative anterior cruciate ligament rehabilitation programs for physically active individuals. Phys Ther. 2000;80(2):128–40.

16. Karagiannopoulos C, Michlovitz S. Rehabilitation strategies for wrist sensorimotor control impairment: from theory to practice. J Hand Ther. 2016;29(2):154–65.

17. Harwood C, Turner L. Conservative management of midcarpal instability. J Hand Surg Eur Vol. 2015;41E(1):102–9.

18. Mesplie G. Instabilités du carpe chez le sportif. Promanu. 2017;1:4–12.

19. Riemann B, Lephart S. The sensorimotor system, part 2: the role of proprioception in motor and functional joint stability. J Athl Train. 2002;37(1):80–4.

20. Chimera NJ, et al. Effects of plyometric training on muscle-activation strategies and performance in female athletes. J Athl Train. 2004;39(1):24–31.

21. Lephart S, Henry T. The physiological basis for open and closed kinetic chain rehabilitation for the upper extremity. J Sport Rehabil. 1996;5:71–87.

Rehabilitation Using Motor Imagery After a Post-Traumatic Cortical Reorganization

François Delaquaize

9.1 Introduction

The mechanisms in brain plasticity and cortical reorganization are becoming increasingly well-known, thanks to the advances made in neurosciences.

The concept of a "fixed" adult brain that can only deteriorate is obsolete. There is a very dynamic brain plasticity. In case of traumatism in the superior limb, the afferent sensorial information and efferent motor command are disturbed. This leads to a remodeling of the superior limb's cortical representation. Medical imagery—especially functional MRI—show very well the brain plasticity becoming worse after an amputation or a complex regional pain syndrome (CRPS). However, this post-traumatic cortical disorganization is reversible. In rehabilitation, we can use brain plasticity to improve and regularize the modifications of the central nervous system.

We intend to quickly review the mechanisms of brain plasticity to better understand and justify the rehabilitation protocols.

We only describe four indications that show promising results in hand rehabilitation: algo hallucinoses in patients with amputation or brachial plexus avulsion, CRPS, segmentary exclusion syndrome (SES), and any immobilization or

underuse of a limb. We will then develop the rehabilitation techniques such as motor imagery (including mirror therapy) that act on the cortical consequences of peripheral traumatic injuries.

We chose to describe these four pathological states only from the perspective of central nervous system modifications and cortical reorganization, in a succinct way. The other aspects of these pathologies are well-known. In neuroscience, the theories and hypotheses explaining cortical mechanisms are complex and constantly evolving.

9.2 Brain Plasticity

"The adult brain is an immutable organ, everything can die, nothing can regenerate." This notion of a "capital of neurons" is outdated. We now know that the brain is a dynamic system, constantly reconfiguring, thanks to brain plasticity phenomena [1].

New neurons are constantly forming from stem cells. Migration and transformation mechanisms are needed for these neurons to be functioning, but they are not well-known. Sprouting mechanisms allow the formation of new synapses and dendrites. The more the brain is stimulated with afferent and efferent information, the more neurons and interconnections are created, leading to new operational circuits. Synaptic plasticity plays an important role in neuroplasticity by modifying its connectivity structure [2]. A

F. Delaquaize (✉)
Hôpitaux Universitaires de Genève,
Genève, Switzerland
e-mail: francois.delaquaize@sfr.fr

Hebbian mechanism reinforces or eliminates the neuronal interconnections depending on their use—or non-use. These mechanisms create functional neuronal network that form a very dynamic cortical map [1, 3–9].

Penfield has mapped the representation of the body parts at the level of the primary sensorimotor cortex and schematized it with his homunculus. The hand area is very large and is adjacent to the face and forearm areas. Penfield's approach has become more nuanced as the homunculus is not fixed; there are large anatomical subregions, with overlapping areas and interconnections. Cortical maps are now seen as dynamic entities whose balance is subjected to permanent modifications acquired through experience [10, 11]. A neuronal connections system forms depending on the function and the activity; this system makes a sensorimotor map adaptable to the needs [5, 7, 8, 12, 13]. Therefore, the cortical areas are remodeled depending on the afferent sensory information and the efferent motor commands [14, 15]. According to Will, "the brain function of an individual under an excessive or lacking stimulation changes its structure, and thereby his future brain function" [2], so "use it or lose it." In an individual, what is important is not the number of neurons, but the quality of its connections and functional network.

9.2.1 Illustrations of Brain Plasticity and Cortical Remodeling

Studies in a patient with bilateral hand amputations and bilateral allografts illustrate these cortical reorganization phenomena, in terms of both deterioration and improvement [16]. After the amputations, the patient has neither afference coming from his hands, nor efference going towards them. A cortical remodeling follows: the hands' cortical representation disappears and is replaced by the adjacent areas—face, forearm, and arm. The adjacent areas colonize and overlap the empty cortical area of the hands. At this point, the reorganization goes in the direction of deterioration.

However, the hand's cortical representation has not completely disappeared. There still is a memory of the sensations and movements in the amputated hand [17–19].

It is encouraging to see that this reorganization can also lead to improvement. Six months after realizing bilateral hand allografts, we can see in this same patient that the cortical representation of the hands regains its initial localization, as information arrives to and comes from the brain again [20].

This reversibility happens in a very progressive way. Five months after the graft, when we touch the face and the hand simultaneously, we note a lack of sensitivity in the hand. However, if we touch only the hand or the hand and another body part, the hand is sensitive [21]. It all happens as if there was a competition between the afferences from the face and the once from the hand.

Other authors [12, 22–25] show a migration of the mouth's somatosensory area towards the hand's somatosensory area in hand amputees. This cortical reorganization can be reversible after retraining the sensory discrimination [22, 26, 27]. The reversibility of the cortical reorganization is very encouraging for the therapist. With these different techniques, and sometimes even visually tricking the brain, we try to restore sensory afferences to recreate a coherent body image in the primary sensorimotor cortex.

In amputee patients, this regularization comes with fewer sensations and phantom limb pain. There is a correlation between the importance of the cortical area's migration and the importance of algo hallucinoses [22, 24, 26, 28, 29].

Another example of the reversibility of cortical reorganization: a patient with a high radial nerve palsy with a quadruple extensor tendons transfer [30]. The functional MRI shows a functional recovery 6 months after the surgery. The analysis of the brain activity shows activity emerging in specific motor and somatosensory areas during fingers extension, thumb extension, and wrist extension.

The positive development of cortical reorganization can happen a long time after the initial event. In patients with congenital syndactylia, the study of the fingers' cortical representation shows that the areas are overlapped and grouped together. Surgically separating the fingers at an adult age leads to the fingers becoming autonomous. The cortical interdigital distance increases, which can be seen as early as a week after surgery [31, 32].

These phenomena of overlapping cortical areas are also found when surgically creating artificial syndactylia in monkeys, as well as in patients immobilized with a cast or with CRPS. They can even happen after a very short period: stimulating the tips of two fingers at the same time causes their cortical areas to get together after a few hours [5, 31, 33].

Brain plasticity also plays a major role in the cortical over- or underrepresentation of the hand, depending on its level of use [33]. A violinist has a hypertrophied cortical representation of his left hand's fingers, especially the fifth finger with the vibrato. However, the left thumb has a normal representation as it does not have a major activity. The importance of this representation is influenced by the number of years of training and by the age at which the musician began to practice [5, 34, 35]. A braille reader also has a hypertrophied cortical representation of the finger he uses to read [5, 36]. This notion of cortical over- or underrepresentation had already been approached by Levame in 1976 [37], before modern imagery techniques. In his concept of "hand-image" and "hand-object," a pianist's "hand-image" had more segments, proportionally to his virtuosity. With the existing knowledge of his time, he recommended a rehabilitation that is no longer adapted. It consisted in saying that if the patient had a "mitten hand," there was no point in working on finger dissociation as it would have been too difficult, especially after a finger traumatism. At times, he even recommended exercises with a glove with fingers sewn together depending on the level of digital independence. This did not consider the potential evolution, thanks to brain plasticity.

Cortical activity depends on the complexity of the task. During the opposition between the thumb and the fingers, several cortical areas are recruited. The recruitment depends on the opposition: it is more important if the thumb opposes the fingers one after the other than if it opposes all the fingers together, and it is the most impor-

tant when we change the order of the opposed fingers—it can even generate activity in the homolateral cortex [38].

Cortical representation is also proportional to the focus on one area or the other. The cortical area representation moves depending on the focused area. The attention given to a task increases the efficiency of the connections between the prefrontal cortex and the premotor cortex, while the absence of attention decreases this efficiency [39]. A sustained attention achieves long-term plastic modifications. This focus is essential in motor imaging therapy.

Painful stimuli can also cause the cortical representation to move [14, 15].

We therefore see that the brain's functional modification is permanent. Neuron plasticity can be very quick as seen when applying a numbing cream on the forearm: in the following hour, there is a cortical expansion of the hand, along with an improvement of the hand sensitivity [40]. The speed of these changes does not seem to be caused by the creation of new circuits but by lifting the inhibitions in preexisting circuits in the hand. The balance between excitatory and inhibitory influences on neurons is lost, a latent connectivity is uncovered [10, 11].

In case of definitive deafferentation, new circuits appear over the long term, thanks to synaptic reinforcement mechanisms (Hebb's theory) and axonal terminal sprouting followed by synaptogenesis.

9.3 Mirror Neurons and Canonical Neurons

The discovery of mirror neurons has been an essential step forward in understanding the neuronal excitability mechanisms [41–44]. Mirror neurons are neurons activated in the premotor cortex when observing a task realized by another person. A motor resonance is produced in the observer, with an increase of the excitability of nervous structures involved in the realization of this task.

These neurons are more active when observing an interaction between the hand and a familiar object. The motor action must be a part of our internal "library" of motor experiences and of our behavioral repertoire [43]. These mirror neurons build a mental representation allowing us to understand the purpose and the motor intention of the observed action. The context of the action is important: it must have a meaning, a purpose. Observing a transitive action oriented towards an object causes a more important activation of the premotor cortex [45]. The motor resonance is not automatic: observing an absurd action in an unrealistic context can even decrease the corticospinal excitability [46]. The more the subject controls an action, the easier the activation of his mirror neurons will be when seeing this action. The mirror neurons can be activated during the construction of an internal representation of a motor action. The subject does not have to see the action, the sound of an identified action alone can activate mirror neurons [47]. An amount of information sufficient so that the subject understands the purpose of the action is enough.

They also play a role in learning mechanisms. The activation of mirror neurons happens very early: babies' mimicry of facial expressions is a good example. The "contagious yawn" also illustrates the activation of mirror neurons.

There are several systems of mirror neurons, for the touch [48], the hearing, the smell, the pain. Seeing a person suffering a painful stimulation activates the same painful circuits in the observer. Fortunately, a "healthy" observer does not feel pain as inhibitory circuits come into action to stop the painful activation [44, 49–52].

There also is a mirror system in the limbic cortex that manages the emotions. We are receptive to feelings of suffering, disgust, pleasure, sadness, fear. The mirror neurons are responsible for empathy, which is the basis of all human relationships. An embodied simulation occurs that places us in a shared neuronal state where we are "in the other's skin and mind."

The discovery of motor neurons is important for rehabilitation. We can exploit their properties in mirror therapy [53–55], they can trick the brain with artificially normal visual information. They are also involved in motor observation and motor imagery.

There are also canonic neurons that work in a similar way. They are activated when seeing a graspable object or food, as if the brain anticipated a potential interaction [56].

They help the hand preparing for grabbing an object depending on its shape and function. A manipulable object oriented in the right direction automatically activates a motor program associated with its use [57]. When working on imagined gripping actions, we must integrate various everyday objects from the patient's daily life. We do not anticipate the same grip when seeing a plastic cup of hot coffee that can crumple and burn us, or when seeing an insulated mug that we can firmly grab. The context of the observed or imagined action is important: it is difficult to imagine grabbing a glass to drink if the film footage shows an empty glass [46].

9.4 Phantom Limb

Described by Mitchell in 1872, the illusion of a phantom limb is frequent as 90% of amputee patients experience it. The perception of a limb as if it still existed comes with pain of various intensities in 70% of cases. The patients sometimes feel like they can move this limb through space. It can feel like it is normal, deformed, or telescoped [58, 59].

Patients with brachial plexus avulsion have the same perceptive illusions. These sensations are disabling and can sometimes bring the monoplegic patients to ask for an amputation. However, an amputation usually does not settle the phantom limb phenomenon. During a brachial plexus avulsion, a phenomenon of "learned paralysis" occurs. This phenomenon explains the fact that after a secondary limb amputation, the phantom limb is felt as paralyzed in the preoperative position [59].

The phantom limb would be a component of the mental representation of the body schema. Melzack [11, 59–61] proposes the concept of "neuro-matrix," responsible for the body schema. This neuro-matrix is made of a neural network localized in several brain structures (cortex, brain stem, thalamus, limbic system, cerebellum). It manages sensory information, emotions, and cognitive activities, including memories of past experiences. This neuro-matrix also produces an individual "neuro-signature" indicating that the sensations concern "my body." It is mostly pre-wired at birth. The innate aspect of the neuro-matrix gives an explanation to the phenomena of phantom limb felt by children with limb agenesis. In case of amputation, the lack of afference projected on the neuro-matrix induces a remodeling of the somesthetic maps; however, the feeling of integrity of the body schema contained in the neuro-matrix is still present.

A painful sensation is not only the direct consequence of a nociceptive signal coming from the periphery towards the superior brain centers. This signal must also go through the subjective filter of experiences, behavior, emotions, and the aspect of purpose. In the end, the painful stimulus is modulated by a variety of interactions and information exchanges at various levels of the neuro-matrix. It is then incorporated as a painful perception specific to each individual [62]. The cognitive aspect also plays a significant role in the perception development.

Many patients experience referred sensations at the level of the phantom limb [25, 59, 63]. Stimulating the cheek or the stump after a transhumeral amputation creates sensations in the phantom hand. Depending on the location of the stimulation, the patient locates the sensations in one finger or the other. These sensations can manifest themselves as pain, paresthesia, or electric shocks. Different stimulations produce distinct types of sensations: applying an ice cube produces a cold sensation, vibrations produce a sensation of vibration [64]. When an amputee patient cringes, he activates the bilateral primary sensorimotor cortical areas of his face and lips, as well as the contralateral primary sensorimotor cortical areas of the hand and arm. This paradoxical activation can be treated with motor imagery (among other things) [5]. Referred sensations can be explained by the colonization of the "empty" cortical area by the adjacent areas.

During a motor activity, the permanent interaction between the motor command and sensory feedback improves the movement's precision and efficiency by readjusting it. It is an unconscious mechanism in most activities. This interaction also alerts and protects the organism when an important discordance is detected: it is the concept of motor cortical control, which regulates all our motor activities [65–71]. Peripheral injuries come with perturbations in sensory afferences and cortical modifications. A conflict will then take place, due to a discordance between the movement feedback and the programmed movement intention (feedforward) and generating pain. In a healthy subject, we can provoke this kind of discordance followed by various problems when the subject simply realizes asynchronous movements opening and closing the hands in a mirror box. Motion sickness is another example of a problem created by a perturbation of the control system when it is under a discordance between the visual, vestibular, and proprioceptive feedbacks. In amputee patients, the lack of proprioceptive and visual information consistent with their intention to mobilize the amputated limb could be the cause of pain and phantom limb sensations [69]. Using a mirror helps reconcile the visual feedback with the motor command by informing the brain that his missing limb can be mobilized correctly [64]. This concept of motor control also explains the disorders occurring in CRPS or exclusion syndrome as the same type of discordances happen.

Several peripheral and central mechanisms participate in the genesis and perpetuation of phantom pains. Flor synthetized them [26, 72]: the intensity and duration of pains before the amputation leads to the development of a cortical memory of pain and a hyperexcitability. This, combined with the reorganization of the amputated area in the somatosensory cortex, participates in the development of phantom pains. After an amputation, several phenomena maintain algo hallucinoses: neuroma, abnormal modifications of the dorsal root ganglion and the posterior horn of the spinal cord, degeneration of C fibers, and sympathetic activation.

Let us recall here the correlation between the importance of the migration of the hand's cortical representation area, and the importance of phantom sensations and pain [22, 24, 26, 28, 29].

Phantom pains decrease in intensity and frequency when training to imagine sensations and movements in the amputated limb [73].

In this context of cortical reorganization, motor imaging therapy is fully justified as it exploits brain plasticity.

9.5   Complex Regional Pain Syndrome

The etiology of CRPS is a multifactorial process involving peripheral and central mechanisms. It is a frequent complication and is always difficult and long to treat. The prognosis depends on a rapid diagnosis according to the Budapest criteria [74, 75], which is essential for an early treatment. We will make no difference between the type 1 CRPS, the type 2 CRPS, and the non-otherwise specified (NOS) CRPS, as the treatment is the same [76]. Furthermore, even if the nerve injury does not damage a "big nerve trunk," there is an axonal injury in 99% of the type 1 CRPS [77–79]. Motor imagery is a technique acting on the cortical aspect of this syndrome. Therefore, we treat CRPS "from the top down," as opposed to more classical approaches that go "from the bottom up" [80].

There is a cortical reorganization that can be compared to the one found in amputee patients. For example, at the level of the hemisphere corresponding to the side with CRPS, the cortical representation area of the thumb and fifth finger gets closer to the cortical representation area of the hand and bottom lip [81, 82]. This cortical reorganization can be reversed after a treatment normalizing the distance between the thumb and fifth finger [83].

In patients with CRPS and other chronic pains, the density of gray matter decreases which disorganizes the interactions with the white matter [84].

Pain, discriminative sensitivity, and cortical reorganization are interdependent. During recovery, the somatosensory cortical representation increases while the discriminative sensitivity improves and the pain decreases [28, 29].

The cortical reorganization is the cause and/or consequence of sensorimotor disturbances, it is proportional to the disturbances. The higher the pain, the more important the cortical changes.

In CRPS, allodynias happen very frequently. Allodynia has a peripheral and central etiology, with important cortical remodeling [80, 83, 85]. The representation of the painful areas is wider, stimulating an allodynic zone with a brush disperses the cortical activations—even in the primary motor cortex.

The patients can also feel phantom sensations and pains like those found in brachial plexus injuries and amputations [72, 86].

In CRPS, we frequently find an exclusion syndrome [87–91]. Motor negligence and cognitive negligence can both be observed. With the first type (motor), there is a loss of spontaneous movement, the patient must pay attention to his limb to move it. With a cognitive negligence, the patient feels like his limb is foreign to him, paralyzed, or even missing. In some cases, he can have a feeling of "telescoping": he feels like his hand is directly attached to the elbow or shoulder [27]. He can also feel like his hand is detached and "sails" around his arm. Almost half of patients have both types of negligence in varying degrees.

A spatial hemi-negligence would even exist, with a displacement of the median reference line [92, 93].

Patients with CRPS and a negligence syndrome usually have an important level of pain and more difficulties to realize imagined movements [70, 94]. The mechanisms of this negligence are similar to the segmentary exclusion syndrome (SES) described later. However, pain is not always found in SES. In CRPS, the pain reinforces the vicious circle by modifying the nervous structures and the synapses and by decreasing the movements due to the fear of pain—which will of course have consequences on cortical reorganization. It is important to search for signs of negligence in CRPS, as it can disturb synchronous bilateral movements: the patient is asked questions about his impressions and feelings, especially in case of cognitive negligence, to guide and personalize the treatment.

The body schema is also disturbed [95] with for example difficulties identifying the finger touched with a cotton swab. The patient can also feel like his hand is larger [94]. Left/right discrimination is disturbed in the limb with CRPS. These body pattern disorders are proportional to the pain intensity [95].

As seen in amputee patients, there are also referred sensations in one-third of CRPS [96, 97]. These referred sensations are caused by the cortical areas overlapping, for example, one of the cheeks with one of the hands. They can sometimes be reciprocal. The vision's impact is important as these sensations disappear when we look at the concerned zone. These referred sensations are sought after as they are markers of the CRPS evolution.

Motor imagery therapy is indicated in CRPS treatment along with other more classic techniques. A study [98] of patients with CRPS shows good results on neuropathic pain, edema, and left/right discrimination.

Early diagnosis and treatment are essential in CRPS, as imagined movements can increase pain and edema in chronic CRPS [55]. In this case, we must adapt our treatment with motor imagery.

Vibratory stimulations on tendons are another therapeutic tool to reactivate some cortical sensorimotor sequences [99, 100]. They act on the motor control system and help to correct the discordance between sensorial afferences and motor efferences—just as mirror therapy. Here, visual feedback is replaced by proprioceptive feedback induced by vibratory stimulations on neuromuscular spindles that create an illusion of movement [99].

In CRPS, if we detect a hyposensitivity or mechanical allodynia that hides an underlying hyposensitivity, a sensory rehabilitation must be started as early as possible [77–79]. This specific somatosensory rehabilitation, benefiting from neural plasticity, is a technique of choice in case of neuropathic pain. It is the perfect complement to motor imagery.

9.6 Segmentary Exclusion Syndrome

The segmentary exclusion syndrome (SES) corresponds to an underutilization of a part of a limb, especially the hand or fingers (frequently the index finger). It can be reversible when urged by a third party to use the concerned part. It happens in the absence of any injury of the central nervous system [101]. Segmentary negligence often comes with a body pattern disorder and finger agnosia. An SES must not be mistaken for a hemi-negligence with a central origin, even if some signs are shared by both conditions.

There are many nonspecific circumstances needed for an SES to happen: a traumatism, an infection, a local inflammation. The post-injury inflammation and the immobilization modify the sensory afferences (deafferentation) [102].

The deafferentation triggers a chain of events: the combined inflammation and edema alter the sensorial and proprioceptive receptors that send distorted information to the brain. The brain and its cortical motor control system are tricked by this misinformation, which is followed by inadequate motor responses in the form of non-utilization that can be associated with an absurd position such as an extended index finger. This deafferentation phenomenon comes with a disturbance of the body schema and a cortical remodeling of the somatosensory mapping, due to immobilization and non-utilization [103, 104]. In a way, the movement gets "erased" from the motor pattern, so the patient needs to relearn it as if it were realized for the first time.

The perpetuation of an SES can be explained by an organic injury of the sensory receptors after a sclerosis caused by the initial inflammation: false sensory information keeps being transmitted to the brain. Another explanation is the cortical reorganization: the area corresponding to the excluded segment is colonized by the adjacent areas [105].

Segmentary exclusion can cause pain when the cortical motor control system detects a conflict between the visual afferences and the proprioceptive and sensory afferences.

Focus is particularly important in an SES in order not to forget the excluded limb at a cortical level, and therefore regularizing the cortical reorganization [68]. Motor imagery therapy uses the patient's focus. Visual control is mandatory when relearning a movement.

SES can be isolated, but it can also be combined with reflex vegetative disorders, pain, or CRPS [88, 89, 101].

The classic treatment of an SES starts with the treatment of the inflammation and pain. It continues with a desensitization to obtain a recalibration of the sensations and cortical representations [106]. The patient's motivation is key to get his focus on his movements in his daily life. We must work on the automatization of gestures, by repeating grasps using the excluded segment. Constraint-induced movement therapy may also be associated [102]. Every technique aiming at regularizing brain reorganization and avoiding the decrease of the excluded segment's cortical representation is relevant. Motor imagery therapy is a complementary technique of choice when dealing with SES.

9.7 Consequences of Immobilization and Underutilization

The harmful effects of immobilization are well-known in hand surgery, so the duration of immobilization has been reduced to a minimum to limit the apparition of adhesions, capsular and ligamentous retraction, amyotrophy, and other complications. We must also consider its negative impact on the cortex.

The volume of the representation of an immobilized muscle or hand decreases proportionally to the duration of immobilization [107, 108] or non-utilization. These two situations come with a decrease of discriminative sensitivity [108]. The loss of strength would be partially due to the patient's difficulty to recruit as many motor units as possible [104].

As seen previously, there overlapping and colonization phenomena from the active adjacent areas. Thankfully, the cortical remodeling accompanying the unlearning of the movements is reversible [109].

A similar yet smaller cortical remodeling can be observed in patients with gonarthrosis [110] and rhizarthrosis [111], for example.

Kinesiophobia in athletes has the same harmful effects.

Therefore, motor imagery therapy has its place in fighting against the cortical consequences of the post-traumatic immobilization or underutilization of a limb.

9.8 Mental Imagery and Motor Imagery

Mental imagery is the mental representation of actions or perceptions, from memorized information. It allows building a mental representation of a motor sequence without realizing a movement. It allows reactivating and re-feeling internal representations that have already been experienced.

There are several types of mental imagery [112]: motor, tactile, kinesthetic, visual, auditory, but also olfactory and gustatory, such as Proust's famous madeleine. In therapy, we combine these various mental sensations and perceptions to reinforce the context of the motor imagery. This way, the effects are potentialized at a cortical level. For example, imagining grabbing a glass of orangeade, cool to the touch, refreshing, with its characteristic taste and smell, in a pleasant and known environment such as holidays by the sea. We can also change the emotional contexts and the environment during therapy. We can learn from motor imagery models such as PETTLEP or MIIMS [113, 114], recommended in athletes to act on different components and obtain a multimodal representation of the imagined action.

9.8.1 Motor Imagery Therapy

Motor imagery therapy includes two techniques:

- **Motor imagery** that can be implicit and unconscious with exercises for left/right discrimination, or explicit and conscious with imagined actions with an internal kinesthetic perspective or an external visual perspective. This explicit motor imagery is usually called motor imagery (MI).
- **Motor observation** (MO) that can be realized with the direct vision of an action or through a mirror or a system of derived mirrors as we will see later [115–117].

Motor imagery therapy completes other classic treatments. It is recommended in pathologies described earlier, as well as after a stroke or in athlete rehabilitation. It uses brain plasticity and the reversibility of cortical changes.

Moseley [98, 118] describes three successive stages in his graded motor imagery (GMI) program for treating patients with chronic pain such as CRPS. He stresses the importance of respecting the stages' order to get a sequential activation of the motor cortical network [119]. This way, the brain is retrained by reproducing the activation sequences happening in planning, preparing, and realizing a movement.

The left/right discrimination activates the premotor cortex and the supplementary motor area [120, 121], then the imagined actions activate the premotor cortex as well as the primary sensorimotor cortex. Finally, the mirror therapy (or motor observation) involves the premotor cortex and the primary motor cortex. The sequence of these three phases must not be dogmatic.

It can be interesting to combine MI and MO [122], or to combine MI with a real movement thus realizing dynamic motor imagery (DMI) [110, 123]. DMI makes remembering kinesthetic sensations easier [124]. DMI can also be associated with MO. We also adjust these techniques graduating the level of motor intention: we start with intention with no movement, then the beginning of an effortless and painless movement, then more and more solicitation [125]. We must build an individual program for each patient and adapt it to his improvements and reactions. We should not hesitate to go back or look at the problem from different angles.

9.8.1.1 Implicit Motor Imagery: Left/ Right Discrimination

The patient must identify the visualized hand. A cortical process starts: first the action is observed, then recognized, then the patient unconsciously reproduces it and realizes a mental rotation to determine if it is a right hand or a left hand. Depending on the signification of the observed action, different cortical areas are activated [51, 126]. We focus on the accuracy and speed of response, without any stress. The patient must not move his hand or his head, as it can help him recognize the hand.

In this exercise, we realize a mental rotation of the hand by using the internal representations of our own limbs, the response time depends on everyone's body schema. There is an isochronous connection between the time needed to realize this mental rotation and the one required for the effective realization of the movement [121, 127]. The more important the amplitude of rotation, the longer the response time. This notion can be compared to Fitts's law, the model of human movement. It predicts the time required to quickly go from a starting position to a final position, depending on the distance from the target and the target's size [112, 128]. This isochrony is also found during the realization of imagined actions and can help us evaluate the patient's capacity for MI [129].

As seen before, pain alters the body schema. It is interesting to note that patients with chronic pain in the superior limb take a much longer time to recognize the right from the left in a picture rotated to 180° on the painful side [95]. There is a link between the duration of symptoms and the recognition time. Recognition also seems to be worse on the painful side. On potential explanation is that a wide mental rotation requires the integration and implication of all the superior limb's joints, which are potentially painful. Moreover, the response is less accurate for a recognition in the painful side. We also find a decrease in speed and accuracy after an immobilization or in amputee patients [130–132].

We can draw a parallel between this slowdown in left/right discrimination in patients with chronic pain, and a chronometry study in hemiplegic patients [127]. It shows a slowdown in the realization of imagined movements with the plegic limb, while the same imagined movements are realized in a normal time with the healthy side—compared to a real movement in the healthy side [133]. This MI slowdown can also be found after an underutilization of a limb, which is like an immobilization [131].

To work on the left/right discrimination, we must create a picture database. They can be simple or have context. There must be many images to have a varied and random choice in each session and avoid the patient getting used to the pictures and bored. During a session, we will show around 30 randomly selected pictures of left and right hands in various positions and orientations (Fig. 9.1). The patients who do not own a computer can have the pictures on paper.

Smartphone applications are also suggested by Noigroup [134]. Several body parts are available. This option has a great advantage: we can follow the patient's evolution as his success rate and his response times for each side are indicated. In the hand, the norm is 80% of correct answers in 2 ± 0.5 s [118]. We can start with pictures of a non-painful area, pictures of simple actions, then pictures with a context involving a cognitive aspect.

9.8.1.2 Explicit Motor Imagery: Imagined Actions

Explicit MI is the mental representation of a motor sequence at the level of the working memory with no associated body movement. It is the result of the conscious access to the content of the movement intention, which is usually unconsciously realized during the preparatory phase of the movement. Conscious MI and unconscious motor preparation-programming share mechanisms and are functionally equivalent [120, 126, 127, 135, 136].

Athletes and musicians know very well the mental practice based on repeating imagined action sequences [137]. There is a link between the increase of the cortex activity during MI and the performance improvement. Mental practice creates functional brain modifications like those observed after physically practicing the same movement [120, 128]. For example, when working on a piano score using imagined "strumming," the expansion in the primary motor cortex is the same as in the real exercise [34, 37, 137]. Simply listening activates a pianist's M1 cortical area, this area is usually active during the phase right before actually pressing the finger on the piano key. The cortical activation degree achieved with MO or MI is more important and precise in an expert than in a beginner [138].

The mental practice of MI improves performances as it helps prepare and plan the movement more than realize the movement itself [131, 128].

A study [139] shows a 35% increase of the abductor digiti minimi strength in a group using only imagined abduction of the fifth finger, compared to a control group with no exercise. A group realizing actual isometric abduction against resistance get a 53% strength increase. Another group realizing imagined elbow flexion only gets a 13.5% increase. These variations between MI movements can be explained by the fact that elbow flexor muscles are already

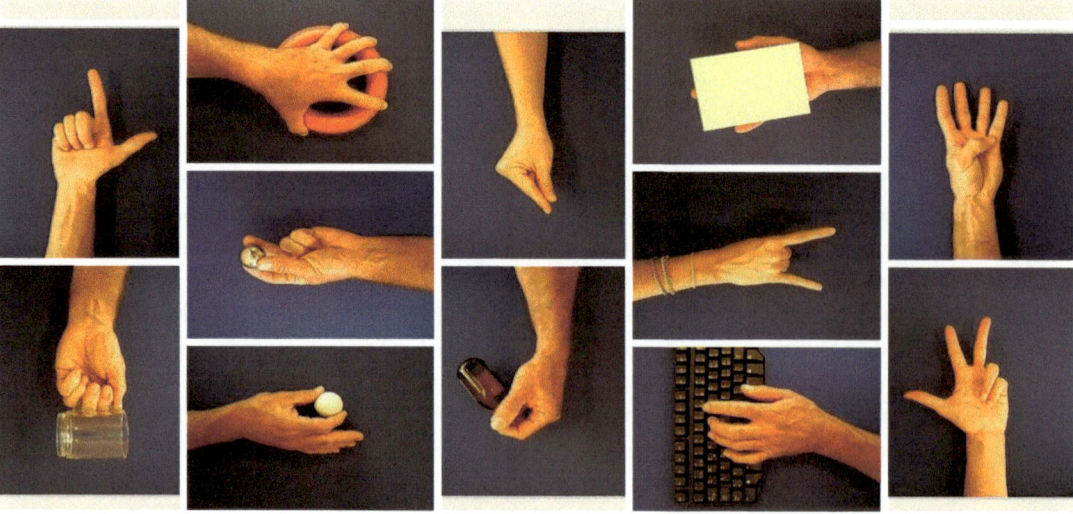

Fig. 9.1 Implied motor imagery: left/right discrimination

"trained" while the abductor digiti minimi is not as it is little used in daily life. The increase in strength is the result of the development of activity in the cortical circuits improving the motor unit's recruitment and increasing their activation frequency. This does not come with muscle hypertrophy.

MI also activates the neurovegetative system [126, 127]. If we imagine swimming a 100 m butterfly, the autonomous system increases the heart and respiratory rates in proportion to the imagined effort, even though the oxygen needs do not change. It is surprising to observe that this ventilation increase can sometimes exceed the metabolic demand required for the real activity [127].

The activated brain areas are different depending on the fact that the observed action has a signification in our internal movement representations repertoire or not. Different brain areas are also solicited depending on the strategy adopted during the observation: recognize the action or imitate it later [51]. In MI, we use pictures with a context that means something to the patient, for example, grabbing objects that he uses in his daily life in a realistic context [46]. In this case, mirror and canonic mirrors are more active. It is easier to imagine an action if it is in our internal representation repertoire, stored during past experiences [140]. Learning a new movement is almost impossible if we only use imagined movements and never realize the action [141].

An inhibition mechanism occurs during an imagined action and in the preparation phase of a real movement to prevent the concerned limb segment from moving.

To realize imagined movements, the patient can choose between two different perspectives [45, 126, 129, 131, 135]:

- **Internal perspective** (Fig. 9.2): "first-person" perspective. It is a kinesthetic imagery where the subject feels and sees himself realizing the action. He imagines, sees, and feels the somesthetic sensations related to this action. This internal perspective is visual and kinesthetic. It shares physiological characteristics with the movement execution and is therefore closer to the real movement [131]. It is more related to

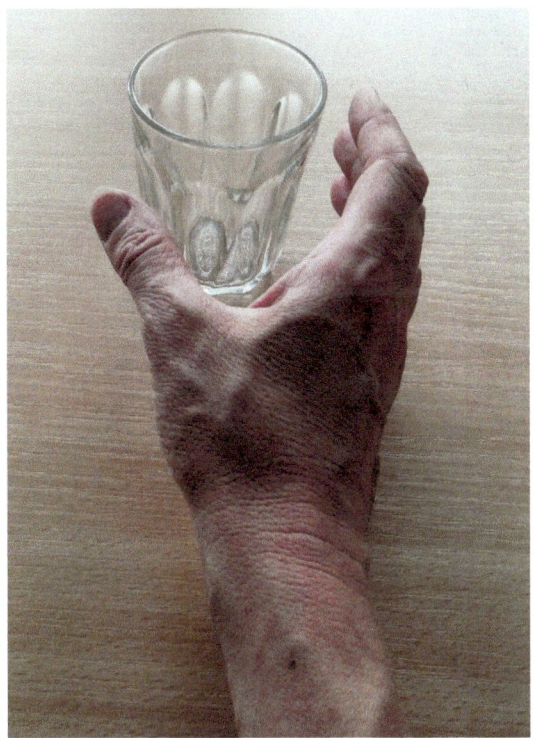

Fig. 9.2 Internal perspective

the sensorimotor system [45]. The corticospinal excitability increases with the kinesthetic imagery (more than with the visual imagery) [142]. The sensorial consequences occurring during a real action are internally stimulated without any sensorial stimulation.

- **External perspective** (Fig. 9.3): "third-person" perspective. It is a visual imagery where the subject watches the action realized by someone else. It seems to increase the cortical excitability by requesting the mirror neurons, as the imagined action is clearly identified as being realized by a third party [143]. This external perspective needs visuospatial transposition and transformation processes, including the occipitotemporal visual areas [45].

The two perspectives have their own characteristics and activate different brain areas, but they are closely linked and coexist within a same person. The separation between them is a little artificial and we can benefit from them both.

Fig. 9.3 External perspective

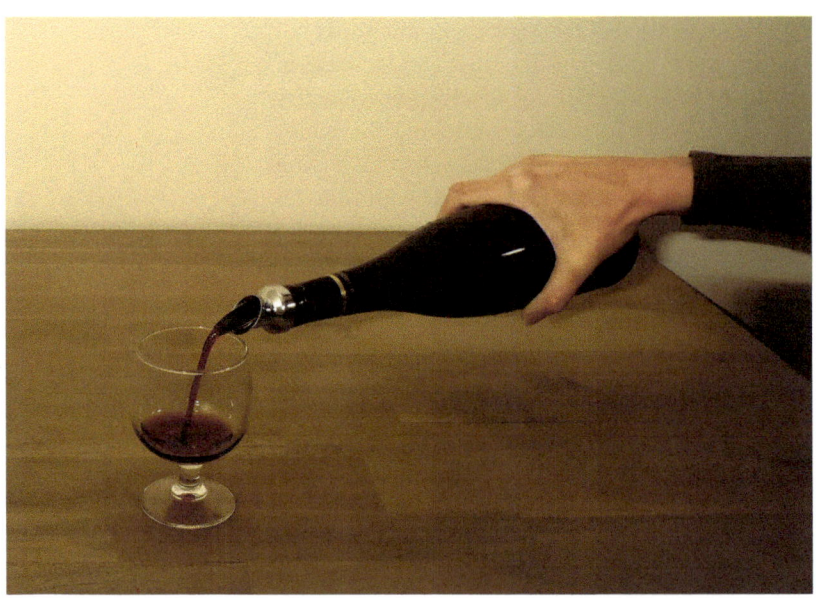

However, we should give the preference to the kinesthetic imagery that is closer to the real movement execution [128].

A good aptitude for kinesthetic imagery combined with high activity in the inferior parietal lobe seems to be a guarantee of performance. On the contrary, a capacity for visual imagery activating the occipital lobe is less promising in terms of MI performance [144].

The capacity for imagery depends on the individual [145]. Patients can have a preferred perspective. It is usually easier to put oneself in an external perspective. Age also seems to play a role, as the elderly are better able to use the external perspective. There are "good imagers" whose cortical recruitment is targeted and focused in specific brain areas, and "bad imagers" who activate many more brain areas and compensate by recruiting the cortico-cerebellar system [145]. This different focus is also noticed in musicians, depending on whether he is a professional or an amateur [137].

There are several ways of evaluating the capacity or motor imagery:

- **Timing the realization**: We must find an iso-chrony between the imagined action and the realization of the action. The closer the times, the better the imager and the more he will adhere to treatment [129]. The duration of MI depends on the length and complexity of the tasks. For the hand, we can time several sequences of object grabbing with the healthy hand. We can also do more automatic activities such as walking and use the Ten Meters test or the Timed Up & Go (TUG) test [146]. The Time Dependent Motor Imagery (TDMI) questionnaire measures the number of movements realized in three different timings (15, 25, and 45 s) [131].

- **Cardio-pulmonary frequency** after the activation of the neurovegetative system, by asking the patient to imagine an action require and important effort.

- **Validated questionnaires** exist to assess the capacity of visual or kinesthetic imagery: The Movement Imagery Questionnaire-Revised (MIQR) [147] and its version adapted to the superior limb (MIQ-RS) [148], the Kinesthetic and Visual Imagery Questionnaire (KVIQ) adapted for the physically impaired [149], and the Vividness of Motor Imagery Questionnaire (VMIQ) [150]. Their goal is to assess the patient's capacity for MI and to guide him towards the perspective best suited for him.

- **Left/right discrimination** requires a mental rotation involving an internal motor simulation. It allows evaluating the degree of cortical reorganization and the capacity for MI [131].

- **Functional MRI and sympathetic cutaneous response** are mostly used in research.

In hand rehabilitation, we try not to exclude any patient as the patients considered as neurologically "healthy" just have better capacities for MI that can still get better with practice [129]. The questionnaires are especially useful to treat patients with brain lesions or pathologies in which we cannot use MI, like injuries of the parietal [151] or premotor cortex.

Before training to imagine actions with the injured hand, we ask the patient to imagine movements with his healthy hand, or even with a completely different body part, to assess his ability to imagine a movement with a non-painful limb which sensorimotor afferences are not disturbed. As we have seen before, pain and negligence make it harder to imagine an action.

During a session working on imagined actions, the patient is in a calm place, conducive to concentration. His hand is placed in a comfortable and pain-free resting position.

Without any muscle contraction or movement, the patient imagines making a movement that can be easily replicable and is in his internal repertoire of activities.

To make this exercise easier, we can use various visual supports closest to the patient's daily life. They can be the pictures of actions in a context used before for the left/right discrimination, but it would probably be less efficient as it takes great effort to imagine a movement from a static image. Moreover, the effects of MO and MI are potentialized if the image or film is in line with the imagined action [152].

They can also be tools and graspable objects the patient will imagine taking or using [56] to use the canonical neurons as seen earlier.

Using films decreases the effort of imagination required from the patient. We use simple films sequences, or even personalized filmed sequences of actions realized by the patient's healthy hand. Then, they are turned digitally to create the illusion if the injured hand moving normally. These films are also used in MO, which we

can combine with MI to potentialize their effect by increasing the corticospinal excitability—compared to each technique used separately [152–154]. This is even more true in beginners relative to an expert who knows how to use his own motor program to realize the MI of an action [155].

Combining MO and MI frees the patient's attention as he does not have to create a visual image of the movement. With MI, he can concentrate on the kinesthetic aspect of the imagined action [122].

The patient can practice both kinds of imageries, knowing that visual imagery is easier than kinesthetic imagery at first. Some patients find it easier to close their eyes from time to time to visualize their hand better. Motivation and adherence to treatment are essential. We must avoid any discouragement by starting with the easiest exercises, the difficulty will then be progressively increased. The patient does not always have a computer or a smartphone, so he can also imagine activities he does in his daily life from his memory.

MI modalities are many and varied (Fig. 9.4). For example, the patient chooses to grab an ample, take a mug, cut bread, run a washcloth over his face, strum. He imagines the weight, texture, temperature, contact. The activity can also require both hands. Sound, ambiance, and smell are also elements that can complete MI.

When the injured hand is the dominant one, we use every imagined movement based on writing and graphism. Imagining writing letters, names, short phrases. Imagining drawing all kinds of simple shapes. The patient practices the external and/or internal perspective, depending on his abilities.

9.8.2 Motor Observation

In motor observation (MO), we also use mirror and canonic neurons to create a motor resonance in the patient [41–43, 51]. MI with imagined actions and MO are both motor stimulations that activate the motor system without any motor execution [122, 156]. MO

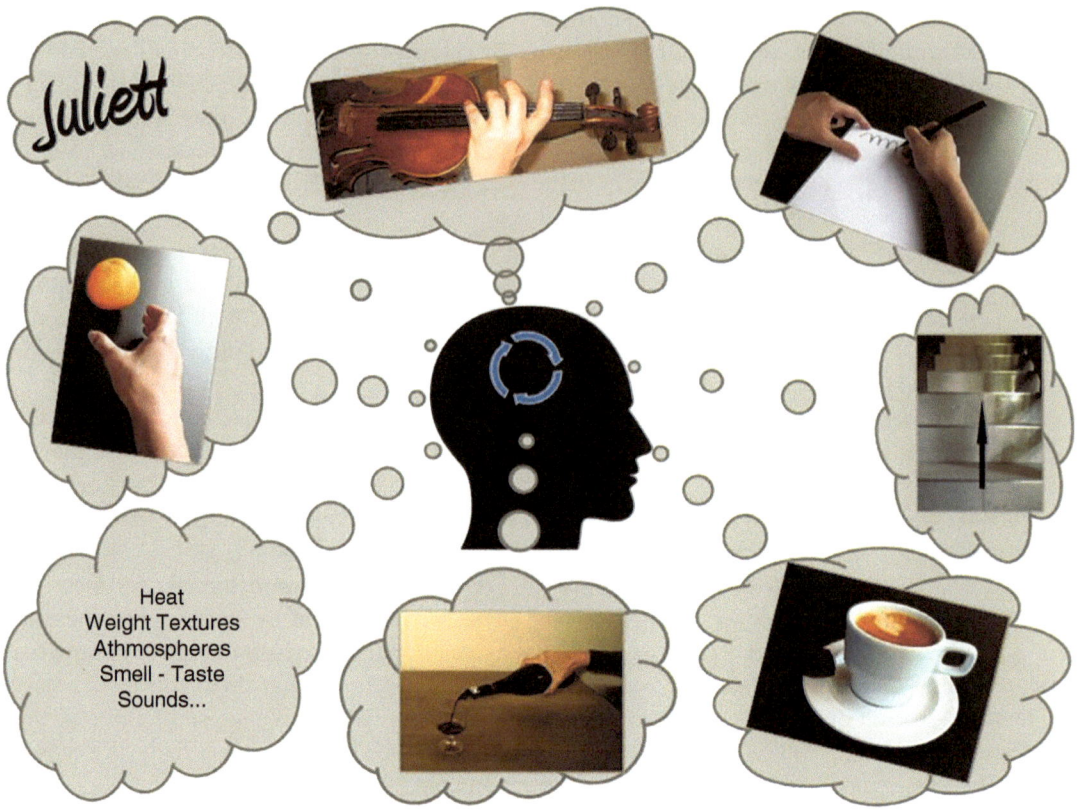

Fig. 9.4 Various modalities for motor imagery

can be done with the direct vision of an action, with mirror therapy, or with a system of derived mirrors.

9.8.2.1 Direct Vision of an Action

The patient concentrates and looks at an action realized by someone else with the same hand as the patient's injured one. He can also look at a filmed action. All these observed actions have a meaning, a goal, with familiar objects and tools.

9.8.2.2 Mirror Therapy

Ramachandran [25, 64, 157, 158] has developed mirror therapy by using MO to treat phantom pain by acting at a cortical level. Here, the mirror is used to trick the brain (Fig. 9.5).

The healthy limb's reflection gives the patient normal visual afferences of his injured limb. The mirror tricks the brain so well that the patient can feel like he is looking at his injured hand as if the mirror were transparent [59]. The mirror acts on

the motor control system by informing the brain that his missing or injured limb moves normally. This helps reconcile visual feedback with motor control. This way, we address the discrepancy between the movement feedback and the programmed movement intention that can partially generate the disorders described earlier. This technique helps to correct pathological body schemas and to get back an internal representation consistent with the movements.

This visual trick promotes the correction of cortical reorganization in a "good way" by restoring sensorial afferences. This way, the phantom pain and sensations can distinctly decline [54, 159].

In CRPS, mirror therapy decreases pain at rest, pain during activities, and even mechanic allodynia according to some authors [160, 161]. However, the allodynia assessment would require more precision. Mirror therapy compensates the absence or decrease of often inadequate proprioceptive information, reestablishing a non-painful

Fig. 9.5 Classic mirror therapy

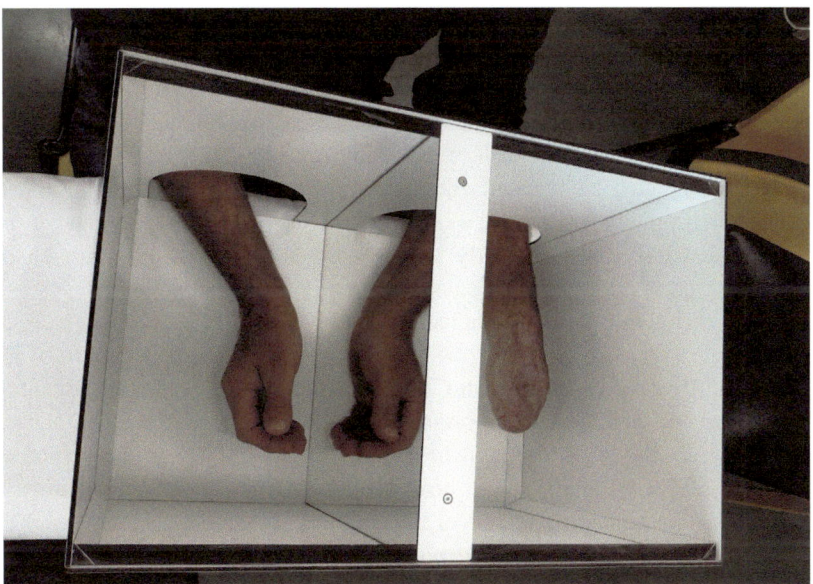

relationship between the sensorial feedback and the motor intention. The mirror helps reducing the memory of pain by showing non-painful movements [68]. This way, we can break the vicious circle partly due to kinesiophobia [70].

It is very easy to trick the brain as visual feedback dominates somatosensory feedback and proprioceptive representation. The patient feels like the hidden limb is in the position reflected by the mirror and not in its real position [55].

Botvinick's experiment [162] illustrates the predominance of visual feedback: a healthy subject attentively observes a fake rubber hand placed on a table next to his "real hand" that is hidden behind a screen. Tactile stimulations are realized with a brush on the same zones of the real and fake hands. After a few minutes, the subject feels like he perceives the stimulations of the visible brush on the fake hand and not the ones on his "real hand." Everything happens as if the rubber hand had become his own and was a part of his body schema, even if he knows he is looking at a rubber hand. Once the appropriation is done, the subject is asked to drag the index of his other hand under the table, with no visual control, at the level of the index of his "real hand." Depending on the degree of appropriation, the experiment shows that he places his index at the

level of the index of the rubber hand that is now an integral part of his body schema.

Along the same lines, a tool can also be an integral part of the body schema and become an extension of the hand. In amputee patients, a myoelectric prosthesis can be integrated in the body schema, unlike a cosmetic prosthesis that has no motor function [132]. Using a prosthesis helps keep the mental representation of the amputated limb [130].

Mirror neurons are highly solicited in mirror therapy and when visualizing an action. Some mirror neurons are activated when seeing an action, even more if the action is directed towards an object and has a goal. Other mirror neurons exist only for the touch [159]. Simply seeing the reflect of the healthy hand being touched by the therapist in the mirror causes a tactile sensation in the phantom hand like the one the patient would get if it had really been touched [64].

The mirror neuron power is such that an amputee patient feels a tactile sensation in his phantom hand only looking at the therapist's hand put in place of the phantom hand and being pinched and rubbed. The patient can localize and differentiate several types of stimulations [159].

Various mirror boxes exist. It is important to avoid any exterior visual interference. A simple mirror reflecting a neutral wall can be enough. In hand rehabilitation, we can provide a mirror box for home exercises. If we are treating an entire limb, we prefer a large vertical mirror between both limbs, without limiting the movements and with a good vision of the reflected healthy limb. The patient must be focused and installed in a calm environment during the session. The sessions must take place regularly but be short so that the patient does not lose focus. He must take out any distinctive element that can reflect in the mirror.

When treating a patient with CRPS and signs of negligence or SES, it is important to check the patient's ability to realize synchronized movements with both hands in the box, even if his mobility is incomplete because of his pathology. In fact, studies [70, 71] have shown that healthy subjects realizing asynchronous hand openings and closings create a visual discrepancy that disturbs the motor control system and causes all sorts of disorders: pain, feeling of foreign or missing limb, nausea, disorientation. Therefore, we do not start mirror therapy with active movements if the patient cannot synchronize his movements. We will stay in the previous MO phase with no movement and work on negligence by focusing attention.

The first exercise with the mirror box is the simple observation of the health hand's reflection without moving. The patient then realizes synchronous movements.

Watching one's hand move in the mirror helps to imagine the movement and to potentialize the patient's ability for MI [163]. Moreover, combining MI with real movements (DMI) reinforces the cortical activation when compared with MI alone [110, 123, 129]. Building on these observations, we combine MO with mirror and DMI when it is possible.

As seen earlier, we can add tactile stimulation on the healthy limb. Thanks to the reflection, this stimulation can produce a tactile sensation in the hidden limb in some cases [55]. However, we must not use this visuo-tactile trick in case of allodynia: when we stimulate a reflected area corresponding to a zone with allodynia or paresthesia in the injured hand, the subject feels a nor-mal sensation in the stimulated area but pain or paresthesia in the injured hand, even if it is not tactilely stimulated [164].

If sensitivity is not too affected, we can add object manipulations that will give meaning to the movements, and a tactile stimulation. This way, we create a convergence between the visual, somatosensory, and proprioceptive feedbacks.

9.8.2.3 System of Derived Mirrors

The major disadvantage of the mirror box, augmented reality 3D systems [116], and virtual reality (whose avatars can be perfected [117]), is that the patient must move his healthy hand to create an image and trick the brain. This double cortical task disturbs the focus on the injured limb and can also be tiring.

The parasitic cortical activity of the healthy hand creates potential interferences between the two hemispheres that impact the corticospinal excitability achieved through MO and MI.

If you want to easily realize the effect of removing this double parasitic task, you can use what I call a "poor man's virtual mirror" (Fig. 9.6). You chose a colleague with a hand looking like yours. In front of the mirror, your colleague will generate an image in the mirror with slow movements. You will observe the reflection as if it were your hand, considered as "injured." Your brain will be tricked as with a normal mirror box, but your healthy hand is at rest, and you do not undergo a parasitic influence from a double cortical task. This way, you can fully concentrate on the MO exercises and vary the motor intention.

To address the problem of the healthy hand's parasitic activity, we can use a computerized mirror system (Fig. 9.7). We film personalized action sequences realized by the patient's healthy hand, then we digitally turn them to make it look like it is the patient's injured hand. In MO and MI therapy, the screen showing the filmed sequences is placed in front of the injured hand to work on an internal perspective (Fig. 9.8). This "do-it-yourself" computerized mirror system requires a little ingenuity and

Fig. 9.6 Poor man's virtual mirror

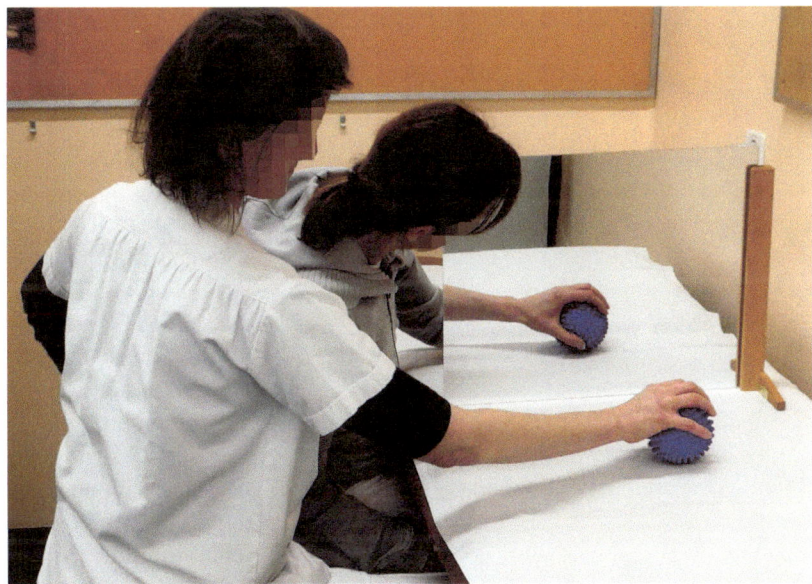

Fig. 9.7 Computerized mirror system: action sequences realized by the patient's healthy hand

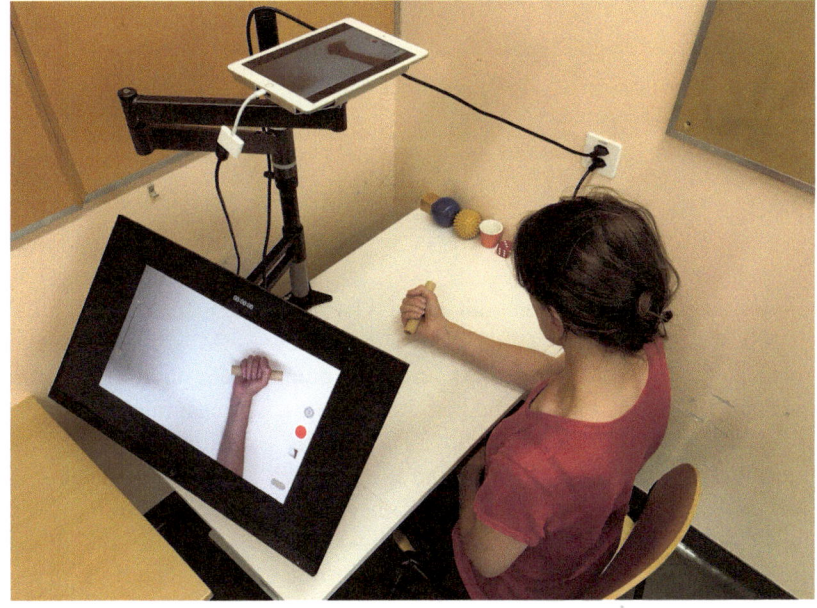

time. It takes a lot of time to create and use personalized films sequences and to have a database adapted to the patient. We add to the database with the patient's evolution.

Another great alternative is to work with the increased visual feedback system IVS3 developed by the Dessintey team [115, 125]. It is quick and convenient to set up, and it has a lot of func-

tionalities to adapt to the patient. The filmed sequences can be slowed down at first for patients with CRPS or a stroke as their chronometry is often low [112, 127, 133].

With these mirror systems, patients have reported a very strong illusion and they appear to perceive the hand movements in a smoother and freer way.

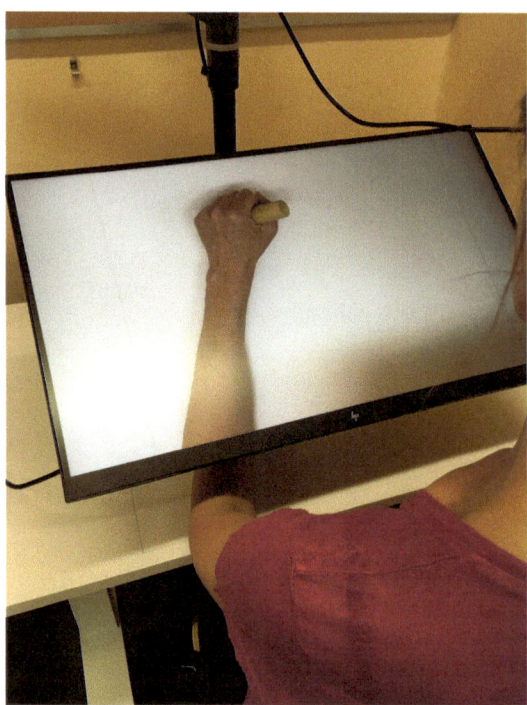

Fig. 9.8 Rehabilitation of the injured hand with a computerized sequence in internal perspective

9.8.3 Precautions and Recommendations

Motor imagery therapy must not be used lightly. If it is badly adapted, it can have a negative impact: increasing the disorders, creating pain and disorientation, making the patient lose confidence, and rejecting any therapy. Therapeutic education is essential to ensure that the patient has understood the process. Even if there is a cortical remodeling and the patient's disorders partially come from his brain, we must get the idea that he is "crazy" and it is "all in his head," out of his mind. This feeling can be very strong in CRPS whose origin is often improperly attributed to a fragile psychological state or a search for secondary benefits. The sincerity postulate is often flouted by the healthcare team.

The complexity of the subject makes it difficult to explain. For the uninitiated, these techniques can appear esoteric or be considered as charlatanism. The therapist must adapt his explanation to the patient's experience and level of understanding. He must remember that the intellectual level is not much help as the patient's cognitive representations interfere considerably on the comprehension of the condition.

An amputee patient can have trouble understanding that using the mirror, we only try to trick his brain with normal visual information. He can think that we try to trick him, thus breaking the relationship of trust. Searching for referred sensations, negligence, and phantom sensations helps the patient become aware of the "weird" things happening in his body. The patient presents talking about these strange sensations as they often come with a negative emotional feeling of rejection or even disgust [94]. The therapist carefully asks him directly about these sensations. He dedramatizes the patient's feeling by showing that these phenomena are well-known and are an integral part of the pathology. Too often, the search for these sensations lacks in the assessment of a CRPS.

MI is not recommended in psychiatric pathologies such as schizophrenia. It is also advised against in people with autism as there would be a dysfunction of the mirror neurons [44].

If the pain and/or disorders increase with MI, the treatment must be adjusted. The patient must be told to do shorter sessions, chose easier images, go back to a previous phase, or go back to observing the mirror with no movement. If the disorders continue, the program must be stopped until he sees the therapist again.

During the sessions, the therapist ensures that the patient does not resist or think about letting his brain getting tricked: the patient should not "intellectualize" or try to "dissect" the mechanism, or it might be less efficient. If the patient feels pain, the therapist controls the movements' synchronization and the patient's good understanding of the instructions. If pain persists even with all the adjustments and verifications, the therapy must be stopped.

We continue the therapy as long as it benefits the patient. If after a fortnight there are no more effects, even if the patient cooperates, the program can be stopped. In amputee patients with algo-hallucinoses or in patients with injuries of the brachial plexus, the patient stops the therapy when he is relieved from pain. He can start again if signs intermittently reemerge, which frequently occurs due to factors such as stress, fatigue, or drinking alcohol. These episodes will become less and less frequent, until they disappear.

We can make a difference between the treatment of an acute CRPS and a chronic CRPS. A study shows that mirror therapy in patients with CRPS for less than 8 weeks decreases pain but has no effect on chronic CRPS [91]. In a CRPS with early diagnosis, if the patient scores well in left/right discrimination, the first phase of GMI can be reduced or even removed to go directly to the following phases. Good results in left/right discrimination can mean that the cortical remodeling is not too settled [165].

It should be noted that these techniques are fairly new, and the protocols are constantly evolving. Based on the experiments described in literature and on our own observations, we must improve our practice. For this purpose, more studies are needed in this field.

The patient's confidence and adherence as well as the treatment success depend on his understanding of the explanations and his visualization and adaptation. The risk of this therapy is to implement an inadequate and counterproductive "push-button" program.

9.8.4   Motor Imagery Therapy in Practice

The patient follows a motor imagery program at home, outside the therapy sessions, which requires him to be available and motivated. Regular and frequent sessions guarantee the treatment efficiency. In practice, we often observe that five 10-min sessions a day appear to be a good compromise. During the first session, we give the patient a "motor imagery set" with an explanation sheet, a mirror box, and a flash-drive with images that can be loaded on a smartphone for the left/right discrimination. The patient can also install the Noir Group app [134]. The smartphone allows more daily sessions and a higher level of adherence from the patient. The sessions must not last longer than 10 min for the patient to stay focused and avoid fatigue. In MO and MI, the patient can use the same images or films as seen earlier. He has a tracking sheet on which he writes the time, frequency, and observations he can have regarding his sensations during the exercises: this allows us to follow and adjust the treatment.

We use the following modalities in motor imagery therapy:

- Implicit MI with left/right discrimination that can first be practiced with another body part if it is too difficult with the hand.
- Simple MO of an action realized by someone else or of a basic filmed sequence.
- MO through a mirror box.
- MO with a system of derived mirrors and personalized filmed sequences, varying the speed of the film if needed.
- MI using all the visualized modalities, perspectives, contexts, objects, and tools.
- Varying the level of motor intention until dynamic MI.
- Combining MO and MI.

The therapist must gradually adapt to the patient's reactions, abilities, advances, and context. He must be creative and not hesitate to go

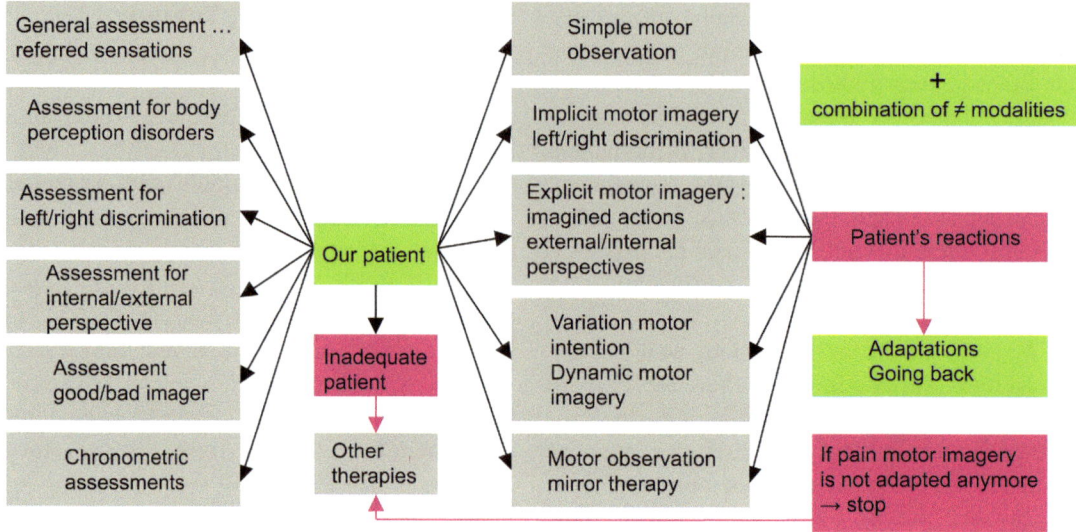

Fig. 9.9 Decision tree

back if needed. A decision tree (Fig. 9.9) helps to choose the technique adapted to the patient and his evolution.

9.9   Other Indications

The motor imagery program can find its place in the treatment of several pathologies inducing a cortical reorganization: strokes, spinal cord injuries, tendon transfers, peripheral nerve injuries, functional dystonia. And, as recommended by Rosèn and Lundborg [166], all the hand conditions.

9.10   Conclusion

Neuroscience has considerably advanced our knowledge of the brain and brain plasticity mechanisms, especially in specific pathologies. The discovery of a previously unsuspected cortical reorganization has allowed to develop new rehabilitation techniques. Motor imagery techniques help normalize the pathological cortical reorganization. In hand rehabilitation, we have selected four indications, but many other indications are developing in other pathologies. As these techniques are fairly new and rapidly developing, we

must pay attention to their evolution and use. The advances in neuroscience will improve our knowledge and confirm or reorient the hypotheses regarding brain plasticity mechanisms and brain function. They are full-fledged techniques that require an extensive and precise knowledge of the cortical mechanisms, despite their apparent simplicity. They do not replace other traditional techniques but advantageously complete them [112].

References

1. Kempermann G, Gage F. La multiplication des neurones chez l'adulte. Pour Sci. 1999;261:30–5.
2. Grangeon M, Guillot A, Collet C. Effets de l'imagerie motrice dans la rééducation de lésions du système nerveux central et des atteintes musculo-articulaires. Sci Mot. 2009;67(2):9–38.
3. Arsenijevic Y. Cerveau et régénérescence. Arch Neurol Psychiatr. 2003;154:86–90.
4. Chen R, Cohen LG, Hallett M. Nervous system reorganization following injury. Neuroscience. 2002;111(4):761–73.
5. Lundborg G, Richard P. Bunge memorial lecture. Nerve injury and repair: a challenge to the plastic brain. J Peripher Nerv Syst. 2003;8(4):209–26.
6. Lundborg G, Rosèn B. Hand function after nerve repair. Acta Physiol. 2007;189(2):207–17.
7. Sanes JN, Donoghue JP. Plasticity and primary motor cortex. Annu Rev Neurosci. 2000;23:393–415.
8. Schaefer M, Flor H, Heinze HJ, Rotte M. Dynamic shifts in the organization of primary somatosensory

cortex induced by bimanual spatial coupling of motor activity. NeuroImage. 2005;25(2):395–400.

9. Spedding M, Lestage P. Plasticité cérébrale et neuropathologies: nouvelles voies pour le médicament. Med Sci (Paris). 2005;21(1):104–9.

10. Xerri C. Plasticité post-lésionnelle des cartes corticales somatosensorielles: une revue. CR Acad Sci Ser III. 1998;321(2–3):135–51.

11. Xerri C. Plasticité des représentations somesthésiques et illusions perceptives: le paradoxe du membre fantôme. Intellectica. 2003;36–37:67–87.

12. Ramachandran VS. Plasticity and functional recovery in neurology. Clin Med. 2005;5(4):368–73.

13. Schaefer M, Flor H, Heinze HJ, Rotte M. Dynamic modulation of the primary somatosensory cortex during seeing and feeling a touched hand. NeuroImage. 2006;29(2):587–92.

14. Buchner H, Richrath P, Grünholz J, Noppeney U, Waberski T, Gobbelé R, et al. Differential effects of pain and spatial attention on digit representation in the human primary somatosensory cortex. Neuroreport. 2000;11(6):1289–93.

15. Noppeney U, Waberski TD, Gobbelé R, Buchner H. Spatial attention modulates the cortical somatosensory representation of the digits in humans. Neuroreport. 1999;10(15):3137–41.

16. Giraux P, Sirigu A, Schneider F, Dubernard JM. Cortical reorganization in motor cortex after graft of both hands. Nat Neurosci. 2001;4(7):691–2.

17. Mercier C, Reilly KT, Vargas CD, Aballea A, Sirigu A. Mapping phantom movement representations in the motor cortex of amputees. Brain. 2006;129:2202–10.

18. Reilly KT, Mercier C, Schieber MH, Sirigu A. Persistent hand motor commands in the amputees' brain. Brain. 2006;129:2211–23.

19. Reilly KT, Sirigu A. Motor cortex representation of the upper-limb in individuals born without a hand. PLoS One. 2011;6(4):e18100. https://doi.org/10.1371/journal.pone.0018100.

20. Vargas CD, Aballéa A, Rodrigues EC, Reilly KT, Mercier C, Petruzzo P, et al. Re-emergence of hand-muscle representations in human motor cortex after hand allograft. Proc Natl Acad Sci U S A. 2009;106(17):7197–202.

21. Farnè A, Roy AC, Giraux P, Dubernard JM, Sirigu A. Face or hand, not both: perceptual correlates of reafferentation in a former amputee. Curr Biol. 2002;12(15):1342–6.

22. Flor H, Elbert T, Knecht S, Wienbruch C, Pantev C, Birbaumer N, et al. Phantom-limb pain as a perceptual correlate of cortical reorganization following arm amputation. Nature. 1995;375(6531):482–4.

23. Grüsser SM, Mühlnickel W, Schaefer M, Villringer K, Christmann C, Koeppe C, et al. Remote activation of referred phantom sensation and cortical reorganization in human upper extremity amputees. Exp Brain Res. 2004;154(1):97–102.

24. Lotze M, Flor H, Grodd W, Larbig W, Birbaumer N. Phantom movements and pain: an fMRI study in upper limb amputees. Brain. 2001;124(Pt 11):2268–77.

25. Ramachandran VS, Hirstein W. The perception of phantom limbs. The D.O. Hebb lecture. Brain. 1998;121(Pt 9):1603–30.

26. Flor H. Phantom-limb pain: characteristics, causes, and treatment. Lancet Neurol. 2002;1(3):182–9.

27. Lewis JS, Coales K, Hall J, McCabe CS. 'Now you see it, now you do not': sensory-motor re-education in complex regional pain syndrome. Hand Ther. 2011;16(2):29–38.

28. Pleger B, Tegenthoff M, Ragert P, Forster AF, Dinse HR, Schwenkreis P, et al. Sensorimotor retuning [corrected] in complex regional pain syndrome parallels pain reduction. Ann Neurol. 2005;57(3):425–9.

29. Pleger B, Ragert P, Schwenkreis P, Förster AF, Wilimzig C, Dinse H, et al. Patterns of cortical reorganization parallel impaired tactile discrimination and pain intensity in complex regional pain syndrome. NeuroImage. 2006;32(2):503–10.

30. Moutet F, Corcella D, Forli A, Martin des Pallières T, Delon-Martin C, Martin O, et al. Réorganisation anatomo-fonctionnelle après transfert tendineux pour réanimation de la main. In: Etude IRM et biomécanique. Poster au congrès de la société française de chirurgie de la main (GEM), Paris; 2009.

31. Blake DT, Byl NN, Merzenich MM. Representation of the hand in the cerebral cortex. Behav Brain Res. 2002;135(1–2):179–84.

32. Mogilner A, Grosmann JA, Ribary U, Joliot M, Volkmann J, Rapaport D, et al. Somatosensory cortical plasticity in adult humans revealed by magnetoencephalography. Proc Natl Acad Sci U S A. 1993;90(8):3593–7.

33. Pascual-Leone A, Amedi A, Fregni F, Merabet LB. The plastic human brain cortex. Annu Rev Neurosci. 2005;28:377–401.

34. Elbert T, Pantev C, Wienbruch C, Rockstroh B, Taub E. Increased cortical representation of the fingers of the left hand in string players. Science. 1995;270(5234):305–7.

35. Watson AHD. What can studying musicians tell us about motor control of the hand? J Anat. 2006;208(4):527–42.

36. Pascual-Leone A, Nguyet D, Cohen LG, Brasil-Neto JP, Cammarota A, Hallett M. Modulation of muscle responses evoked by transcranial magnetic stimulation during the acquisition of new fine motor skills. J Neurophysiol. 1995;74(3):1037–45.

37. Levame JH. Main-image et éducation de la main. Rev Chir Orthop Reparatrice Appar Mot. 1976;62(7):745–8.

38. Lotze M, Erb M, Flor H, Huelsmann E, Godde B, Grodd W. fMRI evaluation of somatotopic representation in human primary motor cortex. NeuroImage. 2000;11(5 Pt):473–81.

39. Rowe J, Friston K, Frackowiak R, Passingham R. Attention to action: specific modulation of corticocortical interactions in humans. NeuroImage. 2002;17(2):988–98.

40. Björkman A, Weibull A, Rosèn B, Svensson J, Lundborg G. Rapid cortical reorganisation and improved sensitivity of the hand following cutaneous anaesthesia of the forearm. Eur J Neurosci. 2009;29(4):837–44.

41. Rizzolatti G, Craighero L. The mirror-neuron system. Annu Rev Neurosci. 2004;27:169–92.

42. Rizzolatti G, Sinigaglia C. Les neurones miroirs. Paris: Odile Jacob Sciences; 2008. 236 p.

43. Gallese V, Fadiga L, Fogassi L, Rizzolatti G. Action recognition in the premotor cortex. Brain. 1996;119(Pt 2):593–609.

44. Ramchandran VS. Le cerveau fait de l'esprit. Enquête sur les neurones miroirs. Paris: Dunot quai des sciences; 2011. 396 p.

45. Jackson P, Meltzoff AN, Decety J. Neural circuits involved in imitation and perspective-taking. NeuroImage. 2006;31(1):429–39.

46. Amoruso L, Urgesi C. Contextual modulation of motor resonance during the observation of everyday actions. NeuroImage. 2016;134:74–84.

47. Kohler E, Keysers C, Umiltà MA, Fogassi L, Gallese V, Rizzolatti G. Hearing sounds, understanding actions: action representation in mirror neurons. Science. 2002;297:846–8.

48. Keysers C, Wickers B, Gazzola V, Anton J-L, Fogassi L, Gallese V. A touching sight: SII/PV activation during the observation and experience of touch. Neuron. 2004;42:1–20.

49. Avikainen S, Forss N, Hari R. Modulated activation of the human SI and SII cortices during observation of hand actions. NeuroImage. 2002;15(3):640–6.

50. Blakemore SJ, Decety J. From the perception of action to the understanding of intention. Nat Rev Neurosci. 2001;8:561–7.

51. Decety J, Grezes J, Costes N, et al. Brain activity during observation of actions. Influences of action content and subject's strategy. Brain. 1997;120:1763–77.

52. Decety J. L'empathie ou l'émotion partagée. Pour Sci. 2003;309:46–51.

53. Funase K, Tabira T, Higashi T, Liang N, Kasai T. Increased corticospinal excitability during direct observation of self-movement and indirect observation with a mirror box. Neurosci Lett. 2007;419(2):108–12.

54. Chan BL, Wittt R, Charrow AP, Magee A, Howard R, Pasquina PF, et al. Mirror therapy for phantom limb pain. N Engl J Med. 2007;357(21):2206–7.

55. Moseley GL, Gallace A, Spence C. Is mirror therapy all it is cracked up to be? Current evidence and future directions. Pain. 2008;138(1):7–10.

56. Chao LL, Martin A. Representation of manipulable man-made objects in the dorsal stream. NeuroImage. 2000;12:478–84.

57. Petit LS, Pegna AJ, Harris IM, Michel CM. Automatic motor cortex activation for natural as compared to awkward grips of a manipulable object. Exp Brain Res. 2006;168:120–30.

58. André JM, Paysant J, Martinet N, Beis JM. Classification et mécanismes des perceptions et illusions corporelles des amputés. Ann Readaptat Med Phys. 2001;44:13–8.

59. Katz J, Melzack R. Phantom limb pain. In: Grafman J, Robertson ICH, editors. Handbook of neuropsychology, vol. 9, Chap. 10, 2nd ed. Amsterdam: Elsevier; 2003. p. 205–230.

60. Melzack R. Phantom limbs and the concept of a neuromatrix. Trends Neurosci. 1990;13(3):88–92.

61. Melzack R. Les membres fantômes. Pour Sci. 1992;176:48–55.

62. Piccut S. L'imagerie motrice et l'observation motrice influencent-elle la douleur fantôme chez les amputés du membre inférieur? Mémoire de master en kinésithérapie. Charleroi: Haute Ecole Provinciale de Hainaut Condorcet; 2010. 163 p.

63. Katz J, Melzack R. Referred sensations in chronic pain patients. Pain. 1987;28(1):51–9.

64. Ramachandran VS. Sensation referred to a patient's phantom arm from another subjects intact arm: perceptual correlates of mirror neurons. Med Hypotheses. 2008;70(6):1233–4.

65. Fink GR, Marshall JC, Halligan PW, Frith CD, Driver J, Frackowiak RSJ, et al. The neural consequences of conflict between intention and the senses. Brain. 1999;122(Pt 3):497–512.

66. Frith CD, Blakemore SJ, Wolpert DM. Abnormalities in the awareness and control of action. Philos Trans R Soc Lond Ser B Biol Sci. 2000;355(1404):1771–88.

67. Harris AJ. Cortical origin of pathological pain. Lancet. 1999;354:1464–6.

68. McCabe C, Lewis J, Shenker N, Hall J, Cohen H, Blake D. Don't look now! Pain and attention. Clin Med. 2005;5(5):482–6.

69. McCabe CS, Haigh RC, Halligan PW, Blake DR. Simulating sensory-motor incongruence in healthy volunteers: implications for a cortical model of pain. Rheumatology. 2005;44(4):509–16.

70. McCabe C. Mirror visual feedback therapy. A practical approach. J Hand Ther. 2011;24(2):170–8.

71. Roullet S, Nouette-Gaulain K, Brochet B, Sztark F. Douleur du membre fantôme: de la physiopathologie à la prévention. Ann Fr Anesth Réanim. 2009;28(5):460–72.

72. Flor H, Nikolajsen L, Jensen TS. Phantom limb pain: a case of maladaptive CNS plasticity? Nat Rev Neurosci. 2006;7(11):873–81.

73. MacIver K, Lloyd DM, Kelly S, Roberts N, Nurmikko T. Phantom limb pain, cortical reorganization and the therapeutic effect of mental imagery. Brain. 2008;131(Pt 8):2181–91.

74. Harden RN, Bruehl S, Galer BS, et al. Complex regional pain syndrome: are the IASP diagnostic criteria valid and sufficiently comprehensive? Pain. 1999;83:211–9.

75. Harden RN, Bruehl S, Stanton-Hicks M, Wilson PR. Proposed new diagnostic criteria for complex regional pain syndrome. Pain Med. 2007;8:326–31.

76. Harden RN, Oaklander AL, Burton AW, et al. Complex regional pain syndrome: practical diagnostic and treatment guidelines, 4th edition. Pain Med. 2013;14:180–229.

77. Spicher C. Manuel de rééducation sensitive du corps humain. Genève, Paris: Médecine & Hygiène; 2003.

78. Spicher CJ. Handbook for somatosensory rehabilitation. Montpellier, Paris: Sauramps Médical; 2006. 204 p.

79. Quintal I, Noël L, Gable C, Delaquaize F, Bret-Pasian S, Rossier P, Annoni JM, MaupasnE SCJ. La méthode de rééducation sensitive de la douleur. In: Encyclopédie Médico-Chirurgicale (EMC), Kinésithérapie-Médecine physique-Réadaptation, vol. 26-469-A-10. Paris: Masson; 2013. p. 1–14.

80. Flor H. Cortical reorganization and chronic pain: implications for rehabilitation. J Rehabil Med. 2003;41(Sup):66–72.

81. Maihöfner C, Handwerker HO, Neundörfer B, Birklein F. Patterns of cortical reorganization in complex regional pain syndrome. Neurology. 2003;61(12):1707–15.

82. Juottonen K, Gockel M, Silen T, Hurri H, Hari R, Forss N. Altered central sensorimotor processing in patients with complex regional pain syndrome. Pain. 2002;98(3):315–23.

83. Maihöfner C, Handwerker HO, Neundörfer B, Birklein F. Cortical reorganization during recovery from complex regional pain syndrome. Neurology. 2004;63(4):693–701.

84. Geha PY, Baliki MN, Harden RN, et al. The brain in chronic CRPS pain: abnormal gray-white matter interactions in emotional and autonomic regions. Neuron. 2008;60(4):570–81.

85. Maihöfner C, Handwerker HO, Birklein F. Functional imaging of allodynia in complex regional pain syndrome. Neurology. 2006;66(5):711–7.

86. Giraux P, Sirigu A. Illusory movements of the paralyzed limb restore motor cortex activity. NeuroImage. 2003;20(Suppl 1):S107–11.

87. Förderreuther S, Sailer U, Straube A. Impaired self-perception of the hand in complex regional pain syndrome. Pain. 2004;110(3):756–61.

88. Galer BS, Butler S, Jensen MP. Case reports and hypothesis: a neglect-like syndrome may be responsible for the motor disturbance in reflex sympathetic dystrophy. J Pain Symptom Manag. 1995;10(5):385–91.

89. Galer BS, Jensen M. Neglect-like symptoms in complex regional pain syndrome: results of a self-administered survey. J Pain Symptom Manag. 1999;18(3):213–7.

90. Lewis JS, Kersten P, McCabe CS, McPherson KM, Blake DR. Body perception disturbance: a contribution to pain in complex regional pain syndrome (CRPS). Pain. 2007;133(1–3):111–9.

91. McCabe CS, Haigh RC, Ring EF, Halligan PW, Wall PD, Blake DR. A controlled pilot study of the utility of mirror visual feedback in the treatment of complex regional pain syndrome (type 1). Rheumatology. 2003;42(1):97–101.

92. Rossetti Y, Jacquin-Courtois S, Legrain V, et al. Le syndrome douloureux régional complexe à la lumière des troubles de la cognition spatiale: des opportunités physiopathologiques et thérapeutiques? In: Syndromes douloureux chroniques en médecine physique et de réadaptation. Paris: Springer; 2013.

93. Filbrich L, Alamia A, Verfaille C, et al. Biased visuospatial perception in complex regional pain syndrome. Sci Rep. 2017;7(9712):1–12.

94. Lewis JS, McCabe CS. Correcting the body in mind: body perception disturbance in complex regional pain syndrome and rehabilitation approaches. Pract Pain Manag. 2010;10:60–6.

95. Schwoebel J, Friedman R, Duda N, Coslett HB. Pain and the body schema: evidence for peripheral effects on mental representations of movement. Brain. 2001;124(Pt 10):2098–104.

96. Maihöfner C, Neundörfer B, Birklein F, Handwerker HO. Mislocalization of tactile stimulation in patients with complex regional pain syndrome. J Neurol. 2006;253(6):772–9.

97. McCabe CS, Haigh RC, Halligan PW, Blake DR. Referred sensations in patients with complex regional pain syndrome type 1. Rheumatology. 2003;42(9):1067–73.

98. Moseley GL. Graded motor imagery is effective for long-standing complex regional pain syndrome: a randomised controlled trial. Pain. 2004;108(1–2):192–8.

99. Gay A, Parrate S, Salazard B, et al. Apport de la rééducation proprioceptive vibratoire dans la prise en charge du syndrome douloureux régional complexe de type I. Rev Rhum. 2007;74:861–7.

100. Roll JP. Rééducation proprioceptive par vibration tendineuse. Profession Kinésithérapeute. 2009;23:11–6.

101. André JM, Vielh-Ben Meridja A, Beis JM, Gable C, Martinet N. Le syndrome d'exclusion segmentaire de la main et des doigts. Comportement de négligence d'origine périphérique? Ann Readapt Med Phys. 1996;39:433–42.

102. Fraser A. Syndrome d'exclusion segmentaire et technique contrainte. Thèse de docteur en médecine. Nancy: Université Henri Poincaré Nancy I; 2006. 187 p.

103. Moisello C, Bove M, Huber R, Abbruzzese G, Battaglia F, Tononi G, et al. Short-term limb immobilization affects motor performance. J Mot Behav. 2008;40(2):165–76.

104. Zanette G, Manganotti P, Fiaschi A, Tamburina S. Modulation of motor cortex excitability after upper limb immobilization. Clin Neurophysiol. 2004;115(6):1264–75.

105. Merzenich MM, Jenkins WM. Reorganization of cortical representations of the hand following alterations of skin inputs induced by nerve injury, skin island transfers, and experience. J Hand Ther. 1993;6(2):89–104.

106. Colteu C. Le phénomène d'exclusion du membre supérieur chez l'adulte: description et approches thérapeutiques conventionnelles et par miroir. Thèse docteur en médecine. Nancy: Université H. Poincaré Nancy I; 2010. 184 p.

107. Liepert J, Tegenthoff M, Malin JP. Changes of cortical motor area size during immobilization. Electroencephalogr Clin Neurophysiol. 1995;97(6):382–6.

108. Lissek S, Wilimzig C, Stude P, Pleger B, Kalisch T, Maier C, et al. Immobilization impairs tactile perception and shrinks somatosensory cortical maps. Curr Biol. 2009;19(10):837–42.

109. de Jong BM, Coert JH, Stenekes MW, Leenders KL, Paans AM, Nicolai JP. Cerebral reorganisation of human movement following dynamic immobilisation. Neuroreport. 2003;14(13):1693–6.

110. Sacheli LM, Zapparoli L, Preti M, et al. A functional limitation to the lower limbs affects the neural bases of motor imagery of gait. NeuroImage Clin. 2018;20:177–87.

111. Gandola M, Bruno M, Zapparoli L, et al. Functional brain effects of hand disuse in patients with trapeziometacarpal joint osteoarthritis: executed and imagined movements. Exp Brain Res. 2017;235:3227–41.

112. Jackson PL, Lafleur MF, Malouin F, Richards CL, Doyon J. Potential role of mental practice using motor imagery in neurological rehabilitation. Arch Phys Med Rehabil. 2001;82(8):1133–41.

113. Holmes PS, Collins DJ. The PETTLEP approach to motor imagery: a functional equivalence model for sport psychologists. J Appl Sport Psychol. 2001;13(1):60–83.

114. Guillot A, Collet C. Construction of the motor imagery integrative model in sport: a review and theoretical investigation of motor imagery use. Int Rev Sport Exerc Psychol. 2008;1(1):31–44.

115. Gruest JP. Projet Optimove. La thérapie miroir réinventée. Kiné Actualité. 2017;1491:27.

116. Mouraux D, Brassinne E, Sobczak S, et al. 3D augmented reality mirror visual feedback therapy applied to the treatment of persistent, unilateral upper extremity neuropathic pain: a preliminary study. J Man Manip Ther. 2017;25(3):137–43.

117. Sato K, Fukumori S, Maruo T, et al. Nonimmersive virtual reality mirror visual feedback therapy and its application for treatment of complex regional pain syndrome: an open-label pilot study. Pain Med. 2010;11(4):622–9.

118. Moseley GL, Butler DS, Beames TB, Giles TJ. The graded motor imagery handbook. Adelaide, Australia: Noigroup Publications; 2012.

119. Moseley GL. Is successful rehabilitation of complex regional pain syndrome due to sustained attention to the affected limb? A randomised clinical trial. Pain. 2005;114(1–2):54–61.

120. Jeannerod M. Mental imagery in the motor context. Neuropsychologia. 1995;33(11):1419–32.

121. Parsons LM. Integrating cognitive psychology, neurology and neuroimaging. Acta Psychol. 2001;107:155–81.

122. Eaves DL, Riach M, Holmes PS, et al. Motor imagery during action observation: a brief review of evidence, theory and future research opportunities. Front Neurosci. 2016;10(614):1–10.

123. Guillot A, Moschberger K, Collet C. Coupling movement with imagery as a new perspective for motor imagery practice. Behav Brain Funct. 2013;9:8.

124. Malouin F, Richards CL. Clinical applications of motor imagery in rehabilitation. In: Lacey S, Lawson R, editors. Mutisensory imagery. New York: Springer; 2013. p. 397–419.

125. Giraux P. Thérapie miroir dans la main traumatique. In: 46ème entretiens de médecine physique et de réadaptation; 2018. http://empr.fr/EMPR2018/2_56_P%20Giraux/index.html.

126. Decety J. The neurophysiological basis of motor imagery. Behav Brain Res. 1996;77(1–2):45–52.

127. Decety J. Do imagined and executed actions share the same neural substrate? Brain Res Cogn Brain Res. 1996;3(2):87–93.

128. Jackson PL, Lafleur MF, Malouin F, Richards CL, Doyon J. Functional cerebral reorganization following motor sequence learning through mental practice with motor imagery. NeuroImage. 2003;20(2):1171–80.

129. Dickstein R, Deutsch J. Motor imagery in physical therapist practice. Phys Ther. 2007;87(7):942–53.

130. Malouin F, Richards CL, Durand A, Descent M, Poiré D, Frémont P, et al. Effects of practice, visual loss, limb amputation and disuse on motor imagery vividness. Neurorehabil Neural Repair. 2009;23(5):449–63.

131. Malouin F, Richards CL. Mental practice for relearning locomotor skills. Phys Ther. 2010;90(2):240–51.

132. Nico D, Daprati E, Rigal F, Parsons L, Sirigu A. Left and right hand recognition in upper limb amputees. Brain. 2004;127(Pt 1):120–32.

133. Sirigu A, Cohen L, Duhamel JR, et al. Congruent unilateral impairments for real and imagined hand movements. Neuroreport. 1995;6(7):997–1001.

134. Noigroup: accès aux applications tests de latéralité recognise™. http://www.noigroup.com/en/Product/BTRAPP.

135. Jeannerod M. The representing brain: neural correlates of motor intention and imagery. Behav Brain Sci. 1994;17:187–245.

136. Lotze M, Halsband U. Motor imagery. J Physiol Paris. 2006;99(4–6):386–95.

137. Lotze M, Scheler G, Tan HRM, Braun C, Birbaumer N. The musician's brain: functional imaging of amateurs and professionals during performance and imagery. NeuroImage. 2003;20(3):1817–29.

138. Mizuguchi N, Kanosue K. Changes in brain activity during action observation and motor imagery: their relationship with motor learning. Prog Brain Res. 2017;234(10):189–204.

139. Ranganathan VK, Siemionow V, Liu JZ, Sahgal V, Yue GH. From mental power to muscle power – gaining strength by using the mind. Neuropsychologia. 2004;42(7):944–56.

140. Courtine G, Papaxanthis C, Gentili R, Pozzo T. Gait-dependent motor memory facilitation in covert movement execution. Brain Res Cogn Brain Res. 2004;22(1):67–75.

141. Mulder T, Zijlstra S, Zijlstra W, Hochstenbach J. The role of motor imagery in learning a totally novel movement. Exp Brain Res. 2004;154(2):211–7.

142. Stinear CM, Byblow WD, Steyvers M. Kinesthesic, but not visual, motor imagery modulates corticomotor excitability. Exp Brain Res. 2006;168:157–64.

143. Fourkas A, Avenanti A, Urgesi C, Aglioti SM. Corticospinal facilitation during first and third person imagery. Exp Brain Res. 2006;168(1–2):143–51.

144. Lebon F, Horn U, Domin M, Lotze M. Motorimagery training: kinesthetic imagery strategy and inferior parietal fMRI activation. Hum Brain Mapp. 2018;00:1–9.

145. Guillot A, Collet C, Nguyen VA, Malouin F, Richards C, Doyon J. Functional neuroanatomical networks associated with expertise in motor imagery. NeuroImage. 2008;41(4):1471–83.

146. Van der Meulen M, Allali G, Rieger SW, Assal F, Vuilleumier P. The influence of individual motor imagery ability on cerebral recruitment during gait imagery. Hum Brain Mapp. 2014;35(2):455–70.

147. Lorant J, Nicolas A. Validation de la traduction française du Movement Imagery Questionnaire-Revised (MIQ-R). Sci Mot. 2004;53:57–68.

148. Gregg M, Hall C, Butler A. The MIQ-RS: a suitable option for examining movement imagery ability. Evid Based Complement Alternat Med. 2010;7(2):249–57.

149. Malouin F, Richards CL, Jackson PL, et al. The kinesthetic and visual imagery questionnaire (KVIQ) for assessing motor imagery in person with physical disabilities. J Neurol Phys Ther. 2007;31(1):20–9.

150. Isaac A, Marks DF, Russell DG. An instrument for assessing imagery of movement: the vividness of movement imagery questionnaire (VMIQ). J Ment Imagery. 1986;10(4):23–30.

151. Sirigu A, Duhamel JR, Cohen L, et al. The mental representation of hand movements after parietal cortex damage. Science. 1996;273:1564–8.

152. Sakamoto M, Muraoka T, Mizuguchi N, Kanosue K. Combining observation and imagery of an action enhances human corticospinal excitability. Neurosci Res. 2009;65:23–7.

153. Wright DJ, Williams J, Holmes P. Combined action observation and imagery facilitates corticospinal excitability. Front Hum Neurosci. 2014;8:951.

154. Romano-Smith S, Wood G, Wright DJ, Wakefield CJ. Simultaneous and alternate action observation and motor imagery combinations improve aiming performance. Psychol Sport Exerc. 2018;38:100–6.

155. Tsukazaki I, Uehara K, Morishita T, et al. Effect of observation combined with motor imagery of a skilled hand-motor task on motor cortical excitability: difference between novice and expert. Neurosci Lett. 2012;518:96–100.

156. Jeannerod M. Neural simulation of action. A unifying mechanism for motor cognition. NeuroImage. 2001;14:S103–9.

157. Ramachandran VS, Rogers-Ramachandran D. Synaesthesia in phantom limbs induced with mirrors. Proc Biol Sci. 1996;263(1369):377–86.

158. Ramachandran VS, Altschuler EL. The use of visual feedback, in particular mirror visual feedback, in restoring brain function. Brain. 2009;132:1693–710.

159. Ramchandran VS, Brang D. Sensations evoked in patients with amputation from watching an individual whose corresponding intact limb is being touched. Arch Neurol. 2009;66(10):1281–4.

160. Cacchio A, De Blasis E, De Blasis V, Santilli V, Spacca G. Mirror therapy in CRPS type 1 of the upper limb in stroke patients. Neurorehabil Neural Repair. 2009;23(8):792–9.

161. Cacchio A, De Blasis E, Necozione S, di Orio F, Santilli V. Mirror therapy for chronic complex regional pain syndrome type 1 and stroke. N Engl J Med. 2009;361(6):634–6.

162. Botvinick M, Cohen J. Rubber hands 'feel' touch that eyes see. Nature. 1998;391(6669):756.

163. Fukumura K, Sugawara K, Tanabe S, Ushiba J, Tomita Y. Influence of mirror therapy on human motor cortex. Int J Neurosci. 2007;117(7):1039–48.

164. Acera NE, Moseley GL. Dysynchiria: watching the mirror image of the unaffected limb elicits pain on the affected side. Neurology. 2005;65(5):751–3.

165. Delaquaize F. Réorganisation corticale posttraumatique et plasticité cérébrale: rééducation par les techniques d'imagerie motrice. In: GEMMSOR; dir. par Boutan M, et al., editors. Rééducation de la main et du poignet. Anatomie fonctionnelle et techniques, Chap. 19. Paris: Elsevier Masson; 2013. p. 187-203.

166. Rosèn B, Lundborg G. Training with a mirror in rehabilitation of the hand. Scand J Plast Reconstr Surg Hand Surg. 2005;39(2):104–8.

Doriane Parmentier

10.1 Fundamental Concepts

Self-rehabilitation has an increasingly important role in rehabilitation. However, there are very few data regarding the methodology for creating a self-rehabilitation program available in the literature.

Implementing such a program requires a personalized expertise from the therapist who evaluates the risk factors regarding the patient's pathology and the patient himself. This expertise fits right in the biopsychosocial model "ICF" (International Classification of Functioning, Disability, and Health) of the WHO (Fig. 10.1).

This model describes the way the biomechanical impairment caused by the pathology leads to activity limitation (the action is difficult to realize) and participation restriction (it is difficult to participate in a situation). It also includes a psychological and social dimension, with personal and environmental factors that can affect the treatment plan [1].

The therapist has theoretical knowledge of every pathology, such as healing time, contraindications, and possible complications. The assessment he makes targets impairments coming from the injured anatomical or organic structures. This is the basis for planning the treatment

and reducing the "biomechanical" risks possibly threatening a self-rehabilitation program.

However, this assessment is not enough, the therapist must also assess the patient as a whole to understand his needs and expectations: the "psychosocial" dimension. Internal (personal context) and external (environmental context) factors interact in a positive or negative way and affect the way the patient manages his pathology, and therefore the treatment [2, 3].

The therapist must know several information: age, gender, hobbies, job, life experiences, level of education, comprehension skill, psychological state (anxiety, depression), comorbidities (other pathologies or medical treatments). He must also check how much the patient knows about his pathology and its consequences, how he manages it and looks at the notion of the patient's self-efficiency in the treatment.

The therapist should also understand the patient's environmental context, which means his physical, social, and attitudinal environment. This helps highlighting the possible obstacles and facilitators for a self-rehabilitation treatment.

Bringing out all these elements during the assessment participates in creating a relationship of mutual trust between the patient and the therapist, leading to taking joint decisions about a self-rehabilitation protocol combining the patient's expectations and needs with the therapist's conclusions.

D. Parmentier (✉)
Institut Sud Aquitain de la Main et du Membre Supérieur, Biarritz, France

© The Author(s), under exclusive license to Springer Nature Switzerland AG 2022
G. Mesplié (ed.), *Hand and Wrist Therapy*, https://doi.org/10.1007/978-3-030-94942-6_10

Fig. 10.1 ICF model: International classification of functioning, disability and health [1]

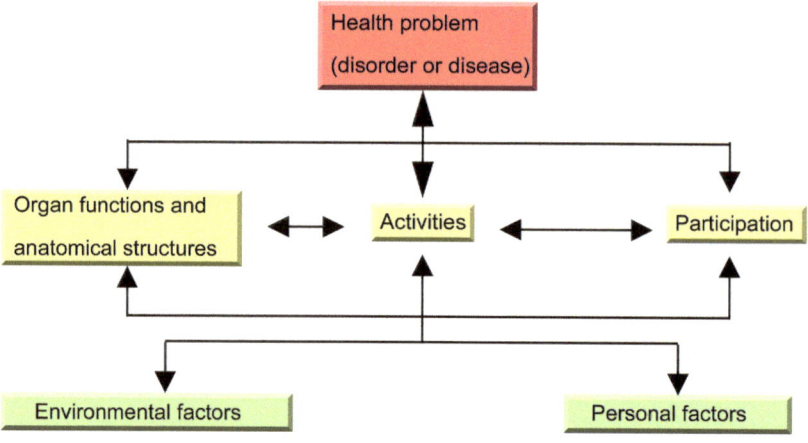

10.1.1 Treatment Plan

First, we must pick several rehabilitation goals, depending on the patient's impairments and activity limitations spotted during the therapist's assessment. They should be adapted, relevant, and achievable. They result in the choice of different techniques for various therapeutical exercises.

A therapeutical exercise is a systematic execution of movements, postures, or activities. It aims at helping the patient correcting or preventing an impairment, improving his function, reducing risks, optimizing his overall health, and improving his fitness and well-being [4].

A complete care includes educational, behavioral, and psychological parts. For and adapted physiotherapy treatment, all those parts can be implemented by a multidisciplinary team.

They appear to have a positive impact of the patient's health, especially in chronic diseases, as the patient plays an active role in his treatment.

The notion of self-efficacy is crucial in self-rehabilitation. This term refers to the belief that someone can have in his ability to conduct a task. The greater the patient's feeling of self-efficacy, the higher the goals he sets for himself and the better his involvement in pursuing them.

To prevent the impairment from worsening, the patient should be taught the right movements and positions to be included in his daily life, especially when doing the activity responsible for the impairment (if there is one).

It may be noted that some adaptation strategies might be in order when some activity limitations cannot be recovered even at the end of the treatment. We can use some devices and gears to realize the activities in question.

10.1.2 Multidisciplinary Care for Patient Education

It is important that the patient knows about his pathology. When he has some anatomical and physio-pathological knowledge about his pathology, he understands better how his system works and can correct or adapt his behavior.

The therapist should implement a pain coping skill training. Some strategies exist to teach the patient cognitive and behavioral skills that help him cope with pain. They also help him getting a more positive perception of his pathology [5].

10.1.3 Physiotherapy Treatment for Treating Impairments and Function (Program Implementation and Progression According to Brody and Hall's Work [6])

The initial program must provide a stable basis from which the therapeutic exercises can evolve. As the patient's symptoms may not progress in a linear way, the treatment cannot be predicted to be linear either. That is why the therapist's role is also to spot and foresee possible changes in the patient's symptoms and to create an adapted initial program. That way, he can create a clear basis for a program adapted to the patient's possibilities and the known obstacles to the rehabilitation. This stability helps clarifying the added effect of the self-rehabilitation program on the patient's general state and adjusting the initial program if needed [6].

The initial program is created based on the patient's impairments and activity limitations. One could think that treating the impairments automatically leads to an improved function, but it is not always the case, especially in chronic or degenerative diseases.

For example, when dealing with hand arthrosis, the patient can realize daily activities, thanks to specific tools and adapted movements. In this case, if the patient has a lack of joint mobility, the primary goal will not be to recover this mobility, but to teach the patient how to adapt his movements and how to use suitable tools in his daily life. Here, the activity limitation takes precedence over the impairment.

The impairments we chose to treat must be related to an activity limitation or a participation restriction, making them a priority [7].

10.1.3.1 What Is the Optimal "Dosage" for Self-Rehabilitation Exercises?

The principle of Specific Adaptations to Imposed Demands (SAID) based on the Physical Stress Theory (PST) gives some advice about the prescription and progression of the initial exercise [8, 9]. This concept suggests that the muscle and other connective tissues are remodeled when stressed. The PST indicates that biological tissues have five ways of dealing with physical stress: decreasing the stress tolerance (atrophy), maintaining the stress tolerance, increasing the stress tolerance (hypertrophy), injury, or death.

For each prescribed exercise, choices must be made regarding several variables putting stress on these tissues. There are lots of variables, such as the frequency, intensity, duration, type of muscle contraction, movement amplitude, stability, speed of movement [10–13]. Among these variables, the most common are the frequency (of the exercise), the intensity (strength or resistance needed to

realize the exercise), and the duration (number of series or duration of the exercise) [14, 15].

However, these adjustments cannot be made randomly. The overall volume of exercises should be considered to determine the right dose of physical stress.

The overall volume of exercises is the total amount of physical exercise realized by the patient in one session. To adjust this global volume, we can increase or decrease the total number of exercises made in one session or adjust the variables of each exercise individually (intensity, duration, frequency, and rest period).

The goal when applying the PST is to get enough physical stress to produce a structural adaptation, but not so much so that it would cause tissue injury [6].

The principle of optimal load provides extra advice. The optimal load is the stress a tissue can bear during a period. This load is neither over nor under-evaluated [6]. For example, if the patient's daily activities or job put great stress on the healing tissue, the rehabilitation exercises should be adapted to keep an optimal overall load.

Furthermore, the tissue tolerance is different in each patient, so the load must be adjusted to the patients' individual specificities.

The management of the applied stress also varies depending on the pathology. For example, in case of stiffness in the fingers, the recommended treatment includes the application of physical stress via a dynamic orthosis, 6 h a day [16]. Self-rehabilitation is then in order, as no patient spends 6 h a day in the physical therapist's office. Moreover, in this case, the patient is the one who adjusts the intensity: He must feel tension but no pain [16].

Educating the patient on this notion of optimal load, and on the adjustment of the different variables for each exercise is key to keeping a good balance and achieving the most efficient recovery possible without creating injuries.

10.1.3.2 Which Activities and Exercises Can Be Recommended?

There are many different treatments for one pathology. That is why identifying the main impairments and activity limitations is essential to define clear treatment goals as a basis for implementing exercises.

Impairments such as pain, edema, and inflammation are usually treated with massage and physiotherapy techniques (see Chap. 3). In self-rehabilitation, the most accessible techniques are massage, thermotherapy, cryotherapy, and sometimes electrotherapy.

Prescribing exercises appears to help patients with musculoskeletal and rheumatic pathologies, having an anti-inflammatory effect, even if there is little scientific evidence [17].

Moreover, educating the patient to treat his activity limitations can have positive effects on his symptoms (especially pain).

There are two other impairments usually found when treating the upper limb: lack of mobility and neuro-muscular deficiency.

Mobility can be impaired by pain and/or a several tissues (joint, muscle, tendon, connective tissue) if their extensibility has been abnormally altered [18].

In case of tendon or ligament injury, the newly synthetized extracellular matrix is not organized properly, leading to a stiff tissue with a resistance lower than normal [19–21]. Building on this, a study showed that applying a mechanical stress by stretching the injured structure helps the matrix fiber align better and improves healing [22].

In any case, active and passive joint mobilizations in all the available range of motion are beneficial, as they nourish the joint surfaces (imbibition), lengthen the tissues surrounding the joint, stimulate the connection between the tissues stressed while moving, and stimulate the mechanoreceptors. An additional benefit comes with an active movement as it activates the muscles, improves circulation, stimulates proprioception, and stimulates the bone activity at the level of the muscle attachment [23].

A lack of mobility is not always a loss of mobility: It can be an excessive pathological mobility creating instability. In this case, the treatment will be based on active joint stabilization, with exercises for conscious and unconscious proprioception [24, 25] (see Chap. 8).

In general, active and passive self-mobilization exercises are interesting in acute pathologies as well as in chronic and degenerative diseases. They must be chosen carefully and meticulously applied by the patient to get the benefit of them.

Neuro-muscular deficits cause instability and require an adapted and progressive proprioceptive protocol (see Chaps. 7 and 8).

10.1.3.3 How to Create a Progression?

According to Brody and Hall [26], two methods are usually used. The first one consists in changing the variables in the exercises without changing the overall volume of exercise, while the second one consists in changing this overall volume (Fig. 10.2).

We must pay attention to the quantity of exercise the patient can tolerate. If the patient's overall daily physical stress is already close to its upper limit, it will be difficult for him to add new exercises: The therapist will have to increase the difficulty of the exercises by changing their variables rather than the number of exercises.

The variables that can be modified are the complexity of the task, the mode of the muscle contraction, the speed, the stability, the feedback, the environment, the order of the exercises, the range of motion, and the cognitive control [26].

For example, the speed of the exercise can be easily changed during the concentric and eccentric contraction. It helps the muscle adapting better to stress. Increasing the speed increases the muscle fatigue and the co-contraction and helps reaching a functional movement speed by the end of rehabilitation. Modifying the range of motion by changing the starting and ending positions allows working on different modes of muscle contraction, and therefore getting closer to functional movements.

Changing these variables does not influence the overall volume of exercise but creates physiological changes at a muscular level [27]. These physiological changes should be considered in the program progression in order not to create too much physical stress.

When the patient can tolerate the initial overall volume of exercise, the program can be modified by increasing this volume.

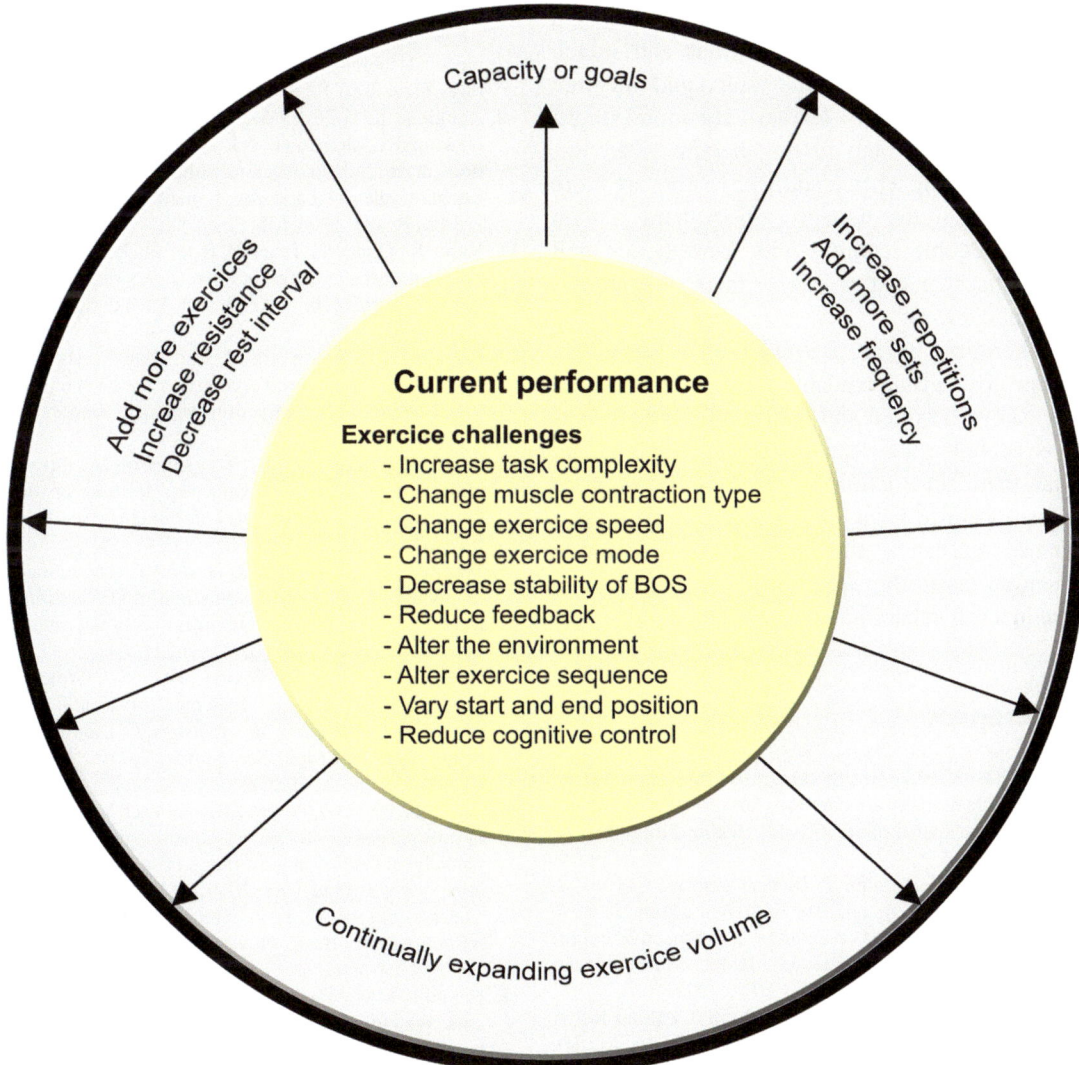

Fig. 10.2 Exercise progression according to Brody and Hall [26]

The frequency, intensity, and duration are the most used variables, as they are easy to change. The increase must be progressive and adapted to the patient's capacities. For example, if the patient needs a day to recuperate between sessions, increasing the frequency would overload the tissues [6], while decreasing the rest period between exercises or mildly increasing their intensity would be more appropriate.

Creating a program with a variety of modalities helps preventing overload, as the patient can alternate between "difficult" days and "easy" days, simply changing the intensity or the duration of the exercise [6]. It is harder to implement but it leads to a program that is better tolerated, more complete, and more effective. Moreover, the fact that it is not repetitive can have a motivational effect on the patient.

10.1.3.4 What Medium Should Be Used to Give the Program to the Patient?

Learning patterns are different for everyone. The VARK evaluation determines the ease of learning with a Visual, Auditive, Read/write, and Kinesthetic approach [28, 29].

Visual learners will be more stimulated by a graphic approach with illustrations and sketch drawings themselves to understand and integrate information. Auditive learners are more stimulated when listening to the therapist's advice. People learning when reading or writing are more stimulated if the therapist gives them written advice. People learning with kinesthetics will need the therapist to show them movements ("practical work").

Therefore, we suggest using different media. Paper gives visual/readable information that can be easily consulted and displayed. Video is less accessible but has visual, auditive, readable, and kinesthetic instructions. Interactive smartphone apps appear to have a positive effect on performances and can be stimulating [30], which makes them an interesting medium for the therapist to use in a self-rehabilitation program.

References

1. WHO. World Health Organization International classification of functioning, disability and health. Geneva, Switzerland: World Health Organization; 2001.
2. Feleus A, van Dalen T, Bierma-Zeinstra SM, et al. Kinesiophobia in patients with non-traumatic arm, neck, and shoulder complaints: a prospective cohort study in general practice. BMC Musculoskelet Disord. 2007;8:117.
3. Ryall C, Coggon D, Peveler R, Poole J, Palmer KT. A prospective cohort study of arm pain in primary care and physiotherapy - prognostic determinants. Rheumatology (Oxford). 2007;46:508–15.
4. American Physical Therapy Association. American Physical Therapy Association Interactive guide to physic. Alexandria, VA: American Physical Therapy Association; 2003.
5. Williams AC, Eccleston C, Morley S. Psychological therapies for the management of chronic pain (excluding headache) in adults. Cochrane Database Syst Rev. 2012;11:CD007407.
6. Brody LT. Effective therapeutic exercise prescription: the right exercise at the right dose. J Hand Ther. 2012;25(2):220–32.
7. McDonough CM, Jette AM. The contribution of osteoarthritis to functional limitations and disability. Clin Geriatr Med. 2010;26:387–99.
8. Kegerreis S. The construction and implementation of functional progressions as a component of athletic rehabilitation. J Orthop Sports Phys Ther. 1983;5:14–9.
9. Mueller M, Maluf K. Tissue adaptation to physical stress: a proposed "physical stress theory" to guide physical therapy practice, education, and research. Phys Ther. 2001;82:383–403.
10. Hakkinen K, Kallinen M, Linnamo V, Pastinen UM, Newton RU, Kraemer WJ. Neuromuscular adaptations during bilateral versus unilateral strength training in middle-aged and elderly men and women. Acta Physiol Scand. 1996;158(1):77–88.
11. Kubo K, Ohgo K, Takeishi R, et al. Effects of isometric training at different knee angles on the muscle tendon complex in vivo. Scand J Med Sci Sports. 2006;16:159–67.
12. Paddon-Jones D, Leveritt M, Lonergan A, Abernethy P. Adaptation to chronic eccentric exercise in humans: the influence of contraction velocity. Eur J Appl Physiol. 2001;85(5):466–71.
13. Seger JY, Arvidsson B, Thorstensson A. Specific effects of eccentric and concentric training on muscle strength and morphology in humans. Eur J Appl Physiol Occup Physiol. 1998;79(1):49–57.
14. Wernbom M, Augustsson J, Thomee R. The influence of frequency, intensity, volume and mode of strength training on whole muscle cross-sectional area in humans. Sports Med. 2007;37(3):225–64.
15. American College of Sports Medicine. American College of Sports Medicine position stand. Progression models in resistance training for healthy adults. Med Sci Sports Exerc. 2009;41: 687–708.
16. Valdes K, Boyd JD, Povlak SB, Szelwach MA. Efficacy of orthotic devices for increased active proximal interphalangeal extension joint range of motion: a systematic review. J Hand Ther. 2019;32(2):184–93.
17. Metsios GS, Moe RH, Kitas GD. Exercise and inflammation. Best Pract Res Clin Rheumatol. 2020;34:101504.
18. Reinold MM, Escamilla RF, Wilk KE. Current concepts in the scientific and clinical rationale behind exercises for glenohumeral and scapulothoracic musculature. J Orthop Sports Phys Ther. 2009;39(2):105–17.
19. Frank C, Woo SL, Amiel D, Harwood F, Gomez M, Akeson W. Medial collateral ligament healing. A multidisciplinary assessment in rabbits. Am J Sports Med. 1983;11(6):379–89.
20. Woo SL, Takakura Y, Liang R, Jia F, Moon DK. Treatment with bioscaffold enhances the fibril morphology and the collagen composition of healing medial collateral ligament in rabbits. Tissue Eng. 2006;12(1):159–66.
21. Niyibizi C, Kavalkovich K, Yamaji T, Woo SL. Type V collagen is increased during rabbit medial collateral ligament healing. Knee Surg Sports Traumatol Arthrosc. 2000;8(5):281–5.
22. Nguyen TD, Liang R, Woo SL, Burton SD, Wu C, Almarza A, Sacks MS, Abramowitch S. Effects of cell seeding and cyclic stretch on the fiber remodeling in an extracellular matrix-derived bioscaffold. Tissue Eng Part A. 2009;15(4):957–63.

23. Uhl TL, Muir TA, Lawson L. Electromyographical assessment of passive, active assistive, and active shoulder rehabilitation exercises. PM R. 2010;2:132–41.

24. Zelenski NA, Shin AY. Management of nondissociative instability of the wrist. J Hand Surg Am. 2020;45(2):131–9.

25. Mesplié G, Grelet V, Léger O, Lemoine S, Ricarrère D, Geoffroy C. Rehabilitation of distal radioulnar joint instability. Hand Surg Rehabil. 2017;36(5):314–21.

26. Hall C. Patient management. In: Brody L, Hall C, editors. Therapeutic exercise: moving toward function, vol. 3. Philadelphia, PA: Wolters Kluwer/Lippincott Williams & Wilkins; 2011. p. 91–4.

27. Kanehisa H, Nagareda H, Kawakami Y, et al. Effects of equivolume isometric training programs comprising medium or high resistance on muscle size and strength. Eur J Appl Physiol. 2002;87(2):112–9.

28. Prithishkumar IJ, Michael SA. Understanding your student: using the VARK model. J Postgrad Med. 2014;60(2):183–6.

29. Aydın L, Ilhan AŞ, Kızıltan E, Yazıhan N, Yazıcı AC, Gundogan NU. The influence of six-year medical education on learning styles in medical students at Baskent University. Open Access Libr J. 2015;02(04):1–8.

30. Valdes K, Gendernalik E, Hauser J, Tipton M. Use of mobile applications in hand therapy. J Hand Ther. 2020;33(2):229–34.

Part III

Common Hand and Wrist Orthoses

Baptiste Arrate, Chantal Donapetry,
and Grégory Mesplié

Making an orthosis for a patient suffering from a hand injury is a fundamental step in their healing process, should it be aiming to immobilize or to rest injured tissues, or to optimize rehabilitation goals.

There are several categories of orthoses:

- Non-articular orthoses that can either have a proprioceptive role or that can help use additives such as silicone for example.
- Immobilization orthoses that aim to block mobility by the means of an external force
- Mobilization orthoses that aim to increase mobility by the means of an external force.
- Restriction orthoses that limit normal mobility by the means of an external force.
- Torque transmission orthoses that redirect the internal forces of one or several joints.

11.1 Materials

Making orthoses with thermoplastic requires a vat filled with hot w used to deform the material (Fig. 11.1), different types of scissors (Fig. 11.2), a heat gun (Fig. 11.3) and various bands used to close the orthosis and to finish its edges (Fig. 11.4).

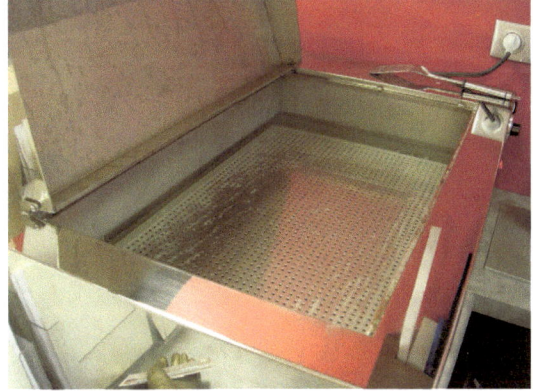

Fig. 11.1 Water vat heated at 60–70 °C

A wide variety of thermoplastics exist that differentiate from each other by their:

- thickness
- elasticity and extensibility
- rigidity
- coating
- color
- stickiness

This immobilization method is suitable for any patient's morphology since the orthosis is molded directly on the patient's skin.

Thermoplastics have many advantages because they make for:

B. Arrate · C. Donapetry · G. Mesplié (✉)
Institut Sud Aquitain de la Main et du Membre
Supérieur, Biarritz, France

© The Author(s), under exclusive license to Springer Nature Switzerland AG 2022
G. Mesplié (ed.), *Hand and Wrist Therapy*, https://doi.org/10.1007/978-3-030-94942-6_11

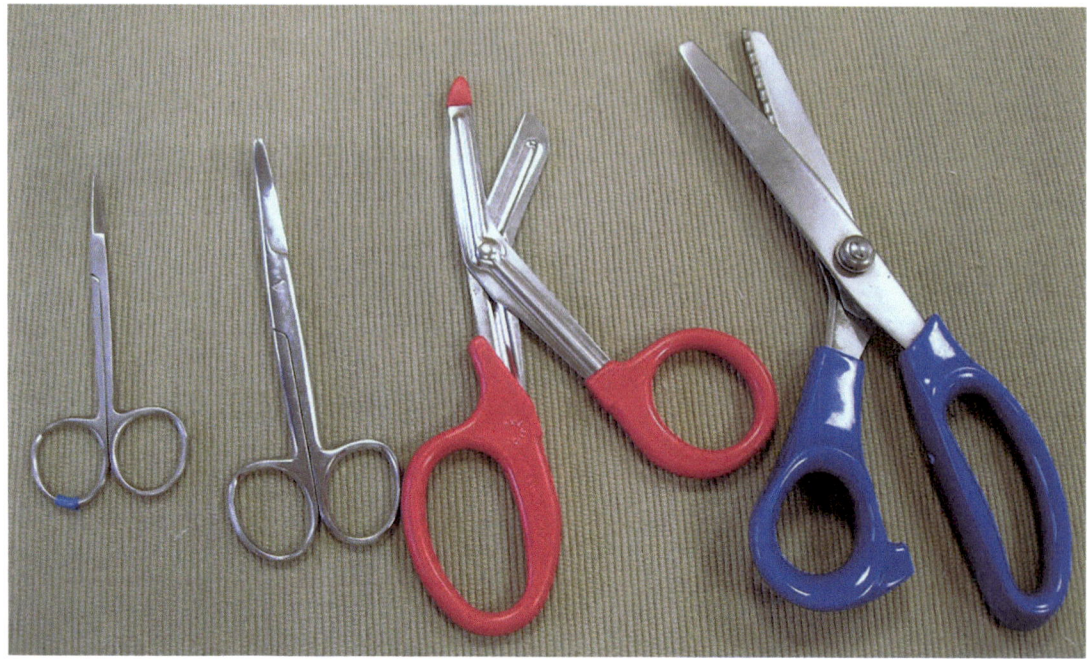

Fig. 11.2 Scissors in different shapes and sizes to adjust to different situations

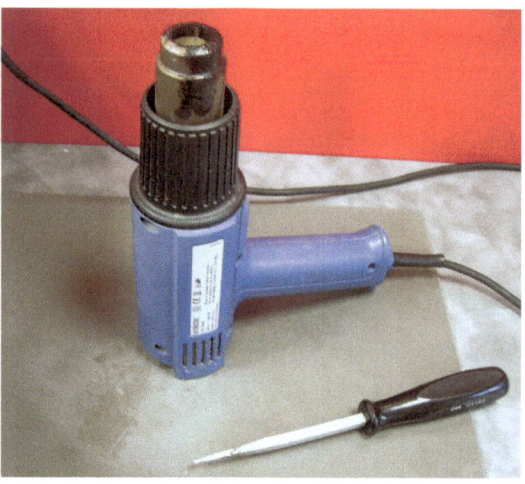

Fig. 11.3 Heat gun

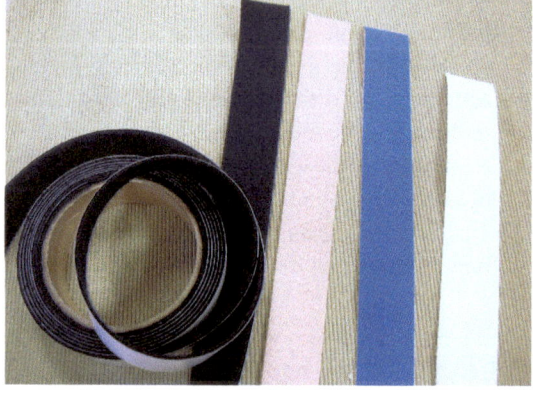

Fig. 11.4 Self-adhesive edges and Velcro straps

- An adjustable molding since the plastic can be reheated and modified according to a potential evolution of the patient's morphology or pathology (decreased swelling, pin rejecting, etc.).
- A precisely sized orthosis limiting only the joints that need to be immobilized and allowing the mobility of all other elements, avoiding stiffness.

- An extremely light-weighted orthosis (six times lighter than resin).
- A breathable orthosis, thanks to the micro-perforations in the plastic, which is better for the skin.
- A hypoallergenic orthosis that can also go under water.
- A radiolucent orthosis.

Guidance sheets are given to each patient that briefly explain the aim of their orthosis, how to

Vous venez de bénéficier d'une orthèse thermoformée pour **rhizarthrose**

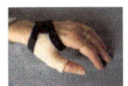 ou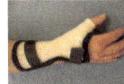

Elle peut être courte ou longue en fonction de vos douleurs et, ou de l'utilisation que vous souhaitez en faire.

Le but de cette orthèse est
- o d'**immobiliser** les articulations touchées par cette arthrose (trapézo-métacarpienne en premier lieu) et donc de soulager inflammation et douleurs.
- o de**prévenir** la déformation du pouce en Z liée à ce rhumatisme.

Vous la portez **la nuit**.
En phase douloureuse, vous pouvez la garder penda
la journée.

L'orthèse ne doit pas être ni trop serrée, ni trop lâche.

En cas d'inconfort, n'hésitez pas à
CONTACTER L'ORTHÉSISTE

En complément, pour reprendre une activité professionnelle ousportive, une orthèse de fonction en néoprène peut vous aider.

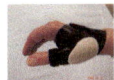 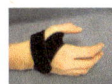

Entretien de l'orthèse :

- o Avec de l'eau tiède et du savon, éventuellement à l'aide d'une vieille brosse à dents.
- o Si votre orthèse contient du silicone, pensez à le couvrir de sa feuille de protection quand vous n l'utilisez pas.
- o Evitez de mettre votre orthèse après avoir mis pommade ou crème sur votre peau (veillez avant à bien sécher votre main et votre poignet).
- o Evitez de laisser votre orthèse sur une source de chaleur (radiateur, plage arrière de voiture etc...) elle pourrait se détériorer

Pour plus de précision, vous pouvez poser vos questions sur notre site : www.isamms.com

Fig. 11.5 An example of a guidance sheet that can be given to each patient according to their injury

clean it, and a few instructions on how to mobilize the free joints (Fig. 11.5).

11.2 Classification

If there is a certain homogeneity between orthosis fabrication methods across the world, we cannot say the same for their classification which is subject to a very big disparity between regions.

11.2.1 Eponymous

This classification uses the name of the inventor of the orthosis. There are numerous examples such as "Duran" and "Kleinert" orthoses for flexor tendon injuries, the "Stack" orthosis for mallet fingers or "Thomine" orthoses for metacarpal fractures. The evident advantage of this classification is its simplicity. The inconvenience

is that, through the years, with the development of knowledge and rehabilitation protocols and according to regions, one same common denomination can correspond to very different orthoses (Fig. 11.6).

11.2.2 Acronymous

This classification uses an abbreviation to define the orthosis. For example, an orthosis that immobilizes the arm, forearm, wrist, and hand can be named EWHO (elbow, wrist, hand orthosis).

11.2.3 Descriptive

This classification method is more precise but also more complex and various authors and organizations have proposed descriptive denominations according to the aim of the orthosis, its

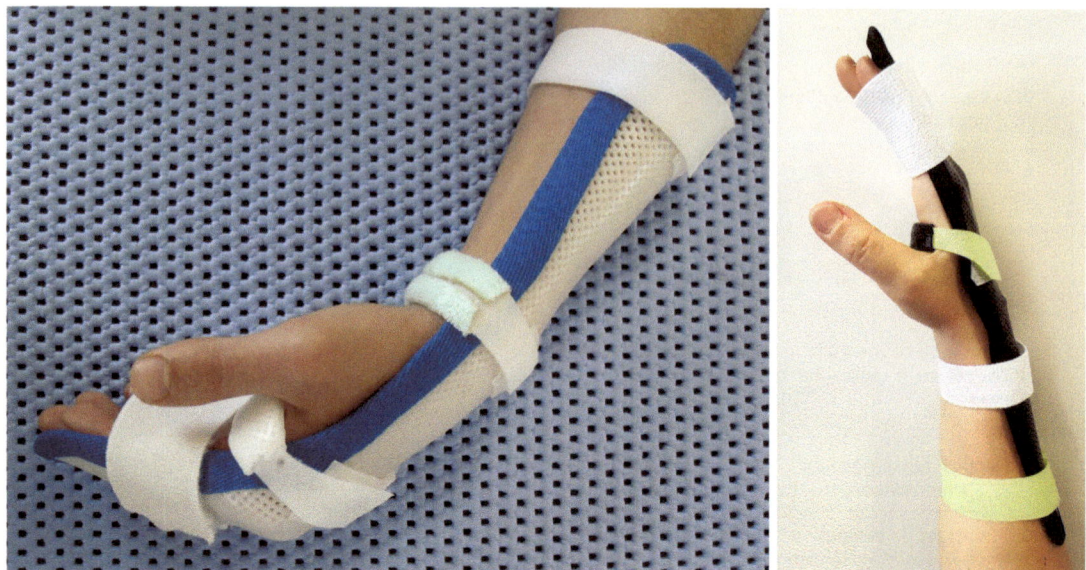

Fig. 11.6 Two examples of "Duran" orthoses. Notice the difference in the positioning of the MCP joints

NON-ARTICULAR ORTHOSES	
Body segment	Examples : humerus, metacarpal, forearm, proximal phalanx, etc …
ARTICULAR ORTHOSES	
Anatomical zone and primary joint	The specific joints aimed by the orthosis, namedby their scientific designation.
Direction	Extension, flexion, radial deviation, ulnar deviation circumduction, abduction, adduction, etc …
Goals	Immobilization, mobilization, restriction, torque transmission.
Type	Number of secondary joints (not always named by their scientific designation). Secondary joints are included to stabilize the extremities of the orthosis. There is no special direction or goal for these joints. They are included to increase the mechanical function of the orthosis.

Fig. 11.7 American Society of Hand Therapy classification criteria

configurations, its mechanical characteristics, or the body segment it contains [1–4].

In 1992, the American Hand Therapy Society proposed a classification [4] that was conducted by Fess et al. in 2004 [3] (Fig. 11.7).

According to this classification, orthoses can be "non-articular" or "articular" depending on if they cover a joint or not.

Non-articular orthoses are named using the body segment they contain.

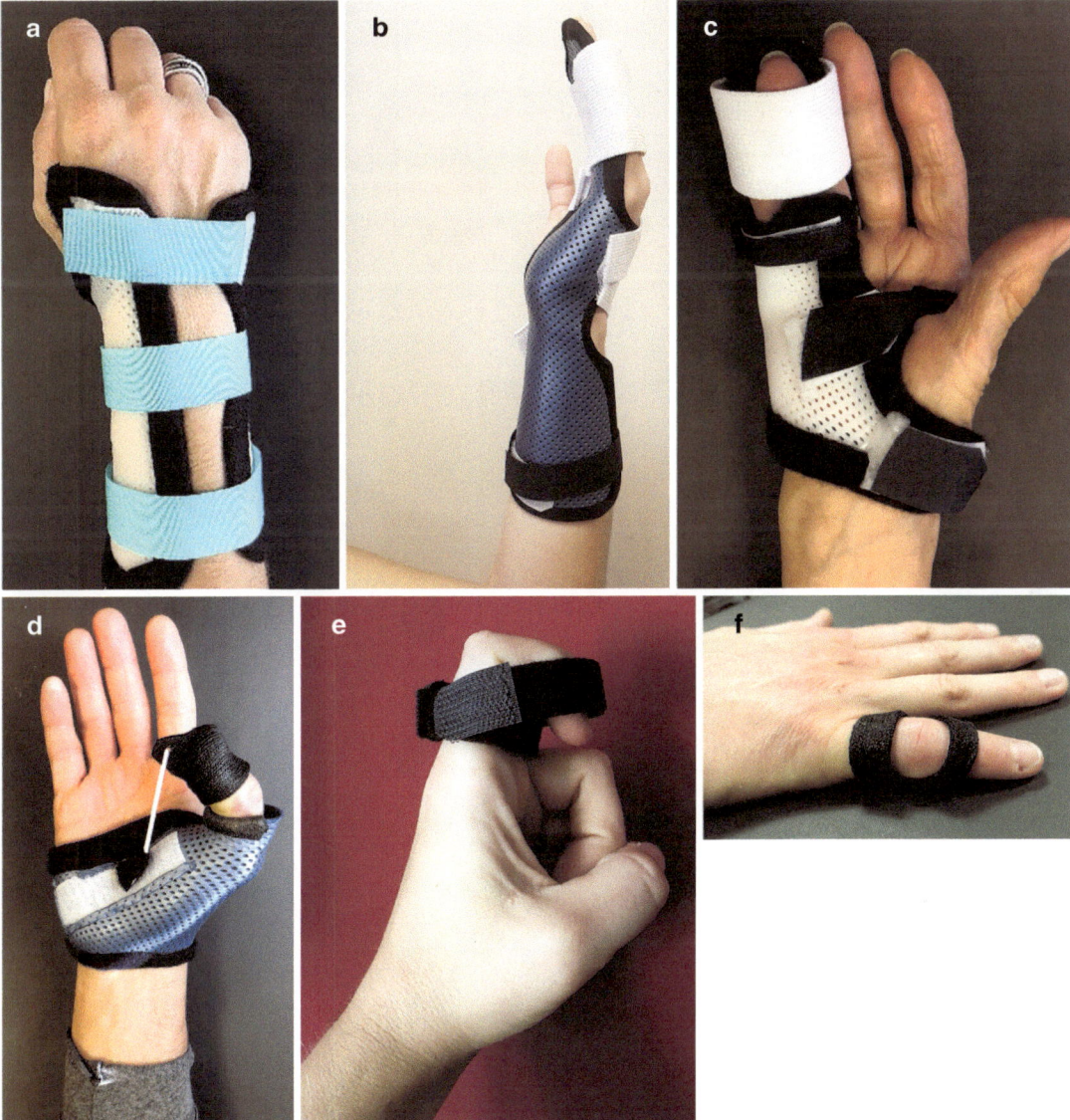

Fig. 11.8 (**a**) Wrist immobilization orthosis; (**b**) Wrist, MP, and finger IP joints immobilization orthosis; (**c**) CM-MP and finger IP joints immobilization orthosis; (**d**) Thumb IP joint flexion mobilization orthosis (dynamic); (**e**) Index IP joints flexion mobilization orthosis (dynamic); (**f**) Small finger PIP joint extension limitation orthosis

Articular orthoses, which are by far the most common, do not carry the term "articular" for convenience. They are ranked according to five subclassifications as follows:

- The purpose of the orthosis which can be immobilization, mobilization, restriction, or torque transmission.
- The direction if it is not an immobilization orthosis.

- The concerned body segment that can be the wrist, a finger, etc.
- The type, corresponding to the number of joints included in the orthosis.

This classification enables different practitioners to have reliable exchanges on a wide variety of orthoses whether they are part of a same team or not (Fig. 11.8).

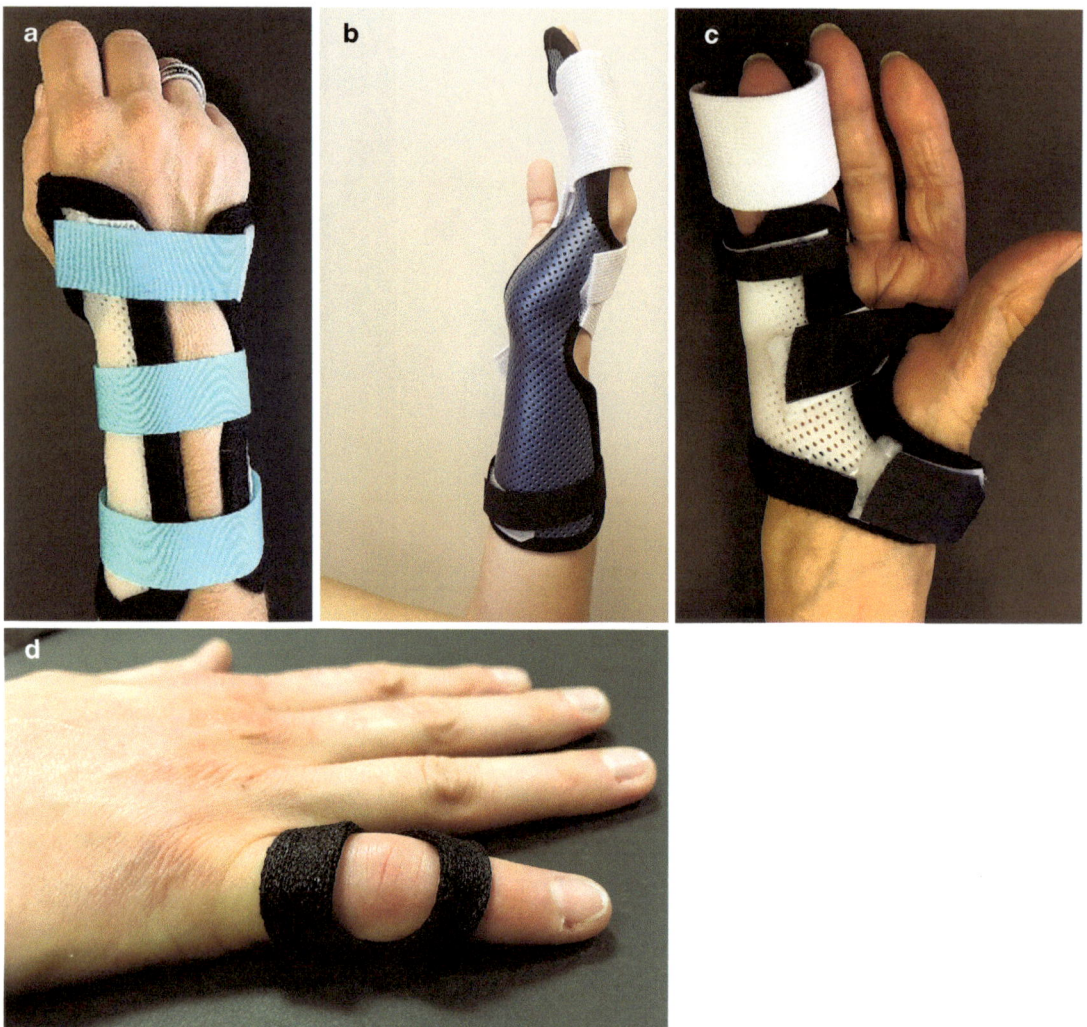

Fig. 11.9 (**a**) Wrist immobilization orthosis (0°); (**b**) Wrist, MP, and finger IP joints immobilization orthosis (ext 30°—flex 70°—ext 0°); (**c**) CM-MP and finger IP joints immobilization orthosis (neutral—70°—straight); (**d**) Small finger PIP joint extension limitation orthosis (−10°)

The exact immobilization position or the imposed limitation can also be added to the name (Fig. 11.9).

11.3 Mechanical Principles

Common knowledge concerning mechanical principles is essential to make an efficient orthosis while limiting the risk of complications due to wearing it.

- **Amount of contact points**: According to the location of the contact points, the applied forces may be poorly tolerated, particularly against a bone or an injured zone (Fig. 11.10).
- **The ratio between contact surface and applied forces**: The more the contact is distributed across a large surface, the easier it will be for the patient to tolerate it since the force is applied to a larger zone (Fig. 11.11).

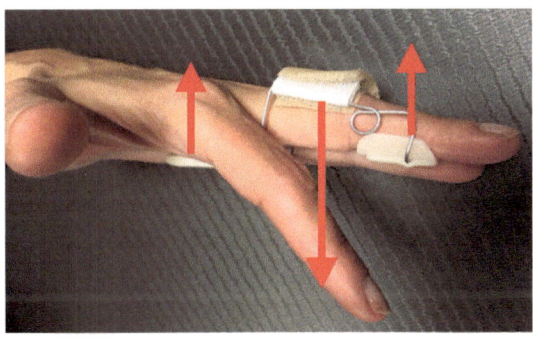

Fig. 11.10 In this example, the contact with the dorsal side of the PIP joint is two times bigger than the palmar contact, which can be sensitive and poorly tolerated

- **Force application angle**: The most efficient direction for a mobilization orthosis is a 90° angle facing the segment that needs to be mobilized. In any other case, the force will be divided between a mobilizing force and a distracting or tightening force according to the angle (Fig. 11.12).
- **Length of the orthosis and forces**: The longer the orthosis is, the more the forces will be distributed across the body segment and the less the orthosis will risk creating a wound due to a contact point (Fig. 11.13).

Fig. 11.11 The dorsal contact point on P1 is larger in (1), which better distributes the forces applied compared to (2), making for a more comfortable and tolerable orthosis (1)

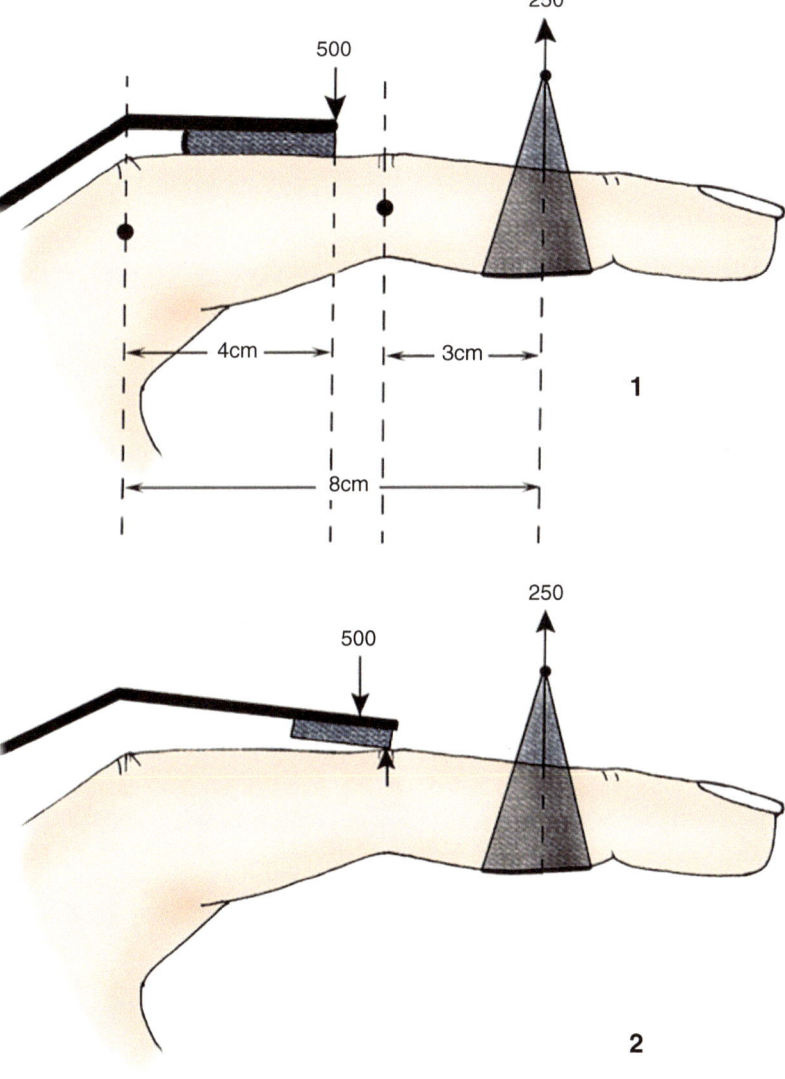

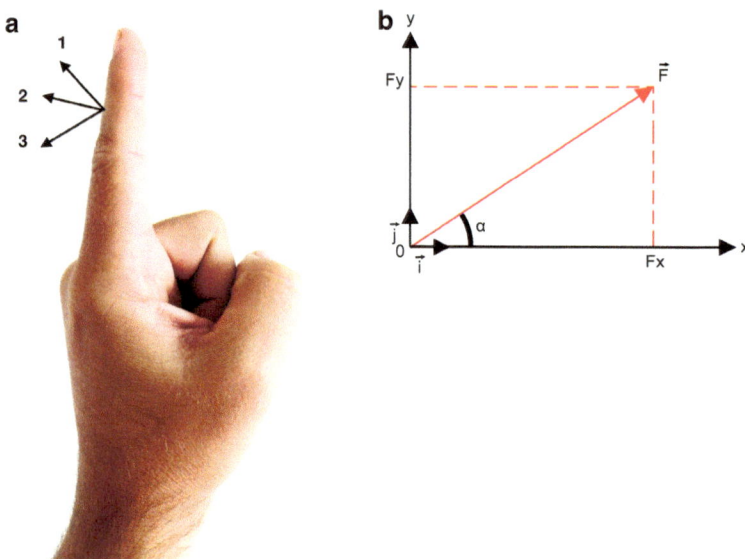

Fig. 11.12 (**a**) The most efficient direction for a mobilization orthosis is a 90° angle facing the segment that needs to be mobilized (arrow no. 2). In any other case, the force will be divided between a mobilizing force and a distracting (1) or tightening (3) force according to the angle. (**b**) This is because the applied force can be broken down into a mobilizing component (Fy) and a tightening/distracting component (Fx) whose value depends on the applied angle

Fig. 11.13 Long orthoses are easier to tolerate because the forces are distributed across a larger surface, limiting the risk of uncomfortable contact points

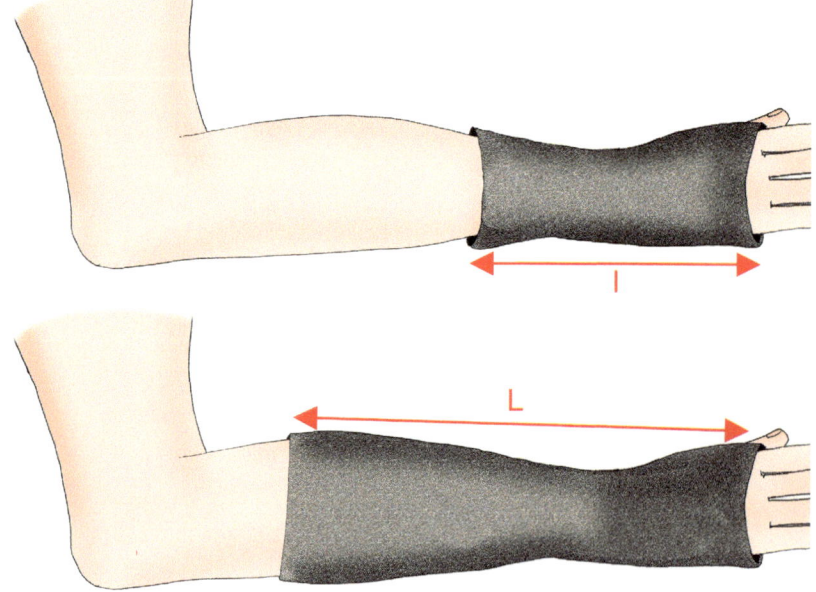

- **Leverage**: The longer the leverage of a force is, the more the moment of the said force increases (Fig. 11.14).
- **Contact localization regarding the joint**: The farther the contact is from the joint center of the joint to mobilize, the more the shear stress increases in the said joint, increasing the risk is to create a premature mechanical "bone to bone" stop (Fig. 11.15).
- **Hing localization**: The hinges must be placed facing the axes of the joint to mobilize (Fig. 11.16).

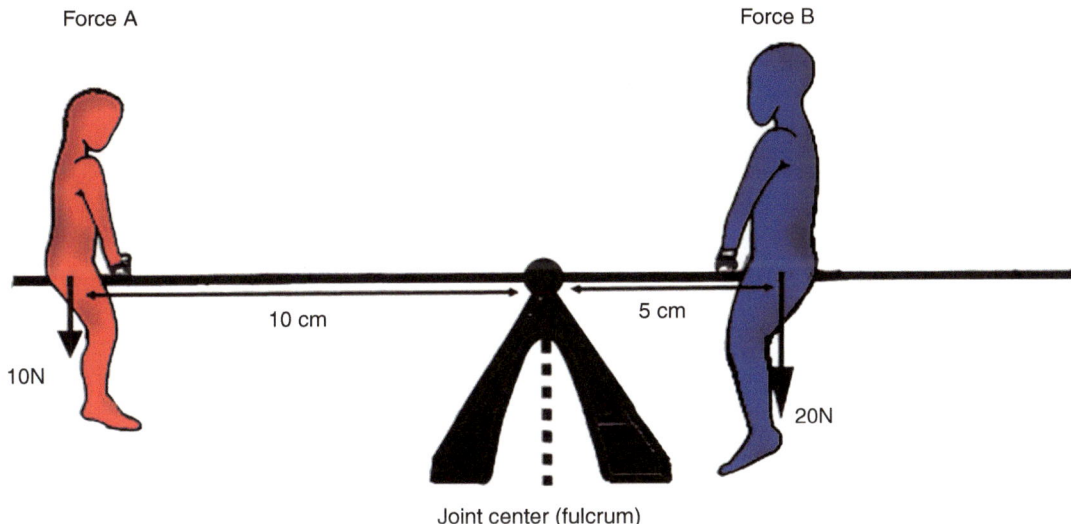

Fig. 11.14   The effect of a 10 N force applied 10 cm from the joint center and the effect of a 20 N force applied 5 cm from the joint center are equal

Fig. 11.15 Mobilizing a joint with a contact close to the joint center limits the shear stress and the risk of creating a premature mechanical "bone to bone" stop

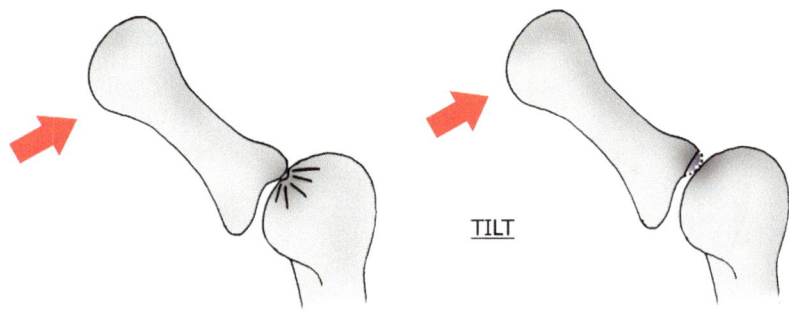

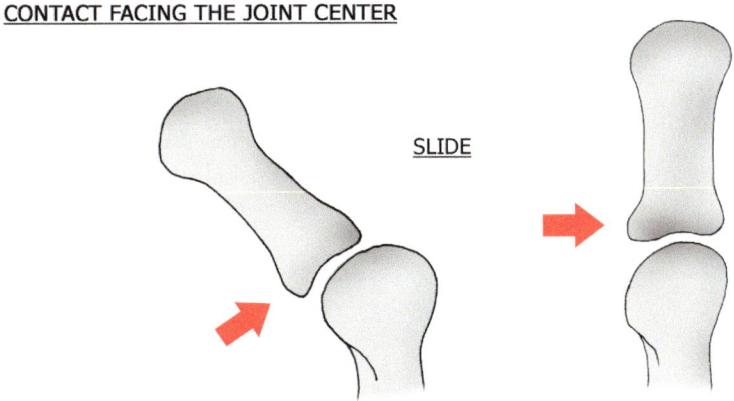

Fig. 11.16 The hinges of the orthosis must be placed facing the axes of the joint

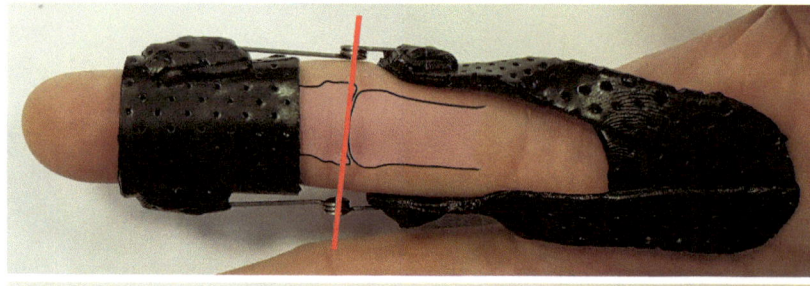

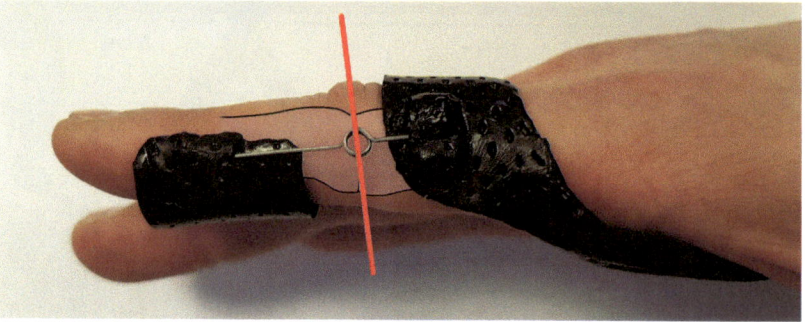

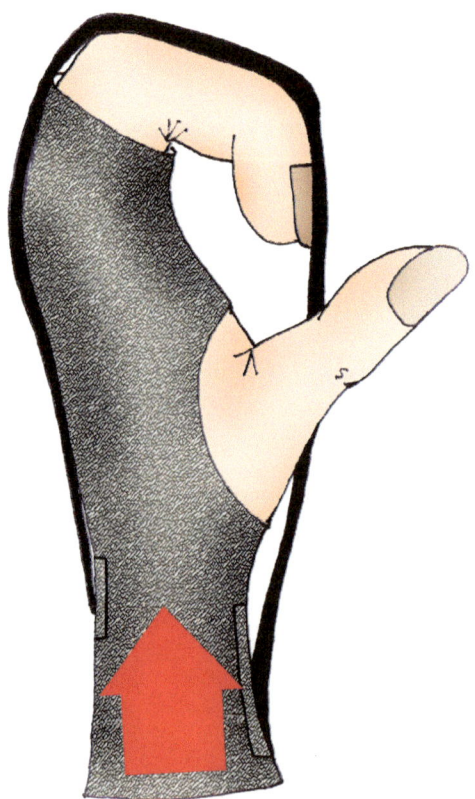

Fig. 11.17 In this example, the orthosis will have a tendency to slip distally if it is not stable enough around the wrist

- **Orthosis' thickness and sturdiness**: With the same type of thermoplastic, the thicker the orthosis is, the sturdier it will be. Folding over the edges will make it even more sturdy.
- **Piston effect**: A mobilization orthosis can cause a piston effect on its fixed portion if the mechanical forces have a longitudinal direction (Fig. 11.17).

11.4 Non-Articular Orthoses

11.4.1 Syndactylies

Their goal is to bond two or more fingers without immobilizing the proximal interphalangeal nor the metacarpophalangeal joints. Flexion and extension remain possible in all fingers, but valgus and varus movements are contained. The syndactylies can be made with non-elastic fabric (Velcro sewed together) (Fig. 11.18), with thermoplastic or with Orficast© (Fig. 11.19). In the case of a bone fracture with a rotary disorder, anti-rotation wedges can be added if surgery is not an option (Fig. 11.20).

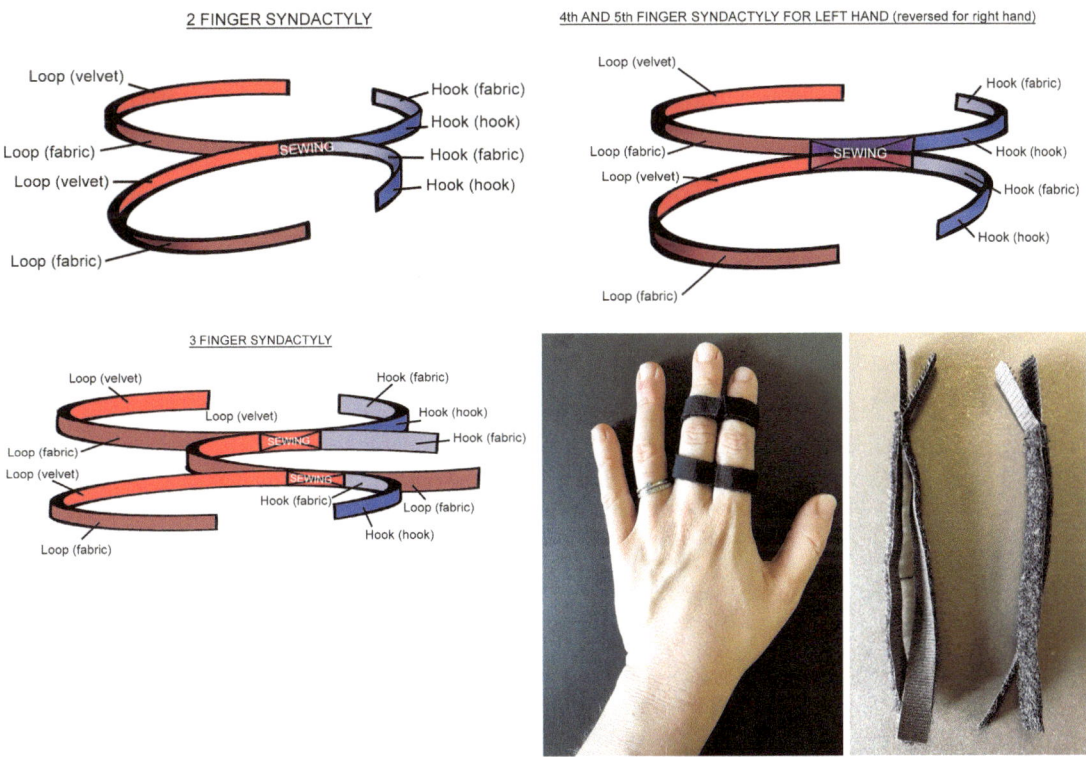

Fig. 11.18   Production method for syndactylies in non-elastic fabric and final product

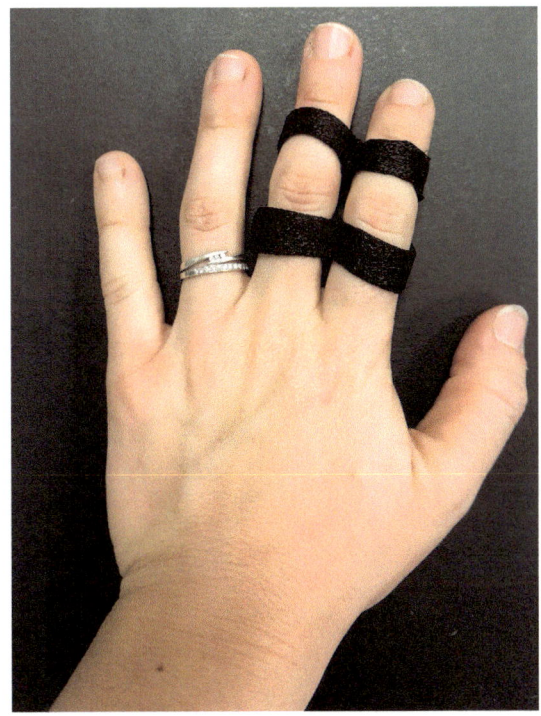

Fig. 11.19   Syndactylies made of Orficast©

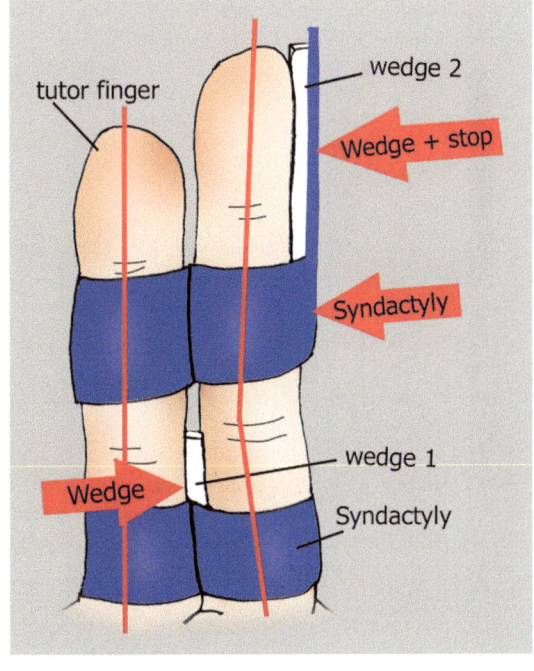

Fig. 11.20   Syndactylies with anti-derotation wedges after a spiral second phalanx fracture where surgery was not an option

11.4.2　Base for Silicone

Non-articular orthoses can be coupled with silicone gel that has a relevant evidence level of efficiency in treating hypertrophic scars [5], thanks to the slight compression against the scar and its anti-inflammatory effects (see Chap. 4).

11.5　Articular Immobilization Orthoses

These orthoses immobilize the mobility of the joints included in the orthosis and can be used for conditions that require strict immobilization (day and night wearing) or rest (alternated wearing).

11.5.1　Articular Wrist Immobilization Orthosis

Characteristics of the orthosis
The orthosis covers the forearm to a greater or lesser extent depending on the case. The MP joints are always free. Depending on the patient's morphology, the thickness of the thermoplastic will be chosen between 1.6 and 2.4 mm
Production method
The plastic is cut into a rectangular shape of which the length matches the distance between the MP joints and the limit desired for the forearm. Once the plastic is malleable, a hole is cut in the upper corner (on the left or right side) leaving about 1 cm above and localized at one-third of the width of the rectangular shape
The patient is asked to rest their elbow on the table with the ulnar side of their hand facing the therapist. The thumb is slipped through the hole and the thermoplastic is wrapped around the hand and the wrist and closed on the dorsal surface of the forearm following the axis of the third metacarpal bone. Depending on the case, the wrist will be placed between 0° and 20° of extension. A straight wrist is the position that causes the least joint pressure (according to Kapandji [6]) and the least stress on the carpal tunnel [7]. The pronosupination position depends on the injury that is diagnosed. The orthosis is cut along the palmar crease to free mobility of the MP and IP joints. The ulnar styloid can be freed by cutting a small notch or the plastic can be puffed out around it. The length of the orthosis depends on the injury. The orthosis is fastened with three Velcro straps across the metacarpals, the wrist, and the forearm

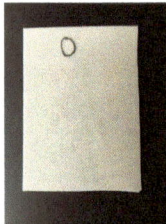 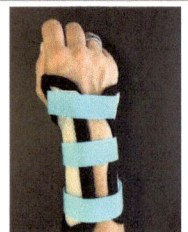 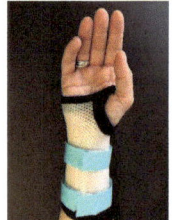

Suitable conditions	*Specific characteristics*
Arthritis in the carpal joints	Straight wrist, length equal to one-third of the forearm
Non-operated carpal tunnel syndrome	Straight wrist, length equal to one-third of the forearm
Lateral epicondylitis	0°–20° wrist extension, slight radial inclination, length equal to one-third of the forearm
Wrist instabilities	Straight wrist, length equal to one-third of the forearm, pronosupination and inclination positions depending on the type of instability
Distal radius fracture with or without an ulnar styloid fracture	Straight wrist, length equal to two-thirds of the forearm
Distal ulna fracture	Straight wrist, length equal to two-thirds of the forearm

Fractures of the carpal bones	Straight wrist, length equal to two-thirds of the forearm
Wrist prosthesis or wrist arthrodesis	Straight wrist, length equal to two-thirds of the forearm
Resection of the first row of the carpus	Straight wrist, length equal to two-thirds of the forearm
Flexor carpi radialis and/or ulnaris tendon sutures with or without nerve or artery sutures	Straight or slightly flexed wrist (if there is nerve or artery damage), length equal to two-thirds of the forearm

Special supervision

It is important that MP joints and elbow mobility are not impeded

The therapist should always make sure the orthosis is comfortable and check for potential contact points that could injure the patient

11.5.2 Articular Wrist and Thumb TM and MP Joint Immobilization Orthosis

Characteristics of the orthosis

The orthosis covers the two-thirds of the forearm and allows mobility in the IP joint of the thumb and the MP joints of the fingers

Depending on the patient's morphology and the condition, the thickness of the thermoplastic will be chosen between 1.6 and 2.4 mm

Production method

The plastic is cut into a rectangular shape of which the length matches the distance between the thumb IP joint and the limit desired for the forearm. A small notch is cut to help mold the thumb. The patient is asked to rest the ulnar side of their arm on the table. Once the plastic is malleable, it is placed at the limit of the head of the proximal phalanx of the thumb. The therapist then wraps the plastic around the patient's arm, closing it on the dorsal surface of the forearm. The thumb is molded in a resting position with a slight flexion-abduction: 25° flexion, 25° abduction, and 15° pronation of the trapezio-metacarpal joint, as well as 10°–15° flexion of the metacarpophalangeal joint [8]. The opening around the thumb must be widened to leave space for the head of the proximal phalanx of the thumb which is wider than its shaft. The orthosis is cut along the palmar crease to free MP and IP joint mobility. The edges of the plastic are folded over around the IP thumb joint to allow comfortable flexion of this joint. The orthosis is fastened with three Velcro straps across the metacarpals, the wrist, and the forearm

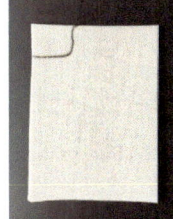 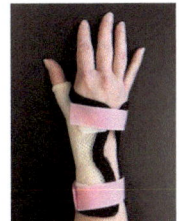 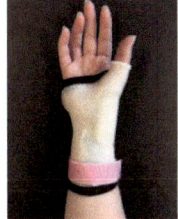

Suitable conditions	Specific characteristics
De Quervain's tenosynovitis	Straight wrist, thumb flexion (25°), and abduction (25°) leaving the IP joint free
Scaphoid fracture	Straight wrist, thumb flexion (25°), and abduction (25°) leaving the IP joint free
First metacarpal diaphysis fracture	Straight wrist, thumb flexion (25°), and abduction (25°) leaving the IP joint free

First metacarpal basis fracture	Straight wrist, thumb flexion (25°), and abduction (25°) leaving the IP joint free
Trapeziectomy-ligamentoplasty	Straight wrist, thumb flexion (25°), and abduction (25°) leaving the IP joint free. Make sure to puff out the zone around the pin
MAIA® prosthesis	Straight wrist, thumb flexion (25°), and abduction (25°) leaving the IP joint free

Special supervision

It is important to free the mobility of the IP thumb joint and the MP joints of the fingers

The therapist should always make sure the orthosis is comfortable and check for potential contact points that could injure the patient

11.5.3 Articular Thumb TM-MP Joint Immobilization Orthosis

Characteristics of the orthosis

The orthosis covers the TM and MP joints of the thumb and allows mobility in the wrist, the thumb IP joint, and the MP joints of the fingers

Depending on the patient's morphology and the condition, the thickness of the thermoplastic will be chosen between 1.6 and 2.4 mm

Production method

The plastic is cut into a rectangular shape of which the width matches the distance between the thumb IP joint and the wrist flexor crease, and the length measures the circumference of the hand including the thumb. A small notch is cut to help mold the thumb

The patient is asked to rest the ulnar side of their arm on the table. Once the plastic is malleable, it is placed at the limit of the head of the proximal phalanx of the thumb. The therapist then wraps the plastic around the patient's hand, closing it on the back. The thumb is molded in a resting position with slight flexion-abduction: 25° flexion, 25° abduction, and 15° pronation of the trapezio-metacarpal joint, as well as 10°–15° flexion of the metacarpophalangeal joint [9]

The opening around the thumb must be widened to leave space for the head of the proximal phalanx of the thumb which is wider than its shaft

The orthosis is cut along the palmar crease to free mobility of the MP and IP joints. The edges of the plastic are folded over around the thumb IP joint to allow comfortable flexion. The orthosis is fastened with one Velcro strap on the back of the hand across the metacarpals

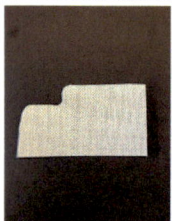 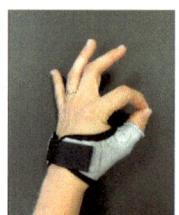 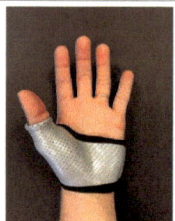

Suitable conditions	*Specific characteristics*
Ulnar collateral ligament sprain	Thumb flexion (25°) and abduction (25°) leaving the IP joint free. The plastic is slightly higher on the radial side of the thumb to go counter thumb valgus
Radial collateral ligament sprain	Thumb flexion (25°) and abduction (25°) leaving the IP joint free. The plastic is slightly higher on the ulnar side of the thumb to counter thumb varus
Trapezio-metacarpal arthritis	Thumb flexion (25°) and abduction (25°) leaving the IP joint free
Carpo-metacarpal arthritis	Thumb flexion (25°) and abduction (25°) leaving the IP joint free
MP joint arthritis	Thumb flexion (25°) and abduction (25°) leaving the IP joint free
MP joint dislocation	Thumb flexion (25°) and abduction (25°) leaving the IP joint free

Special supervision

It is important to free the mobility of the wrist, the thumb IP joint, and the MP joints of the fingers

The therapist should always make sure the orthosis is comfortable and check for potential contact points that could injure the patient

11.5.4 Articular Finger CM-MP Joint Immobilization Orthosis

Characteristics of the orthosis

The orthosis is different depending on the type of fracture and its stability

Depending on the patient's morphology, the thickness of the thermoplastic will be chosen between 1.6 and 2.4 mm

Production method

The plastic is cut into a rectangular shape of which the length and the width vary depending on the decision that is made to immobilize the wrist or the IP joints or not

The patient is asked to rest their elbow on the table with the ulnar side of their hand facing the therapist. For fractures of the fourth and fifth fingers, the therapist wraps the plastic around the ulnar side of the hand, the fingers and the wrist if needed, placing the MP joints at 60° of flexion [9] and the IP joints straight if they need to be immobilized [10]. For fractures of the index and middle finger, a hole is cut in the plastic to slip the thumb through to wrap it around the fingers (and the wrist if necessary), and then the therapist places the joints in the correct position

The orthosis is cut to allow the mobility of all non-injured fingers and joints depending on the fracture (wrist, IP, and/or MP joints). If the wrist is immobilized, the zone around the ulnar styloid can be puffed out or protected with foam if needed

The orthosis is fastened with Velcro straps around the forearm, the wrist and across the MP joints and the fingers according to the case

 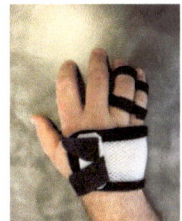 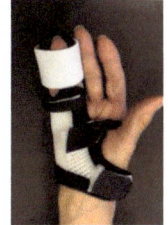 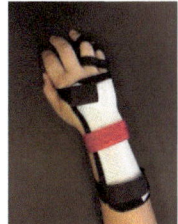

Suitable conditions	Specific characteristics
Finger MP joint sprain	Syndactylies
First phalanx head of shaft fracture (operated or not)	Wrist free, 60° flexion of the MP joints, IP joints straight
First phalanx base fracture (operated or not)	Wrist free, 60° flexion of the MP joints, IP joints free with syndactyly
Metacarpal head fracture (not operated)	Wrist free, 60° flexion of the MP joints, IP joints free with syndactyly
Metacarpal head fracture treated by pinning	Protection shell with wrist free and fingers free with syndactylies
Metacarpal shaft fracture (operated or not)	Protection shell with wrist free and fingers free with syndactylies
Metacarpal base fracture (operated or not)	0°–20° wrist extension, fingers free with syndactylies

Special supervision

It is important to make sure that the orthosis does not impede the mobility of the non-injured fingers and the joints that the therapist chooses to free

The therapist should always make sure the orthosis is comfortable and check for potential contact points that could injure the patient

11.5.5 Articular Finger IP Joint Immobilization Orthosis

Characteristics of the orthosis

The orthosis covers the finger to a greater or lesser extent according to the injury

Depending on the patient's morphology, the thickness of the thermoplastic will be chosen between 1.6 and 2.4 mm

Production method

The plastic is cut into a rectangular shape large enough to wrap around the patient's finger and tall enough to cover the joints that need to be immobilized. Once the plastic is malleable, the therapist folds over the edges of the plastic on what will be the bottom of the orthosis

The patient is asked to rest their elbow on the table with the ulnar side of their hand facing the therapist who then places the hem of the plastic at the base of the finger (or at the base of second phalanx if the PIP joint is left free), wrapping the plastic around the patient's finger and pinching it on the radial or ulnar side as well as at the distal extremity. The PIP joint is set in a straight position (to tighten the radial and ulnar collateral ligaments to avoid stiffness in this joint according to the study of Sandhu et al. [10])

The orthosis is cut along the radial or ulnar side leaving a small slit to make it adjustable (important in case of edema and for the patient's comfort)

The orthosis is fastened with one or two thin circular Velcro straps (about 1 cm large)

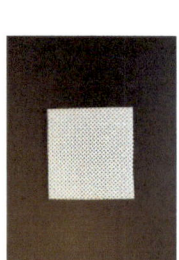 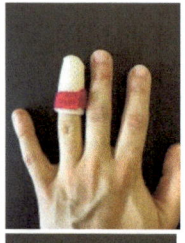 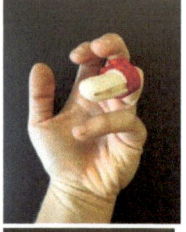 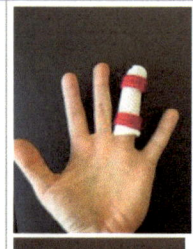
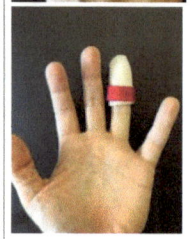 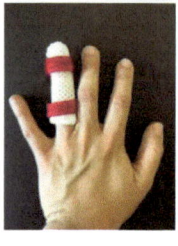 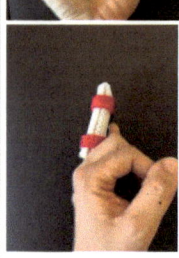

Suitable conditions	*Specific characteristics*
PIP or DIP joint arthritis	PIP and DIP joints extension with radial slit—Do not force the position if there are osteophytes
Volar plate sprain	PIP and DIP joints extension at night/syndactylies during the day
First phalanx head fracture	PIP and DIP joints extension
Second phalanx base or shaft fracture	PIP and DIP joints extension
Second phalanx head fracture of third phalanx fracture	DIP joint extension, PIP joint free
Extensor tendon suture in zone 3 (fingers)	PIP joint extension, DIP joint free
Extensor tendon suture in zones 1 and 2 (fingers)	DIP joint hyper-extension (<15°), PIP joint free
Extensor tendon suture in zone 1 and 2 (thumb)	IP joint extension, MP joint free

Special supervision

It is important to make sure that the orthosis does not impede the mobility of the joints that should be free

The therapist should always make sure the orthosis is comfortable and check for potential contact points that could injure the patient

11.5.6 "Stack" Orthosis—Articular Finger DIP Joint Immobilization Orthosis

Characteristics of the orthosis
The orthosis covers the dorsal side of the second phalanx and the palmar side of the third phalanx, placing the DIP joint in a hyper-extension position that does not exceed 15°
A "thin" thermoplastic is most suitable (1.6 mm)

Production method
The plastic is cut into a rectangular shape large enough to wrap around the patient's finger and tall enough to cover the last two phalanx
The patient is asked to rest their elbow on the table with the ulnar side of their hand facing the therapist who then wraps the plastic around the patient's finger, pinching it on the radial or ulnar side. The DIP joint is set in a hyper-extension position (<15° according to Evans [11])
The orthosis is cut along the radial or ulnar side, leaving the second phalanx free on its palmar side, as well as the fingernail. A piece of plastic can be added to the side where the plastic was cut to reinforce the orthosis. The plastic should be slightly puffed out around the dorsal extremity of the orthosis to avoid compressing the nail bed
The orthosis is maintained with non-stretch surgical tape around the second phalanx making sure to leave the PIP joint free

 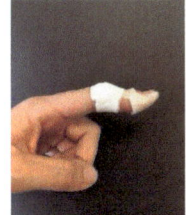 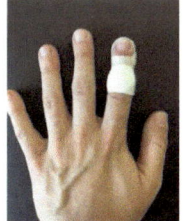 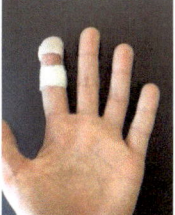

Suitable conditions	*Specific characteristics*
Non-operated tendinous mallet finger (extensor tendon tear in zones 1–2)	Slight hyper-extension of the DIP joint <15°, PIP joint free
Non-operated osseous mallet finger	DIP joint straight

Special supervision
It is important to make sure that the orthosis does not impede the mobility of the PIP joint
The therapist should always make sure the orthosis is comfortable and check for potential contact points that could injure the patient

11.5.7 "Modified Duran" Orthosis— Articular Wrist, Finger MP-IP Joint (or Thumb TM-MP-IP Joints) Immobilization Orthosis

Characteristics of the orthosis
The orthosis is dorsal and covers the distal third section of the forearm and the fingers. If the flexor pollicis longus tendon is damaged, the orthosis covers the thumb, leaving the fingers free
A 2.4 mm thick thermoplastic is most suitable

Production method

The plastic is cut into a rectangular shape with one curved edge. The length matches the distance between the finger extremities and the distal third section of the forearm. A small notch is cut on one side of the rectangle to simplify leaving the thumb free
The patient is asked to rest their elbow on the table with the ulnar side of their hand facing the therapist who places their hand in a protective position with the wrist and the fingers slightly flexed. Once the plastic is malleable, it is placed on the back of the hand and the forearm. The plastic is pinched in two places around the wrist and the forearm and molded around the ulnar side of the hand and the small finger as well as the radial side of the index. The plastic can be puffed out around the ulnar styloid or it can be protected with foam if needed
The orthosis is fastened with four Velcro straps as follows:

- a non-stretch Velcro strap around the forearm
- a thin elastic Velcro strap around the wrist
- a non-stretch Velcro strap reinforced with thermoplastic molded against the transversal metacarpal arch at the palm of the hand made to act as a counter support for the hand to maintain it in the orthosis
- a large elastic Velcro strap around the fingers or the thumb

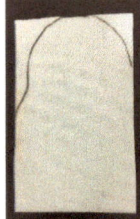 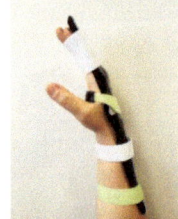 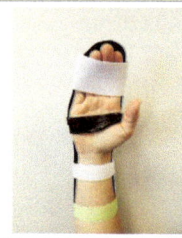

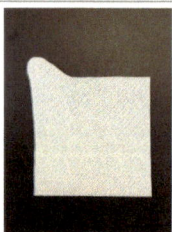 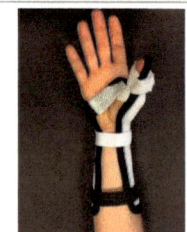 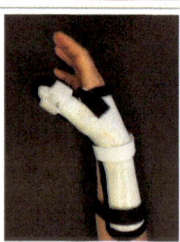

Suitable conditions	*Specific characteristics*
Suture of one or several flexor tendons (superficialis or profundus) of one or several fingers	0°–30° wrist flexion, 15° MP joint flexion [8], PIP and DIP joints straight. Thumb free
Specific case: Suture of the flexor pollicis longus tendon	30° wrist flexion, 30° TM joint abduction, 15°–60° MP joint flexion [12], IP joint straight. Fingers free (except the index finger in the case of Linburg syndrome)

Special supervision

It is important to make sure that the orthosis does not impede the mobility of the thumb for sutures of the finger flexor tendons, and the mobility of the fingers for sutures of the flexor pollicis longus. The elastic Velcro strap around the fingers or the thumb should not be too tight
The therapist should always make sure the orthosis is comfortable and check for potential contact points that could injure the patient

11.5.8 Articular Finger PIP Joint Immobilization Orthosis

Characteristics of the orthosis	
The orthosis covers the first and the second phalanx placing the PIP joint straight and leaving the DIP joint free	
Depending on the patient's morphology, the thickness of the thermoplastic will be chosen between 1.6 and 2.4 mm	
Production method	
The plastic is cut into a rectangular shape large enough to wrap around the patient's finger and tall enough to cover the first two phalanx	
The patient is asked to rest their elbow on the table with the ulnar side of their hand facing the therapist who then wraps the plastic around the patient's finger, pinching it on the radial or ulnar side, making sure to leave the DIP joint free and placing the PIP joint straight (the protective position for the central slip [11])	
The orthosis is fastened with two thin Velcro straps located at each extremity	

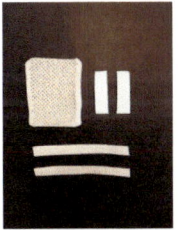 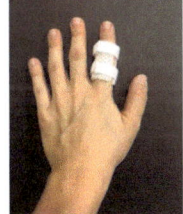 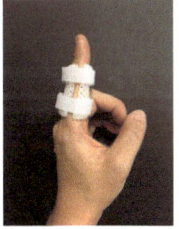

Suitable conditions	*Specific characteristics*
Central slip injury (extensor tendon in zone 3)	PIP joint straight, DIP joint free

Special supervision
The therapist should always make sure the orthosis is comfortable and check for potential contact points that could injure the patient

11.5.9 Articular Wrist, Finger MP-IP Joint Immobilization Orthosis

Characteristics of the orthosis
The orthosis is palmar and covers the wrist and the fingers
A 2.4 mm thick thermoplastic is most suitable
Production method
The plastic is cut into a rectangular shape. A small notch is cut on one side of the rectangle to simplify leaving the thumb free
The patient is asked to rest their elbow on the table with the ulnar side of their hand facing the therapist who places their hand in a protective position. Once the plastic is malleable, it is placed on the palm of the hand and the forearm. The plastic is pinched in two places on the dorsal side of the wrist and the forearm and molded around the ulnar side of the hand and the small finger as well as the radial side of the index. The ulnar styloid can be freed by cutting a small notch or the plastic can be puffed out around it
The orthosis is fastened with four Velcro straps as follows:
• a non-stretch Velcro strap around the forearm
• a thin elastic Velcro strap around the wrist
• a thin elastic Velcro strap across the metacarpals
• a large elastic Velcro strap around the fingers

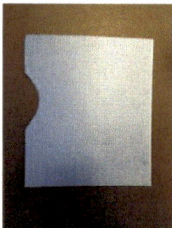 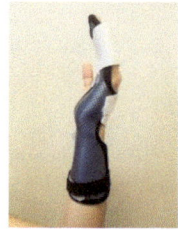 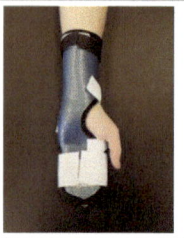 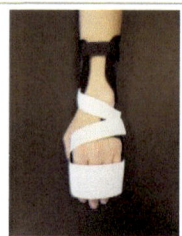

Suitable conditions	Specific characteristics
Suture of one or several extensor tendons (zones 4 to 8)	30° wrist extension, 0°–70° MP joint flexion, IP joints straight [13]

Special supervision

The therapist should always make sure the orthosis is comfortable and check for potential contact points that could injure the patient

11.5.10 Articular Wrist Immobilization and MP Joint (of the Injured Finger) Restriction Orthosis

Characteristics of the orthosis

The orthosis has two components. The first part is a palmar orthosis immobilizing the wrist at 25° of extension, and the second part is a yoke splint that places the MP joint of the injured finger with 15°–20° more extension than the other fingers

A 2.4 mm thick thermoplastic is most suitable

Production method

The plastic is cut into a rectangular shape. The patient is asked to rest their elbow on the table with the ulnar side of their hand facing the therapist who places the wrist in a slightly extended position. Once the plastic is malleable, it is placed on the palm of the hand and the forearm. The plastic is pinched in three places on the back of the hand, the dorsal side of the wrist and the forearm. The ulnar styloid can be freed by cutting a small notch in the plastic around it. The orthosis is fastened with three non-stretch Velcro straps across the metacarpals and around the wrist and the forearm

For the yoke splint, the plastic is cut into a long band as wide as the patient's first phalanx. The molding depends on the finger that is injured. For the annular and the middle fingers, the adjacent fingers will act as support for the orthosis, placing the injured finger with 15°–20° more extension than the others. Start on the palmar side of one of the adjacent fingers to be able to mold the yoke splint in one go, making two rings for the adjacent fingers and a palmar hammock to support the injured finger in the right position. For the index and small fingers, an extension must be made around the radial side (for the index finger) or around the ulnar side (for the small finger). Always make sure to not mold too tightly to avoid compression risks

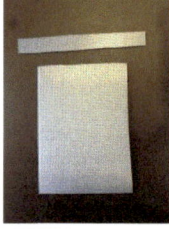 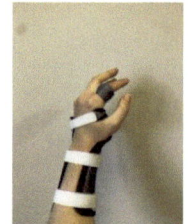 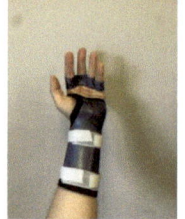 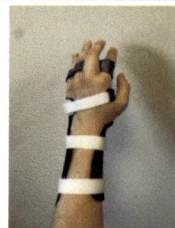

Suitable conditions	Specific characteristics
Suture of one or several extensor tendons (zones 4 to 8)	25° wrist extension, 15°–20° more extension of the MP joints of the injured finger compared to the others [14]

Special supervision

The therapist should always make sure the orthosis is comfortable and check for potential contact points that could injure the patient

11.5.11 Articular Wrist, Thumb TM-MP-IP Joint Immobilization Orthosis

Characteristics of the orthosis	
The orthosis is palmar and covers the wrist and the thumb. The fingers must be completely free	
A 2.4 mm thick thermoplastic is most suitable	
Production method	
The plastic is cut into a shape tailored to follow the thumb's position whose direction is opposite the fingers. The patient is asked to rest their elbow on the table with the ulnar side of their hand facing the therapist who places the wrist and the thumb in an extension. Once the plastic is malleable, it is placed on the palm of the hand, the forearm, and the thumb. The plastic is pinched in three places on the dorsal side of the thumb, the wrist, and the forearm. The ulnar styloid can be freed by cutting a small notch in the plastic or it can be puffed out around it	
The orthosis is fastened with four Velcro straps as follows:	

- a non-stretch Velcro strap around the forearm
- a non-stretch Velcro strap around the wrist
- a thin elastic Velcro strap across the metacarpals
- a thin elastic Velcro strap around the IP joint of the thumb

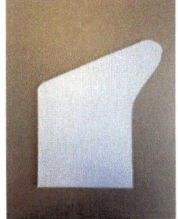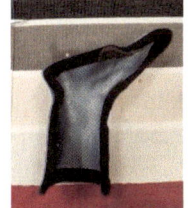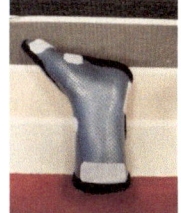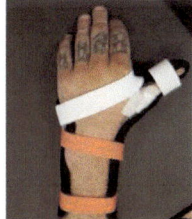

Suitable conditions	*Specific characteristics*
Suture of the extensor pollicis (zones 1 to 7)	30° wrist extension, 20°–30° extension and adduction of the TM joint, MP and IP joints straight
Special supervision	
The therapist should always make sure the orthosis is comfortable and check for potential contact points that could injure the patient	

11.6 Articular Mobilization Orthoses

11.6.1 Range Gaining Orthoses

These orthoses aim to increase mobility by means of an external force. Their efficiency depends on the intensity and the duration of the applied force [15]. The best efficiency that enables tissue growth (and not stretching of existing fibers) is obtained by applying a low intensity force (between 100 and 250 g) during a long period of time (at least 6 h/day) [16, 17] (Fig. 11.21).

Furthermore, the results are maximized if this protocol is established 2–3 months after the injury at the latest [17].

In certain cases of chronic stiffness, particularly for PIP joint flessums, the patient can wear the orthosis non-stop for a few days with satisfying results [18].

Considering that a flexed position can be dangerous on a vascular level, flexion orthoses are worn several times a day for relatively short periods of time (about 20 min), whereas extension orthoses are easier to tolerate all night.

There are four types of range gaining orthoses as follows:

- **Serial static orthoses**: These orthoses are static, molded in a position creating tension in the hypo-expandable tissues. They are regularly modified to adapt to the decline in tissue resistance.
- **Dynamic orthoses**: These orthoses apply a dynamic force to a specific joint in a direction that creates tension in the hypo-expandable

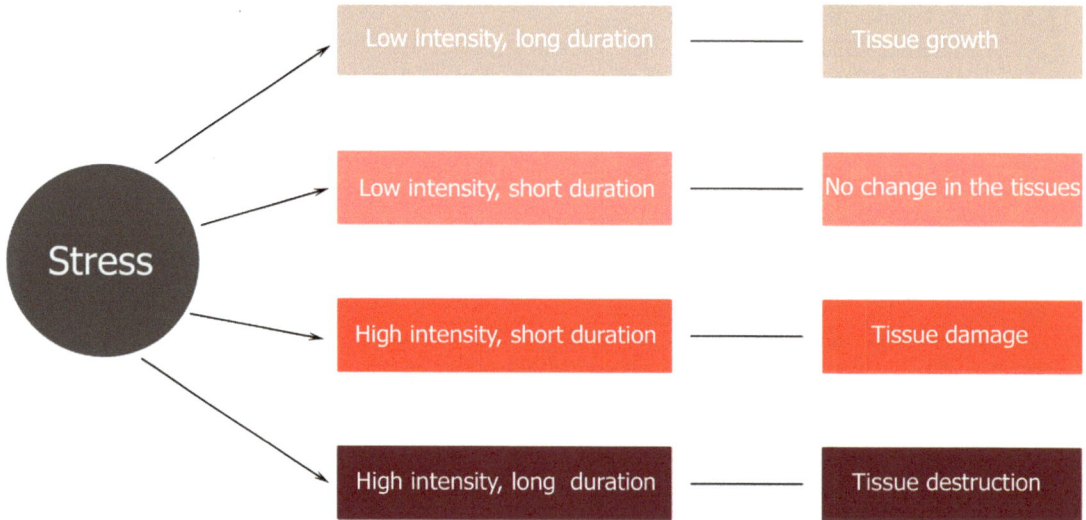

Fig. 11.21 Connective tissue response to applied stress. Tissue growth is obtained using low intensity force applied at least 6 h/day

tissues. The force can be generated by an elastic band, a Levame blade or a piano wire.

- **Static progressive orthoses**: Their design is similar to that of dynamic orthoses, except that the applied force is not dynamic. For example, the force can be conveyed by a worm screw or a non-elastic Velcro strap.
- **Torque transmission orthoses**: The aim of these orthoses is to redirect the internal forces of one or several joints to encourage the effect of one muscular mechanism compared to another. This type of orthosis is not considered as an "articular mobilization orthosis" and will be discussed in the Sect. 11.8, "Torque Transmission Orthoses."

To choose the most suitable orthosis for each case of stiffness, the Weeks test is extremely useful. The test is based on gain in range of motion after a 30-min session consisting of a 15-min warm up (hot bath or heating pads), followed by 10–15 min of passive mobilization by a hand therapist [19]:

- If the gain is superior to 20°, no need for an orthosis
- 15° gain: serial static orthoses
- 10° gain: dynamic orthosis
- If the gain is inferior to 5°: static progressive orthosis

In addition, the ASHT (American Society of Hand Therapists) proposes to choose the most suitable range gaining orthosis based on the injured tissues' stage in their healing process (Fig. 11.22).

11.6.1.1 Serial Static Orthoses

Articular PIP Extension Mobilization Orthoses

This orthosis targets gaining extension in the proximal interphalangeal joint. It can be made of thermoplastic (2.4 mm thick), Orficast© or plaster [20], applying slight strain towards extension while molding. The patient must not feel any pain when molding is done. The orthosis must completely cover the first phalanx to reduce friction and be the most efficient as possible (Fig. 11.23). The orthosis is circular which distributes the mechanical strain not only across the whole surface of the finger but also at three contact points (Fig. 11.24).

The orthosis is remolded frequently to adapt to the decline in tension of the injured tissues and the trophic status of the treated finger.

Articular Finger MP and IP Joint Extension Mobilization Orthosis

This orthosis targets extension in all the finger joints. It is made of thermoplastic that is 2.4 mm

INFLAMMATORY	PROLIFERATIVE	CELL MATURATION
Articular mobilization serial static orthosis		
	Articular mobilization static progressive orthosis	
	Articular mobilization dynamic orthosis	
		Torque transmission orthosis

Fig. 11.22 Choosing the most suitable range gaining orthosis based on the healing phase according to the ASHT (American Society of Hand Therapists)

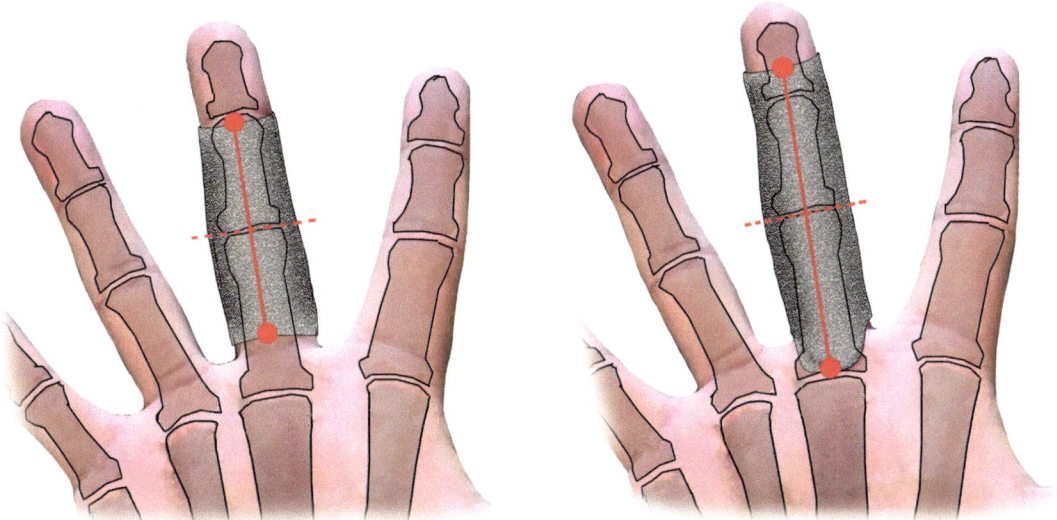

Fig. 11.23 In order to completely cover the first phalanx, the orthosis must be more proximal than the neighboring commissures

thick), applying slight strain towards extension while molding. The wrist can be covered or not according to the leverage needed and the histological origin of the stiffness (see Chap. 2) (Fig. 11.25).

11.6.1.2 Static Progressive Orthoses
Static progressive orthoses are adjustable and use a force applied by the means of a Velcro strap or a worm screw (Fig. 11.26) and not a

"dynamic" force, as articular dynamic mobilization orthoses do.

11.6.1.3 Dynamic Orthoses

Pro-Flexion
To avoid vascular disorders due to a flexed position during a long period of time, this type of orthoses is worn for short amounts of time (around 20 min), several times per day. The

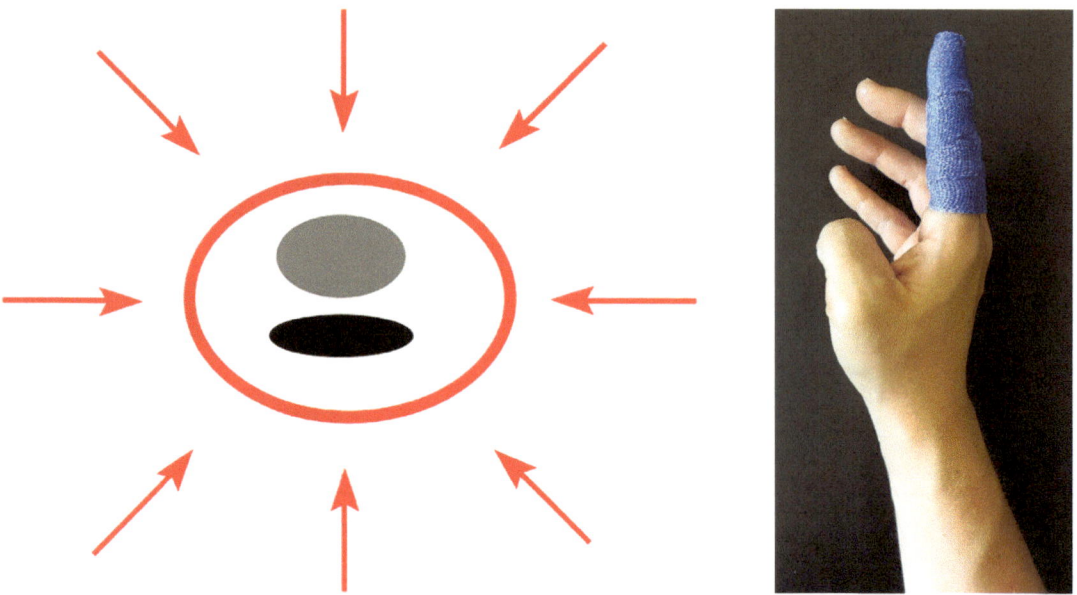

Fig. 11.24 Articular PIP extension mobilization orthosis made of Orficast©. The circular form of this orthosis evenly distributes the mechanical strain across the whole surface of the finger

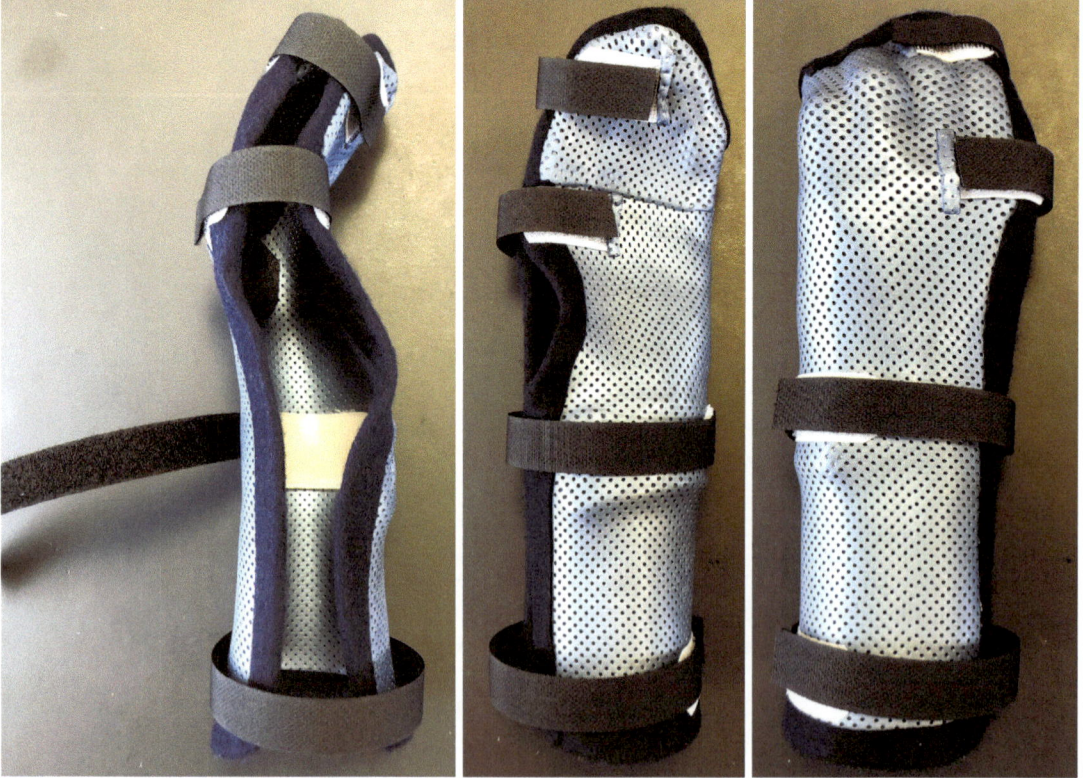

Fig. 11.25 Articular MP and IP finger joints extension mobilization orthosis. In this example, the slight strain applied during the first molding process made for a slightly flexed position of the MP and IP joints

Orthèse statique progressive

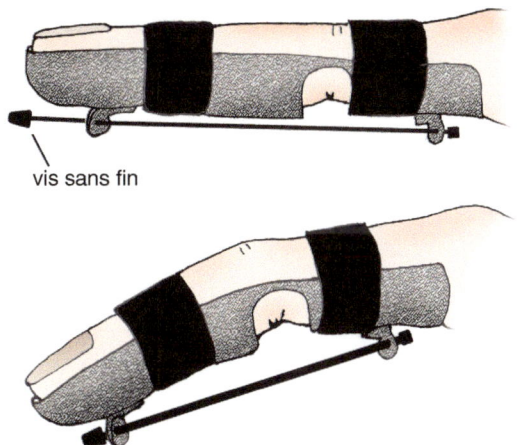

vis sans fin

Fig. 11.26 Static progressive orthosis with a worm screw (articular PIP extension mobilization orthosis)

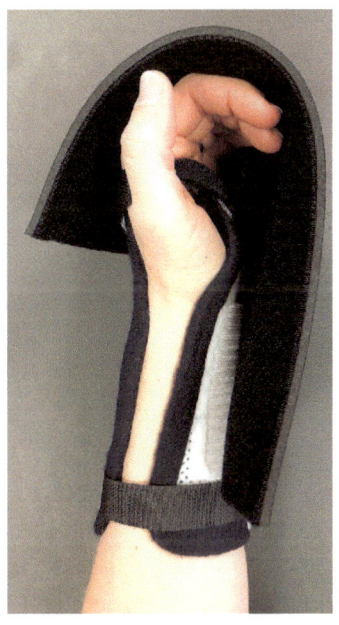

Fig. 11.27 Articular finger MP-PIP-DIP joint flexion mobilization orthosis made of thermoplastic

applied force is defined by the patient's pain: they should feel slight tension without pain to avoid tissue damage. The direction of the strain must follow the flexion axis of the fingers that all merge towards the scaphoid tubercule. The position should be released progressively to avoid pain, and it is recommended that the patients mobilize their fingers after each positioning period.

Articular Finger MP-PIP-DIP Joint Flexion Mobilization Orthosis

This orthosis is addressed to patients presenting global stiffness in one or several fingers. To avoid piston effect, the wrist is included in the static element of the orthosis, made of either a 2.4 mm thick thermoplastic (Fig. 11.27) or neoprene fabric (Fig. 11.28). The orthosis is closed on the ulnar side of the forearm if the three radial fingers are targeted, and on the radial side of the forearm if the two ulnar fingers are aimed. A strap of hook Velcro is glued on the dorsal side of the orthosis to attach a low-resistant band of neoprene fabric that will stretch over the fingers that need posturing. Making sure to follow the flexion axis of the fingers (Fig. 11.29), the neoprene band is attached to a long strap of hook Velcro glued on the palmar

side of the orthosis, adjusting the tension according to the patient's pain.

To adapt to eventual trophic disorders or pain, the neoprene band can be replaced by a less aggressive elastic Velcro strap (Fig. 11.30).

Articular MP Joint Flexion Mobilization Orthosis (Fingers/Thumb)

This orthosis is addressed to patients presenting analytical stiffness in the metacarpophalangeal joints in the fingers or the thumb.

For fingers, the base of the mobilizing strap is an orthosis placing the wrist in a straight position. The distal limit of the orthosis follows the palmar crease, allowing complete metacarpophalangeal joint mobility. The edge can be reinforced by folding over the plastic and should be covered with a protective foam material. To have an impact on the four fingers, the mobilizing strap is fastened to the ulnar side of a piece of plastic fused perpendicularly on the palmar side of the wrist orthosis, then goes across the dorsal side of the first phalanx. It is fastened to the radial side of another piece of plastic with the same direction

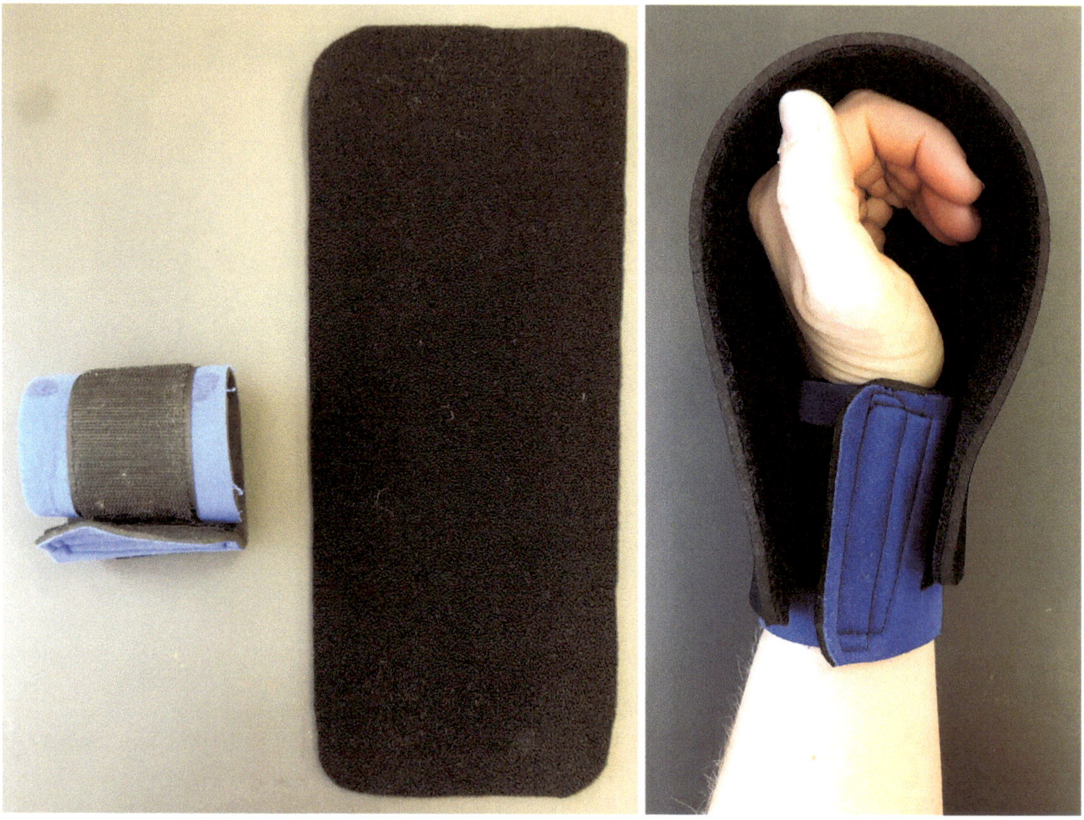

Fig. 11.28 Articular finger MP-PIP-DIP joint flexion mobilization orthosis made of neoprene fabric

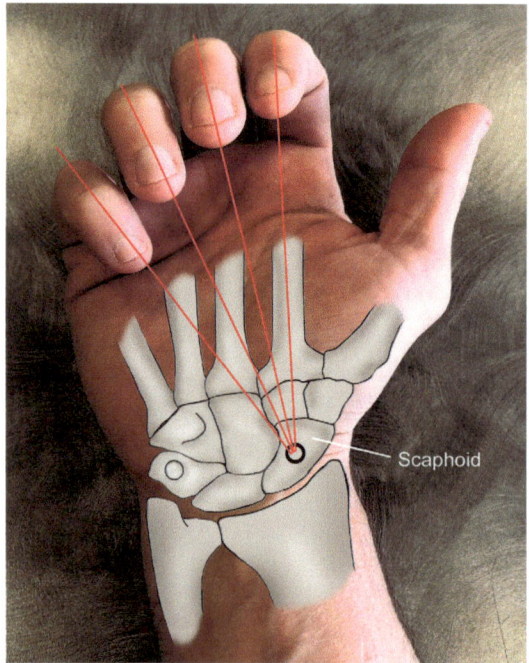

Fig. 11.29 Flexion axis of the fingers

as the first one (Fig. 11.31). If one or more fingers are specifically aimed, the position of the two pieces of plastic must simply be adjusted (Fig. 11.32). The mobilizing strap can be reinforced using a piece of thermoplastic molded across the dorsal side of the first phalanx in order to increase the tension (Fig. 11.33). The same effect can also be obtained by replacing the elastic mobilizing strap with hammocks made of Orficast© tied to elastic strings attached to hooks fused to the palmar side of the wrist orthosis at multiple levels (Fig. 11.34). For each production method, the tensile force must be perpendicular to the first phalanx, making it more efficient while avoiding compressive stress on the metacarpophalangeal joints.

For the thumb, the base of the mobilizing strap is a gauntlet immobilizing the trapeziometacarpal joint allowing metacarpophalangeal and interphalangeal joint mobility.

According to the tension tolerated by the patient, the motor can be either an elastic Velcro

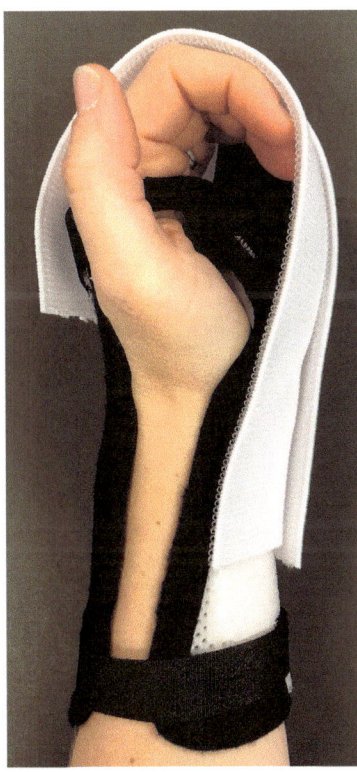

Fig. 11.30 Low-tension articular finger MP-PIP-DIP joint flexion mobilization orthosis made of thermoplastic using elastic Velcro straps.

or neoprene strap fastened to a piece of plastic fused to the orthosis following the flexion axis of the thumb, or a hammock made of Orficast© tied to an elastic string attached to hooks fused to the palmar side of the orthosis at multiple levels (Fig. 11.35).

Articular PIP Joint Flexion Mobilization Orthosis for Fingers (and the IP Joint of the Thumb)

This orthosis is addressed to patients presenting analytical stiffness in the proximal interphalangeal joints of the fingers or the interphalangeal joint of the thumb.

For the fingers, the base of the mobilizing strap is an orthosis immobilizing the metacarpophalangeal joints in a straight position if the stiffness is caused by interossei muscle tightness, and in a flexed position if the stiffness is caused by adhesion of the extensor tendon on the dorsal side of the first phalanx. If the stiffness has and articular origin, the position of the metacarpophalangeal joint is indifferent (see Chap. 2). The distal limit of the orthosis follows the crease of the proximal interphalangeal joint and the edge can be reinforced by folding over the

Fig. 11.31 Articular MP joint flexion mobilization orthosis for all four fingers

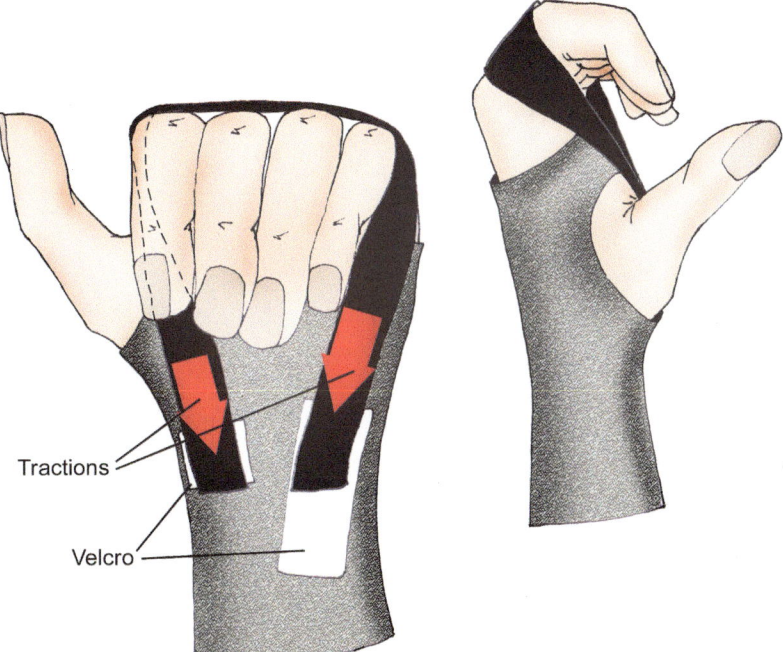

Flexion of the metacarpophalangeal joints

Fig. 11.32 Articular
MP joint flexion
mobilization orthosis for
one finger

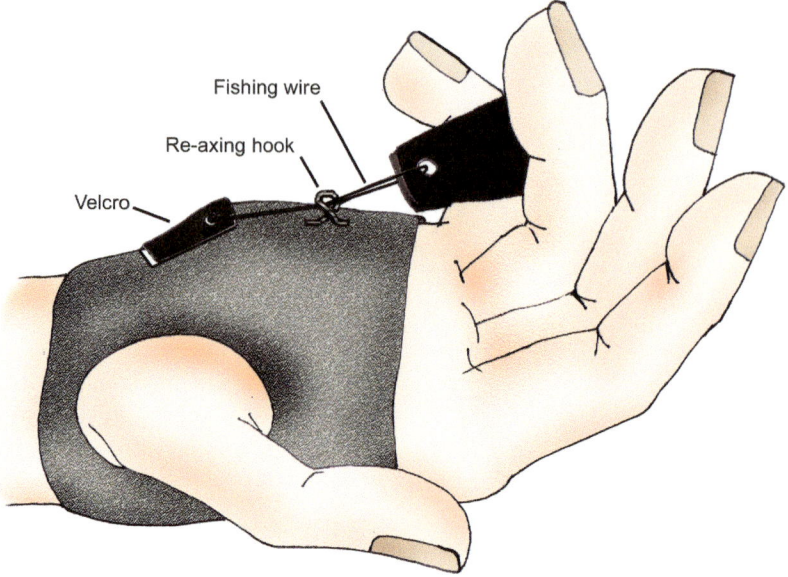

Fig. 11.33 Articular MP joint flexion mobilization
orthosis for all four fingers with a thermoplastic reinforcement across the dorsal side of the first phalanx

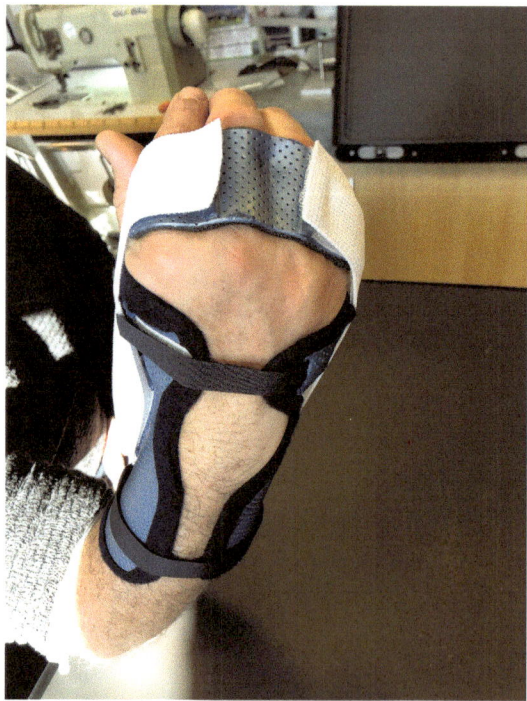

Fig. 11.34 Articular MP joint flexion mobilization
orthosis for all four fingers using hammocks made of
Orficast© tied to elastic strings attached to hooks

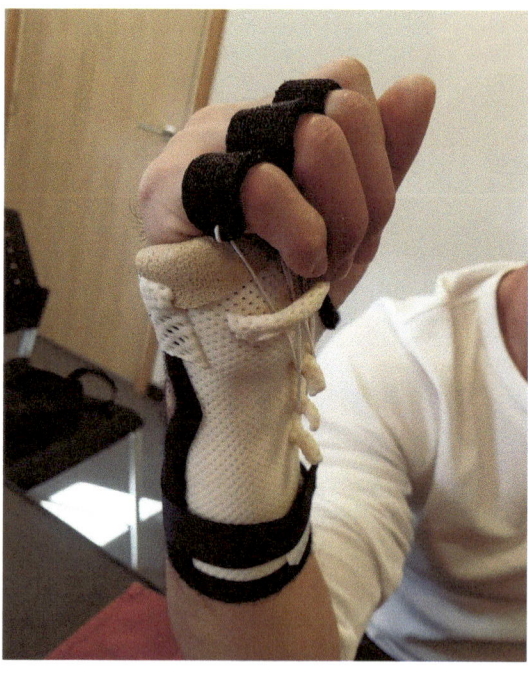

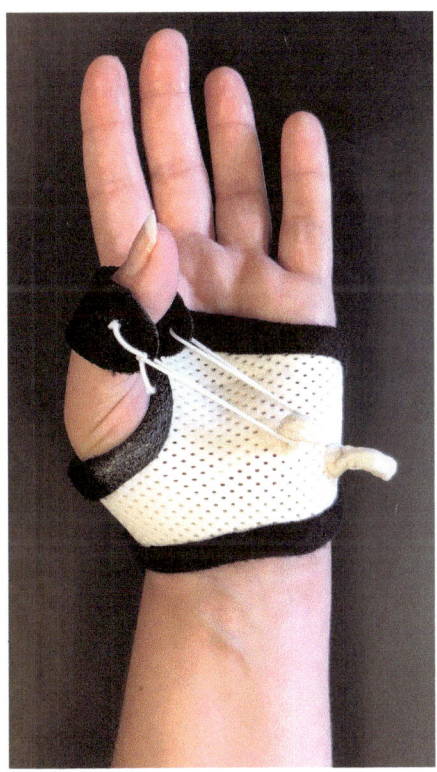

Fig. 11.35 Articular MP joint flexion mobilization orthosis for the thumb

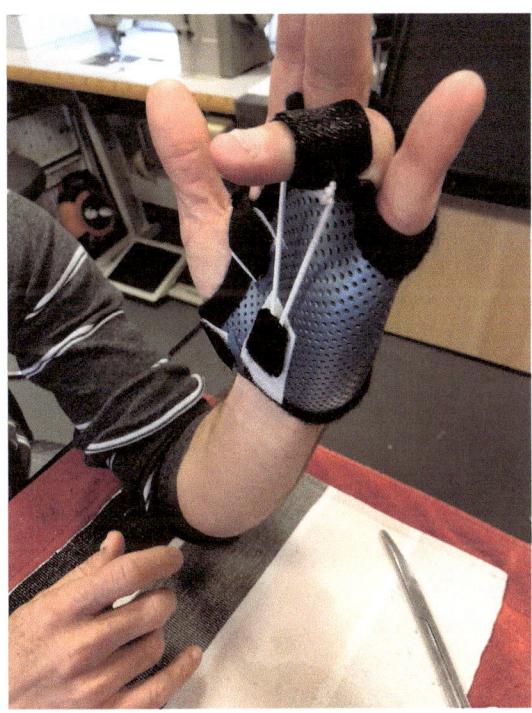

Fig. 11.36 Articular PIP joint flexion mobilization orthosis for one finger

plastic. The mobilizing strap is fastened to the back side of the orthosis, goes across the dorsal side of the aimed finger bringing it to a flexed position, and finishes attached to the palmar side of the orthosis, following the flexion axis of the finger. The mobilizing strap can be an elastic Velcro strap, a band of neoprene or a hammock made of Orficast© tied to an elastic string (Fig. 11.36).

For the thumb, the base of the mobilizing strap is an orthosis immobilizing the trapezio-metacarpal and the metacarpophalangeal joints, allowing complete mobility of the interphalangeal joint of the thumb. According to the tension tolerated by the patient, the motor can be either an elastic Velcro or neoprene strap fastened to a piece of hook Velcro glued to the palmar side of the orthosis following the flexion axis of the thumb, or a cap made of Orficast© tied to an elastic string (Fig. 11.37).

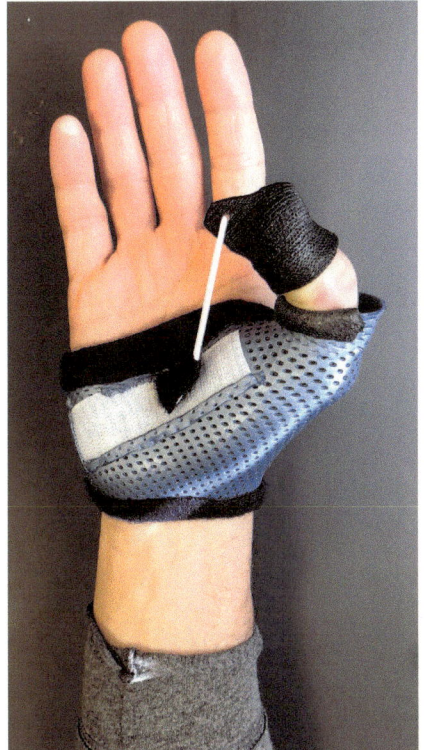

Fig. 11.37 Articular IP thumb joint flexion mobilization orthosis

Articular Interphalangeal Joint Flexion Mobilization Orthosis for Fingers

This orthosis is addressed to patients presenting analytical stiffness in the interphalangeal joints of the fingers.

The orthosis can be made of a 1.6 mm thick thermoplastic or a thin strap of neoprene.

The orthosis made of thermoplastic has two components: a flat plate covering the dorsal side of the first phalanx and a cap around the third phalanx freeing the flexion crease of the distal interphalangeal joint. A piece of hook Velcro is glued to the plate and to the cap across the fingernail (Fig. 11.38). The flexed position is obtained using an elastic Velcro strap that brings the two components together (Fig. 11.39).

The neoprene orthosis is one component made of a 1.5–2 cm wide neoprene band that is about 20 cm long. The band is sewed making a snug loop for the first phalanx whose size is adjusted to each patient, keeping the velvet side of the neoprene fabric on the outside. A piece of

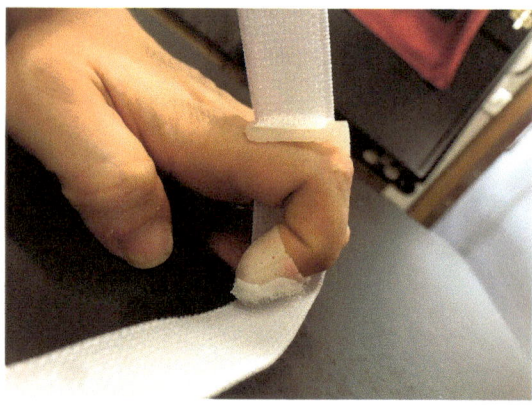

Fig. 11.39 How to set up an articular interphalangeal joint flexion mobilization orthosis for one finger made of thermoplastic

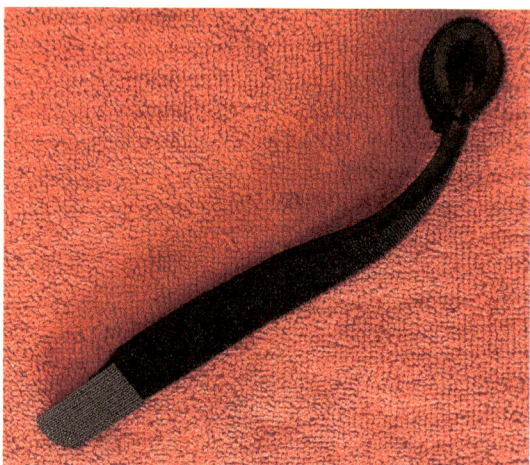

Fig. 11.40 Articular interphalangeal joint flexion mobilization orthosis for one finger made of neoprene

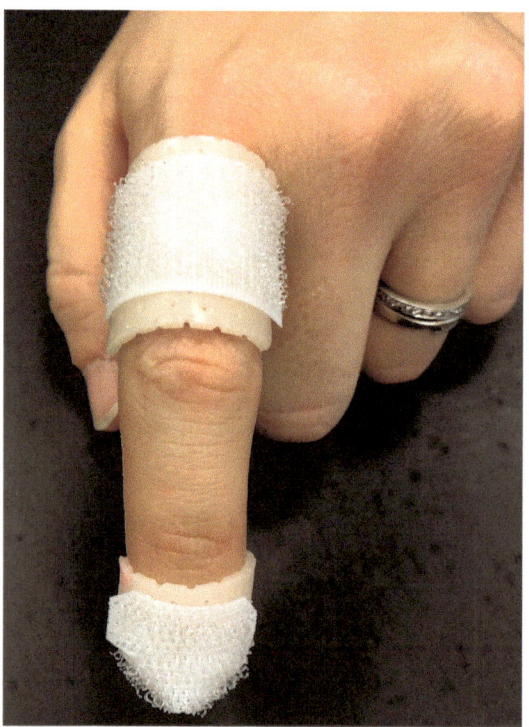

Fig. 11.38 The two components of and articular interphalangeal joint flexion mobilization orthosis for one finger made of thermoplastic

hook Velcro is sewed to the extremity of the leftover strip (Fig. 11.40). The loop is placed around the patient's first phalanx, leaving the leftover strip of the neoprene towards the back of the hand (Fig. 11.41). The strip is then pulled around the third phalanx bringing it more or less towards the first phalanx and fastened to the velvet side of the neoprene loop around the first phalanx (Fig. 11.42).

Pro-Extension

Just like pro-flexion orthoses, the efficiency of pro-extension orthoses depends on the period of time they are worn and not their high tension. The applied stress is defined by the patient's pain: they should feel slight tension without pain to avoid tissue damage. Generally, pro-extension orthoses are worn at night so that the patient's hand can be used normally during the day. The position should be released progressively to avoid pain, and it is recommended that the patient mobilize their fingers after each positioning period.

Articular MP-PIP-DIP Joint Extension Mobilization Orthosis for the Fingers or "Levame" Orthosis

The motor of this dynamic orthosis is a "Levame" blade (the name of its inventor). The base of the blade(s) is a gauntlet that slightly covers the metacarpophalangeal joints. This contact surface is protected with a foam material. A blade is mounted to the back of the orthosis with a rivet for each finger that needs to be treated. It is essential that the blades follow the direction of the fingers' opening axis to respect the physiological architecture of the hand (Fig. 11.43). The blades are cut to match the length of each finger and the extremity must be protected with a foam material. Each finger is secured in an extended position using a Velcro strap fastened across the DIP

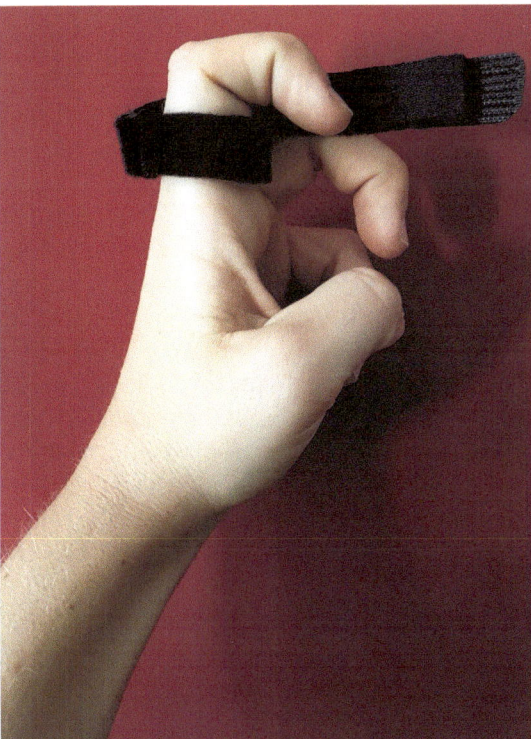

Fig. 11.41 Starting point to set up an articular interphalangeal joint flexion mobilization orthosis for one finger made of neoprene

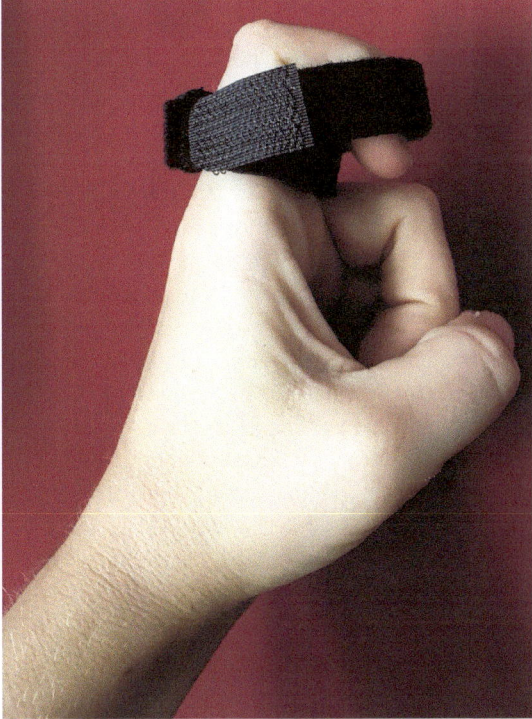

Fig. 11.42 Finished set up of an articular interphalangeal joint flexion mobilization orthosis for one finger made of neoprene

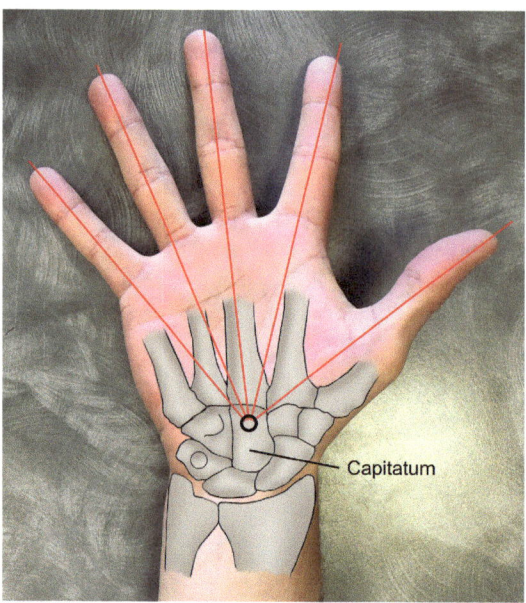

Fig. 11.43 Axis of each finger during the opening of the hand

joint (to avoid its hyper-extension). This orthosis offers global extension action for the whole finger (Fig. 11.44).

In some cases, it can be necessary to mold the base orthosis covering the dorsal side of the finger(s) up to the PIP joint to obtain analytical action on this joint (Fig. 11.45).

Articular PIP Joint Extension Mobilization Orthosis or "Capener" Orthosis

The Capener extension orthosis acts using two palmar contact surfaces and one dorsal counter contact surface. It is designed to address proximal interphalangeal joint flexion deformity. The two palmar contact surfaces are located against the metacarpal head and the head of the second phalanx (Fig. 11.46). The dorsal counter contact surface is located on the dorsal side of the first phalanx (Fig. 11.47). The orthosis is made of 1.6 mm thick thermoplastic and piano string which is the motor of the orthosis (Fig. 11.48).

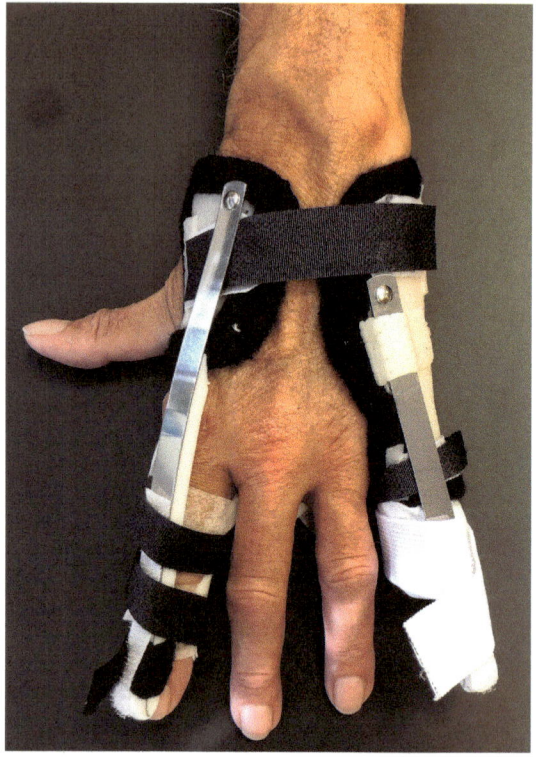

Fig. 11.44 "Levame" orthosis with global extension action

First, two pieces of piano string are cut to match the length of the patient's finger from the head of the second phalanx to the shaft of the first phalanx, with a spiral facing the proximal interphalangeal joint. Using a small rectangle of thermoplastic, a small hole is cut at the third of its length. The patient's finger is passed through the hole leaving the longer side of the plastic against the palm of the hand, and the shorter side against the back of the first phalanx folding over the plastic on the sides (Fig. 11.49). Using a smaller rectangular piece of thermoplastic, a hammock is made to go across the palmar side of the finger facing the head of the second phalanx. The tension can be adjusted by modifying the diameter of the piano string and the number of spirals which is inversely proportional to the stress induced.

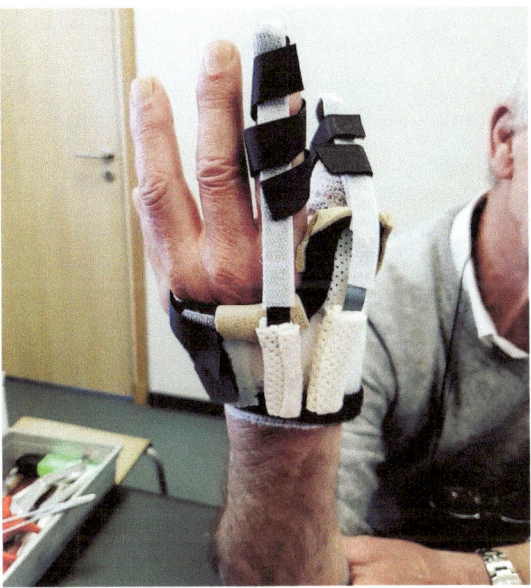

Fig. 11.45 "Levame" orthosis with analytical extension action on the PIP joint of the small finger

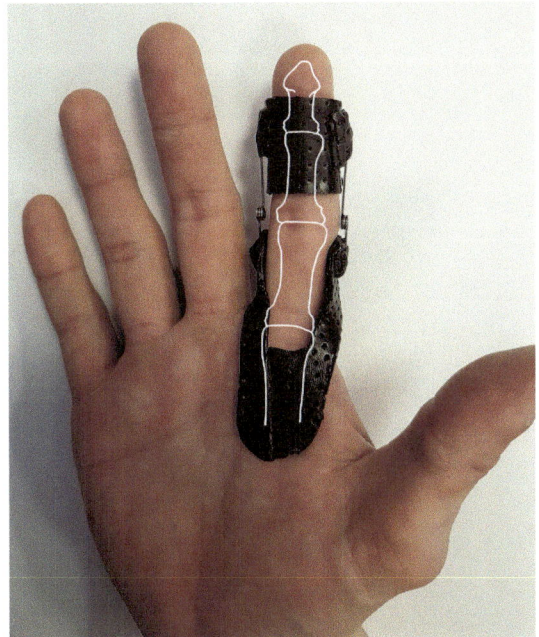

Fig. 11.46 Contact surfaces of a "Capener" orthosis

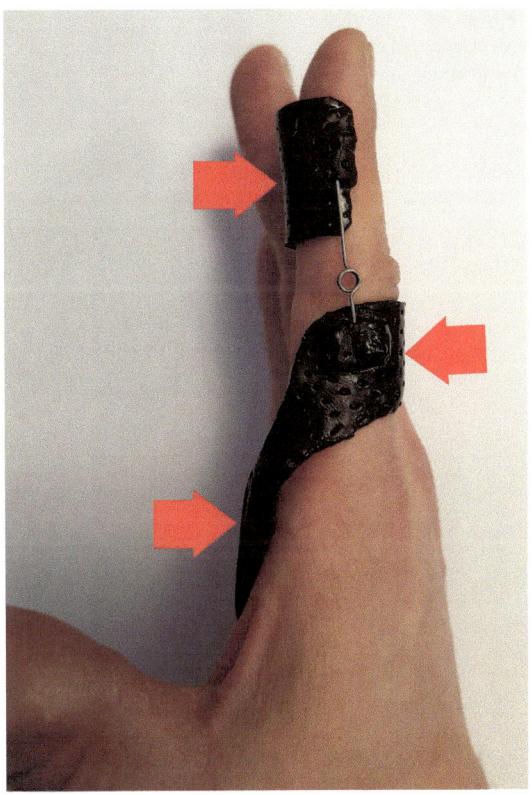

Fig. 11.47 Forces applied by a "Capener" orthosis

11.6.2 Substitution Orthoses

The aim of these orthoses is to supplement muscle weakness to enhance the patient's functional capacity.

11.6.2.1 Articular MP Joint Extension Mobilization Orthosis (Radial Nerve Palsy)

When a patient presents radial nerve palsy, the clinical examination reveals "wrist drop" with impossible wrist and finger extension due to extrinsic muscle damage. Interphalangeal joint extension remains functional by the means of the interossei and lumbrical muscles, innervated by the ulnar and median nerves.

Fig. 11.48 Materials for "Capener" orthosis fabrication

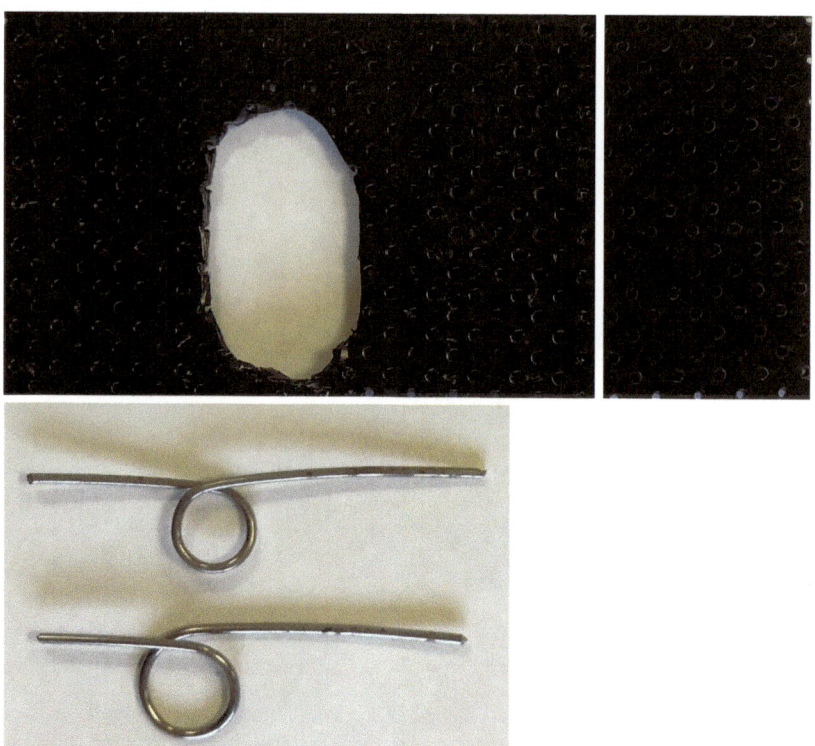

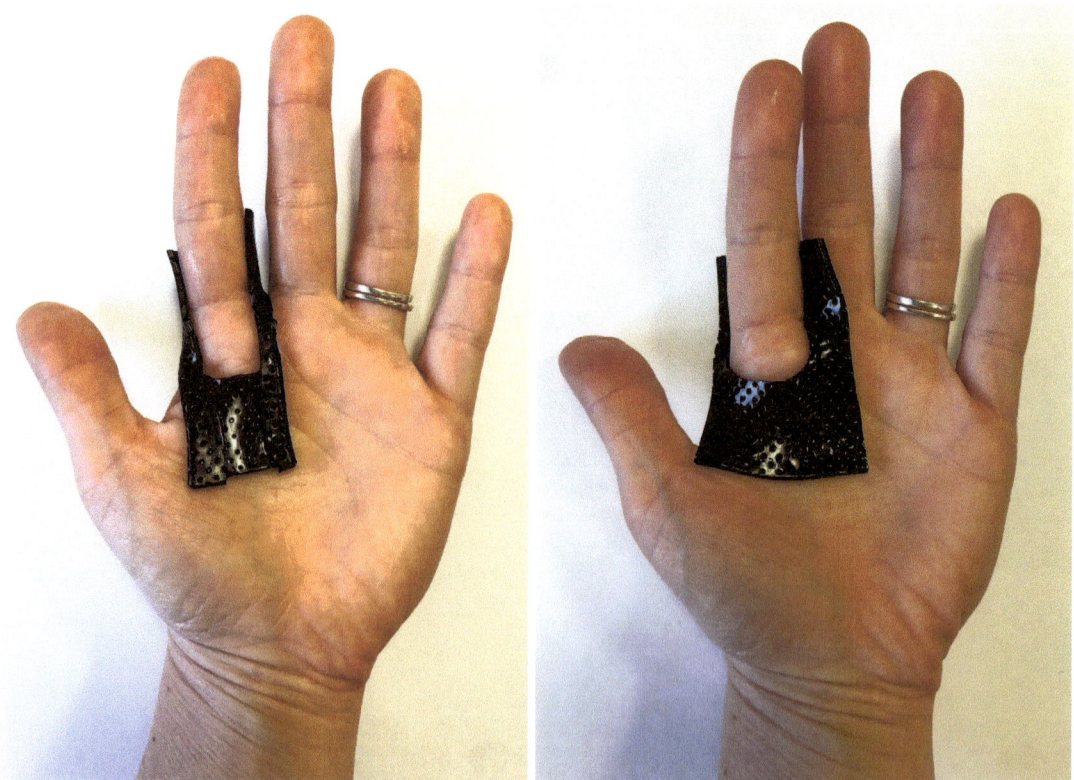

Fig. 11.49 Making of the proximal piece of a "Capener" orthosis

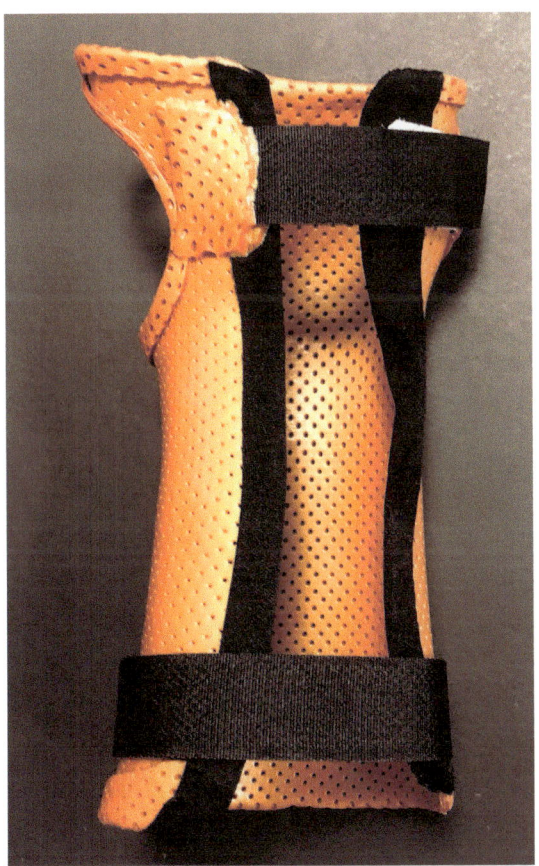

Fig. 11.50 Wrist orthosis (first component of a substitution orthosis for radial nerve palsy)

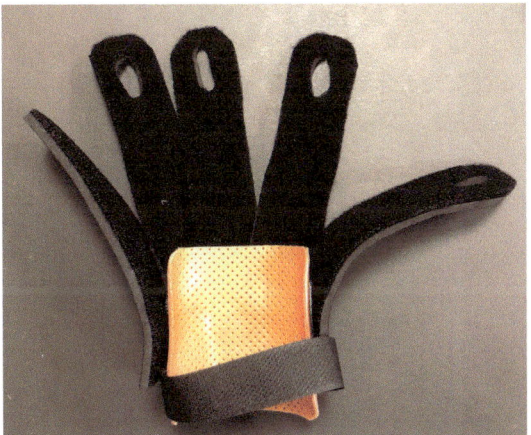

Fig. 11.51 Neoprene bands responsible for finger extension (second component of a substitution orthosis for radial nerve palsy)

The goal of this orthosis is to substitute the action of the muscles innervated by the radial nerve, meaning wrist, and finger extension to offer the patient functional use of their hand during everyday activities. It is made of two components: a wrist orthosis placing the joint in a slightly extended position (Fig. 11.50) and a clip fastened to the back of the forearm where the patient can attach neoprene bands, or any other elastic material, which pull the five fingers back into an extended position (Fig. 11.51). Thus, the patient's wrist is maintained, and he may use active finger flexion while passive finger extension will be induced by the elastic neoprene bands (Fig. 11.52).

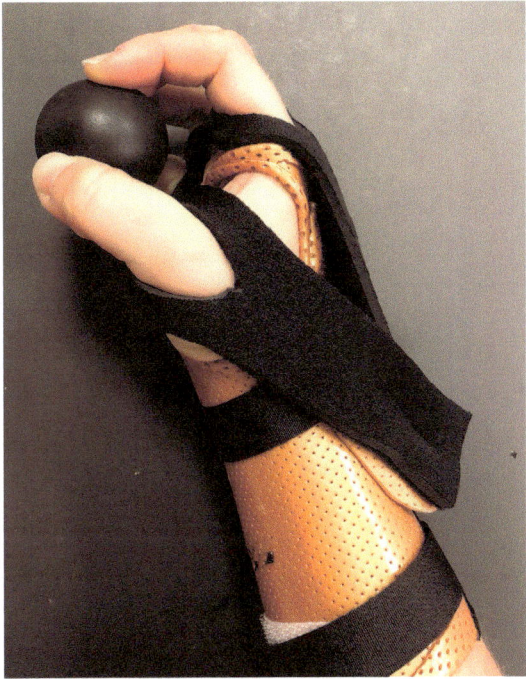

Fig. 11.52 Substitution orthosis for radial nerve palsy

11.7 Restriction Orthoses

11.7.1 Articular PIP Joint Extension Limitation Orthosis

Swan neck deformity is characterized by hyper-extension of the proximal interphalangeal joint and flexion of the distal interphalangeal joint. The anti-swan-neck splint or figure-8 splint places the proximal interphalangeal joint in slight flexion in order or rectify the deformity (Fig. 11.53).

Thus, the patient can bend his finger, but hyper-extension is limited by the orthosis. The orthosis can be made of thermoplastic, Orficast©, or a metal wire. The advantage of plastic and metal is that there is no problem with water, but the disadvantage is that these materials can be uncomfortable due to their stiffness. Orficast© is a softer material, easier to fit onto the finger due to its slight flexibility, but less suitable for water-based activities.

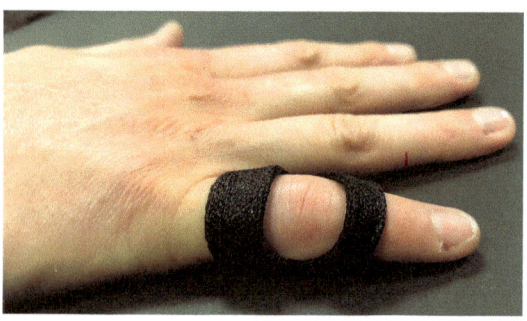

Fig. 11.53 Articular PIP joint extension limitation orthosis for the small finger (−10°)—Anti-swan-neck splint or figure-8 splint

11.7.2 Articular MP Joint Extension Limitation Orthosis for Fingers 4 and 5

This orthosis is addressed to patients presenting an "ulnar claw," meaning hyper-extension of the metacarpophalangeal joints and flexion of the interphalangeal joints of the fourth and fifth fingers, which is often due to ulnar nerve damage. This deformity is related to interossei and lumbrical muscle deficiency in the last two fingers. Since the radial lumbrical muscles are innervated by the median nerve, the index and middle fingers do not present the "claw" effect.

The goal of this orthosis is to substitute the action of the interossei and lumbrical muscles by resisting against the metacarpophalangeal hyper-extension in the last two fingers. It can be made of 2.4 mm thick thermoplastic or Orficast©. The pattern is a long band that is 1 cm wide and about 25 cm long (depending on the size of the patient's hand). The starting point is located on the palmar side of the first phalanx of the small finger. The band then goes around the back of the hand, along the palmar crease, across the back of the first phalanx of the last two fingers and back to the starting point. The molding must be tight enough to resist against the hyper-extension of the metacarpophalangeal joints while allowing IP flexion of all the fingers (Fig. 11.54).

This orthosis can also be classified into the category of torque transmission orthoses considering it optimizes the action of the extensor sys-

Fig. 11.54 Articular MP joint extension limitation orthosis for fingers 4 and 5

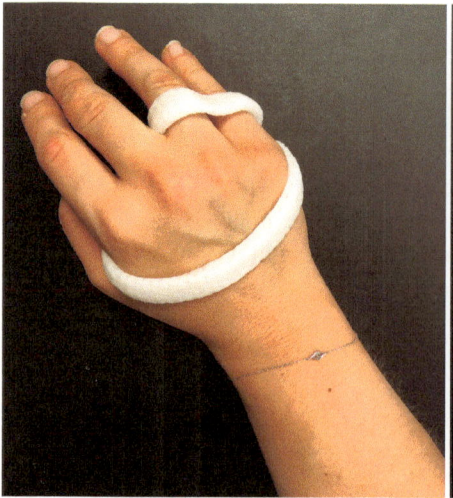
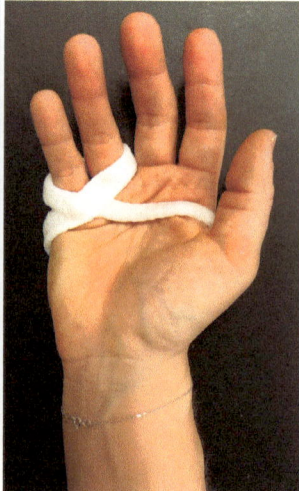

tem on the proximal interphalangeal joints of the fourth and fifth fingers. Thus, it can be used to avoid musculotendinous PIP joint flexion deformity.

11.8 Torque Transmission Orthoses

The aim of these orthoses is to redirect the internal forces of one or several joints to enhance the action of one muscular system versus another. Most frequently, the result is achieved by immobilizing the "normal" joints to redirect muscular power to the stiff joints [21].

11.8.1 Active Redirecting Orthoses

Stiffness can disturb the motor pattern which can itself induce chronification of the stiffness because the stiff joint is not mobilized, or very little, during daily activities [20, 22]. Using an orthosis that goes against this pattern by enhancing the action of the underutilized (or poorly utilized) musculotendinous systems enables the patient to reprogram their motor cortex, while actively and repetitively mobilizing damaged tissues, which helps reorientate their collagen fiber. These orthoses are worn continuously and for a long period of time (often for a few weeks) and removed progressively.

Stiffness in immobilized healthy joints is rarely described in the literature, but it seems preferable to evaluate their range of motion frequently.

In practice, the preference is making nonremovable orthoses in Orficast© (Fig. 11.55), thick thermoplastic (3.2 mm) or plaster.

There are numerous possibilities, and the most suitable choice is made by the therapist according to their clinical examination (Fig. 11.56).

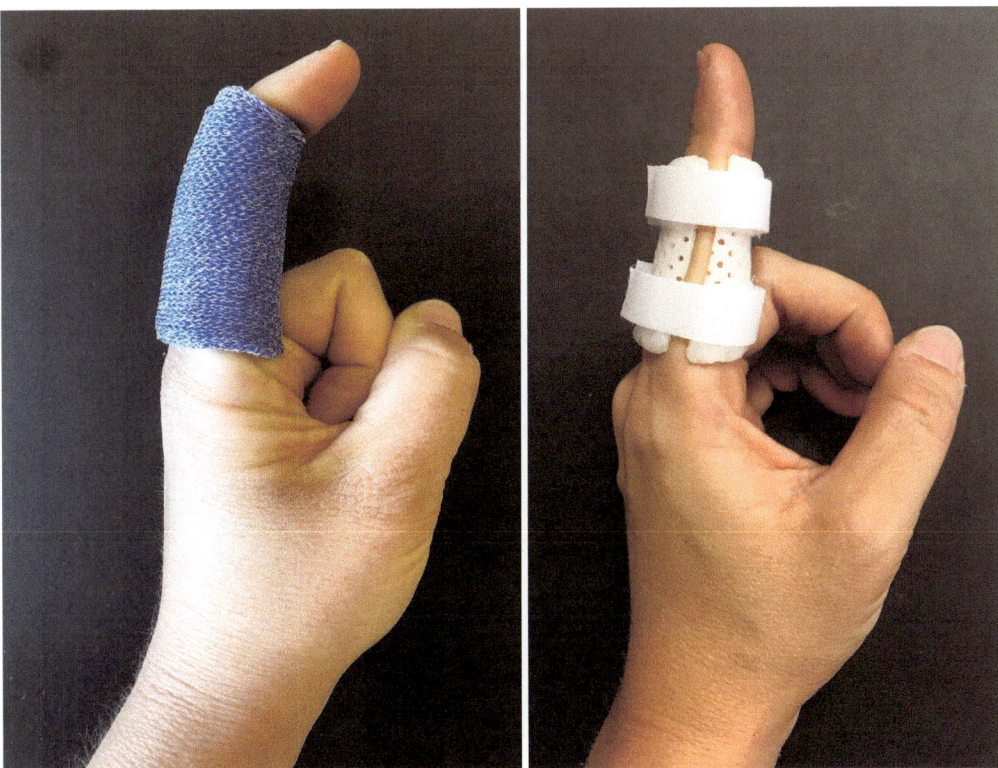

Fig. 11.55 Articular torque transmission orthoses in Orficast© or thermoplastic

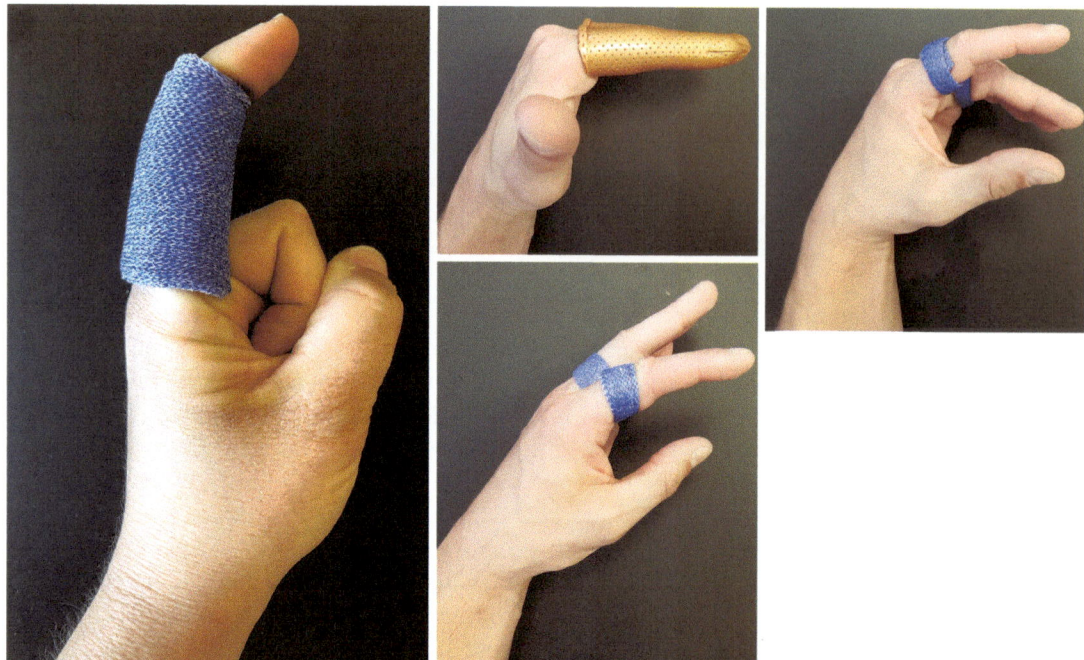

Fig. 11.56 Other articular torque transmission orthoses

These orthoses can also be used as a tool to optimize active mobilization exercises during therapy. The difference between this kind of orthoses and the ones described above is the period of time they are worn.

11.8.2 Casting Motion to Mobilize Stiffness (CMMS)

This orthosis, described by Colditz [23], is a torque transmission orthosis that includes the wrist, the metacarpophalangeal joints, and sometimes the interphalangeal joints of all four fingers. It has an "anti-stiffness" effect due to muscular power transfer, but it also has an impact on edema [24] and cortical reprogramming of deficient mobility [20].

The use of plaster is promoted because it is particularly comfortable, avoids the risk of creating contact points, and has a positive impact on edema.

Depending on the etiology of the stiffness, different molding positions can be imagined (Fig. 11.57).

If the stiffness is due to tense intrinsic muscles (positive Finochietto test—see Chap. 1), the orthosis will be molded placing the wrist in slight extension (to enhance the fingers' flexor tendon action) and the metacarpophalangeal joints in extension. Thus, active flexion of the interphalangeal joints will induce stretching of the interossei and lumbrical muscles. If progression is needed, the extension position can be increased to have a greater stretching effect on the intrinsic muscles (Fig. 11.57a).

All free mobility is allowed, but in this case the patient must focus on interphalangeal joint flexion as a priority exercise.

If finger bending cannot be initiated at the distal interphalangeal joint, the orthosis shall be molded placing the wrist in slight extension, 60°–70° flexion of the metacarpophalangeal joints and slight flexion of the interphalangeal joints with a little more flexion in the distal interphalangeal joints compared to the proximal interphalangeal joints. This position helps the flexor digitorum profundus act on distal interphalangeal joint flexion (Fig. 11.57b).

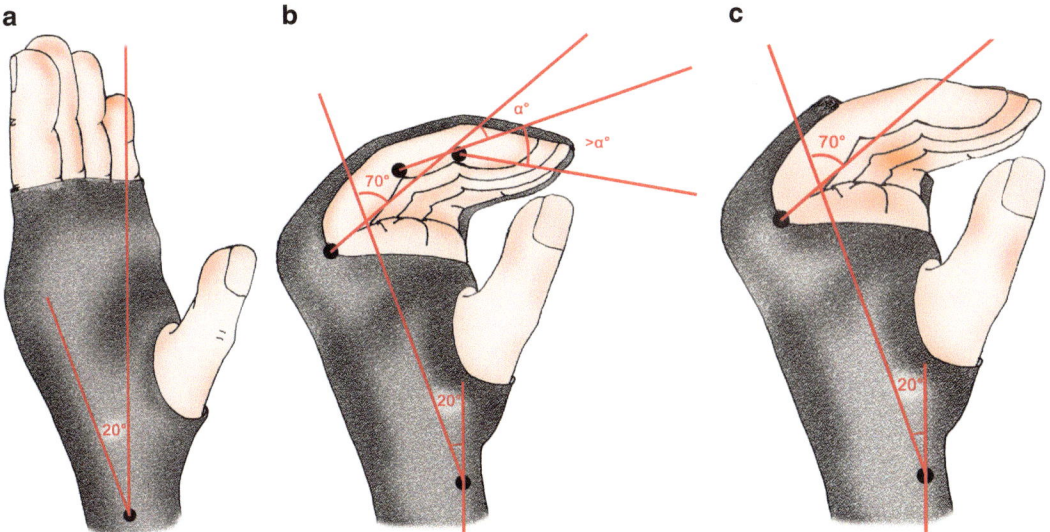

Fig. 11.57 Articular torque transmission orthoses facilitating; extrinsic flexor digitorum action and intrinsic muscle stretching (**a**), flexor digitorum profundus action (**b**), metacarpophalangeal joint flexion by their flexed position and proximal interphalangeal joint extension by their resistance against the dorsal roof (**c**)

All free mobility is allowed, but in this case the patient must focus on finger bending initiated by the distal interphalangeal joint as a priority exercise.

If the limited range of motion concerns proximal interphalangeal joint flexion, the orthosis is molded placing the wrist and the metacarpophalangeal joints in slight extension which helps the flexor digitorum act on the PIP joint, thanks to the tenodesis effect (Fig. 11.57a).

All free mobility is allowed, but in this case the patient must focus on analytical interphalangeal joint flexion as a priority exercise.

If the limited range of motion concerns proximal interphalangeal joint flexion and extension equally, the orthosis is molded placing the wrist in slight extension and 45° flexion of the metacarpophalangeal joints with a dorsal roof covering the first phalanx. This position helps the flexor digitorum act on proximal interphalangeal joint flexion and the dorsal stop facilitates the action of the extensor system on this same joint (Fig. 11.57c).

All free mobility is allowed, but in this case the patient must focus on analytical interphalangeal joint flexion and extension as a priority exercise.

If the stiffness concerns metacarpophalangeal joint flexion, the orthosis is the same with more flexion of the metacarpophalangeal joints that can be modified according to the patient's progress. Nevertheless, the metacarpophalangeal joints shall not be placed in maximal flexion (which would make it an articular mobilization orthosis and not a torque transmission orthosis) to allow their active mobility in the orthosis (Fig. 11.57c).

All free mobility is allowed, but in this case the patient must focus on analytical metacarpophalangeal joint flexion as a priority exercise.

The exercises shall be repeated 15–20 times, once an hour during the day.

The orthoses shall be worn continuously and for a long period of time (often a few weeks) and removed progressively when sought mobility has recovered and is feasible without wearing the orthosis.

11.9   Articular Functional Orthoses

Their role is to help patients return to functional daily activities. The measurements used to design the pattern are taken in an anatomical functioning

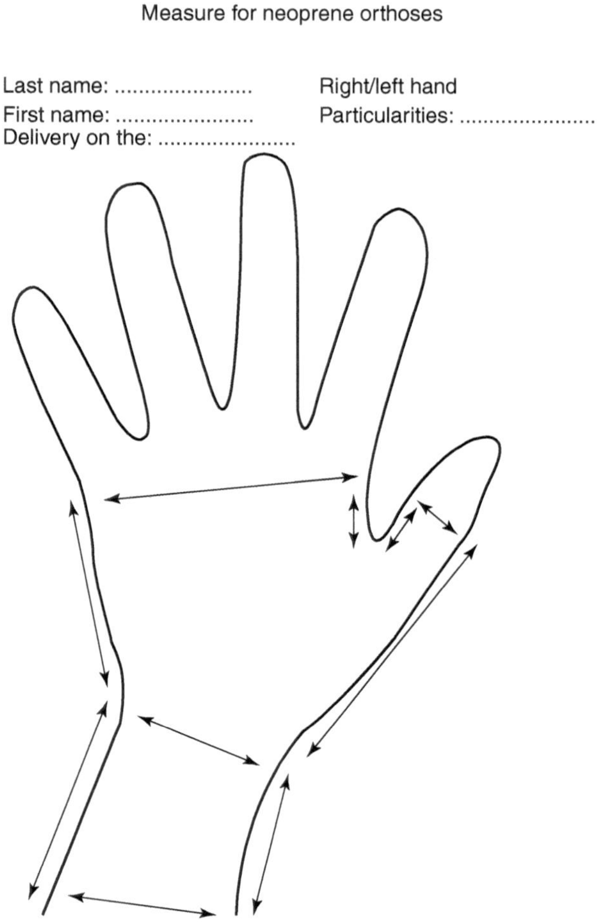

Fig. 11.58 Measuring
sheet for articular
functional neoprene
orthoses

Measure for neoprene orthoses

Last name: ....   Right/left hand
First name: ....   Particularities: ....
Delivery on the: ....

position in most cases. If a certain activity requires a particular grip position, the measurements can be adjusted to the patient's specific needs.

According to the patient's needs and the material chosen (neoprene, leather, etc.), they can be more or less rigid:

- In most cases, functional orthoses are compliant, made of neoprene that is 3 or 4 mm thick. The neoprene is chosen based on the activities that the patient wants to complete and their morphology. Therefore, the orthosis offers flexible support to help gripping become more physiological (in the case of rhizarthrosis, for example).
- Sometimes it can be necessary to reinforce the neoprene orthosis with thermoplastic. This way, it can offer a lock against painful mobility, avoid contact with areas that are fragile, inflammatory, or sensitive because of a scar.

- In rare cases, a functional orthosis can be entirely made of thermoplastic when a joint needs more sturdy support.

Functional orthoses are made from measurements taken on the patient with a soft tape measure and written on a special sheet (Fig. 11.58). These measurements are not exhaustive, and the orthosis shall tempt to adjust to each specific indication. The pattern is then based on the measurements to create the orthosis.

11.9.1 For the Wrist

These orthoses support the wrist and the palm of the hand leaving finger mobility completely free. The pattern is different based on the side of the injury to correctly cover the palm of the hand and to obtain dorsal fastening (Fig. 11.59). The first

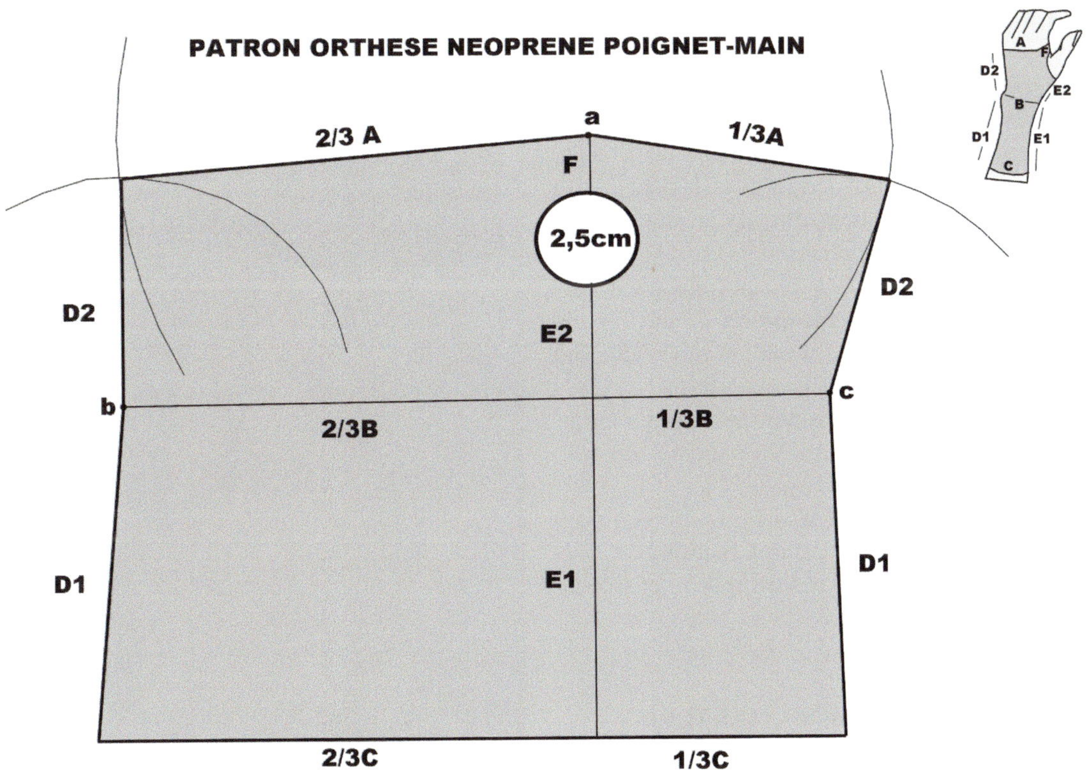

PATRON ORTHESE NEOPRENE POIGNET-MAIN

2/3 A   a   1/3A

F

2,5cm

D2   D2

E2

b   c

2/3B   1/3B

D1   D1

E1

2/3C   1/3C

Fig. 11.59 Pattern for an articular functional neoprene orthosis

step is drawing a line E1-E2-2.5 cm-F vertically. Perpendicularly to that line, lines C and B are drawn respecting the ratio 1/3 and 2/3. Then, from point A, a circle of radius 1/3 of A is drawn. From point C, a circle of radius D2 is drawn next. At the crossing point of the two circles, the superior extremity of the "small side" of the orthosis is thus created. The method is the same for the "large side." A small hole with a 2.5 cm diameter is cut for the thumb that can be adjusted with the patient.

The orthosis is fastened with hook Velcro straps that are either sewn or simply attached to the velvet side of the neoprene material. The straps must be directed in a way that the patient can easily seize them with their healthy hand to fasten the orthosis.

A piece of plastic can be added to limit painful or prohibited mobility if needed (Fig. 11.60).

The same pattern is used to create neoprene gauntlets that free the wrist for painful scars or inflammatory reactions (in the case of pillar pain after carpel tunnel surgery, for example).

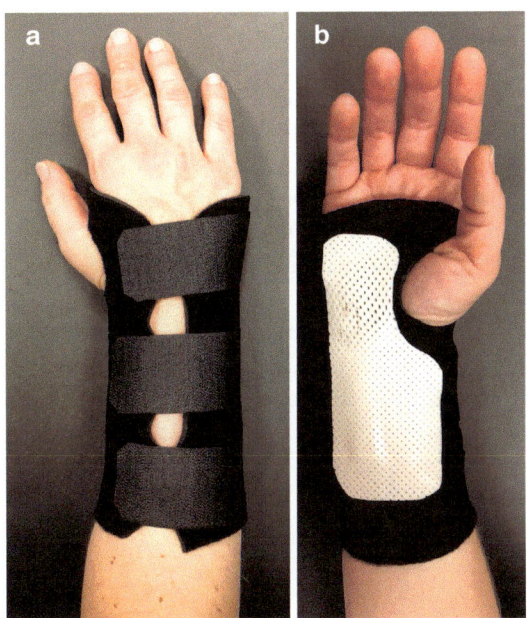

Fig. 11.60 (a) Articular functional neoprene orthosis. (b) Articular functional neoprene orthosis with a palmar thermoplastic reinforcement

11.9.2 Wrist Wrap

A wrist wrap aims to support the wrist joint.

It is made of 3 mm thick slightly elastic neoprene with one smooth side and one velvet side, cut into a trapezoidal shape. It is fastened with three wide Velcro straps directly attached to the velvet side of the neoprene (Fig. 11.61).

Precise measurements are not always necessary and a trapezium measuring 22 cm for the superior width, 19 cm for the inferior width and 13 cm for the height, fits most patients.

Of course, these measurements can be modified according to the size of the patient's forearm, their injury, or their activity.

The wrist wrap can also be reinforced with thermoplastic to limit painful mobility or garnished with silicone to absorb shocks or to protect a scar (Fig. 11.62).

11.9.3 For the Wrist and the Thumb TM-MP Joints

The measurements are taken with the patient's hand in a functional position to design the pattern (Fig. 11.63).

Two symmetrical patterns are cut and glued, then sewn together along the radial side, and glued together at the first commissure (Fig. 11.64). Three Velcro straps are used to fasten the orthosis on the ulnar side. They can be sewn or simply attached to the velvet side of the neoprene material (Fig. 11.65). Speaking from experience, it seems that fastening the Velcro straps from the bottom to the top is easier for patients. According to the side of the injury, the direction of the Velcro straps must be adjusted.

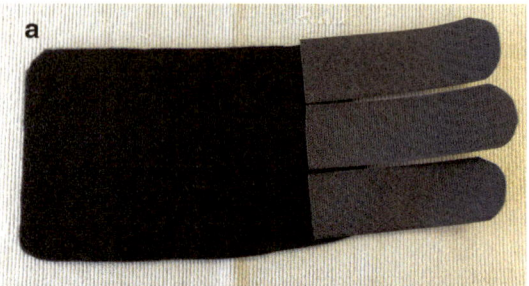

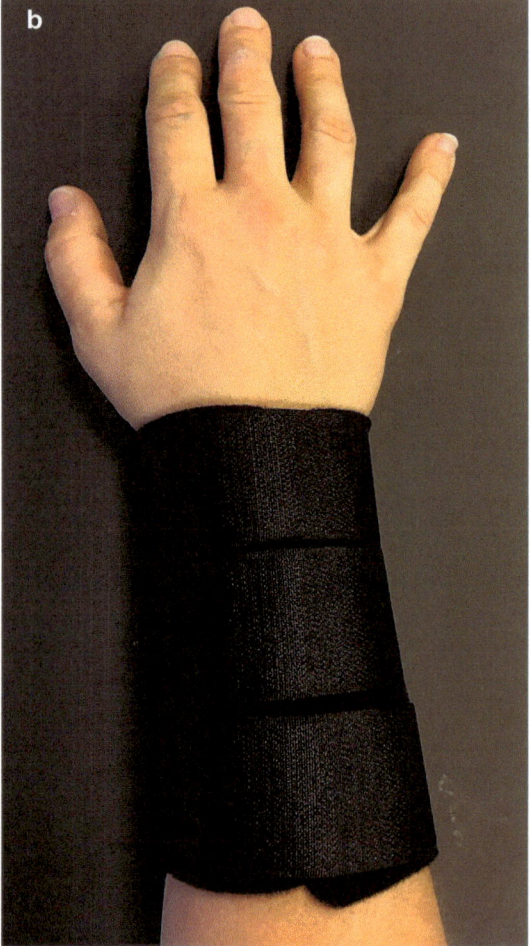

Fig. 11.61 Wrist wrap alone (**a**) and worn (**b**)

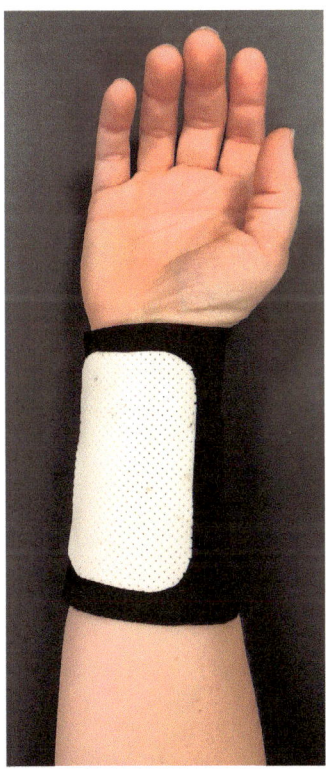

Fig. 11.62 Wrist wrap reinforced with thermoplastic

A small patch of thermoplastic can be glued to the neoprene with a heat gun to protect an inflammatory zone or to limit mobility if needed. The orthosis can also be garnished with silicone to absorb shocks or to protect a scar.

11.9.4 For the Thumb TM Joint

These orthoses are mainly used for patients with rhizarthrosis. They offer support to patients that experience pain during professional or leisure activities that use pinch grip (sewing, modeling, etc.).

11.9.4.1 Neoprene Straps

The concept of these straps is to go against the subluxation of the first metacarpal basis by maintaining abduction of the thumb, thanks to the strap that goes over the first commissure and counters the subluxation by being pulled snugly against the trapezio-metacarpal joint (Fig. 11.66). They are made of a band of 4 mm thick slightly elastic neoprene with one smooth side and one

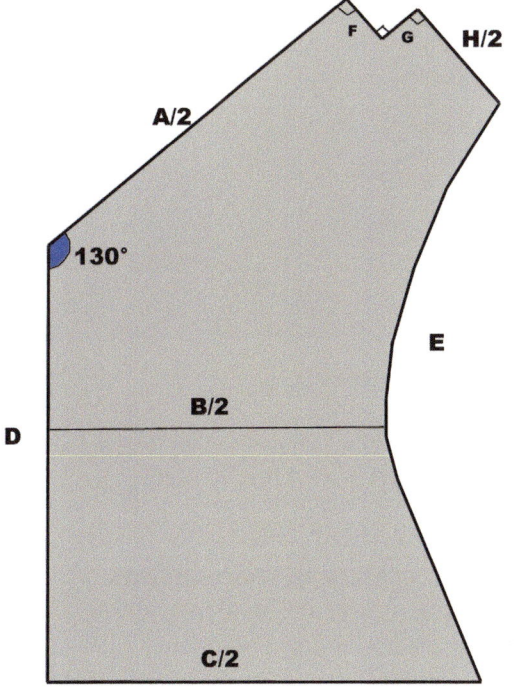

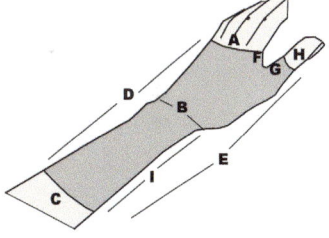

ORTHESE NEOPRENE POIGNET-POUCE

Fig. 11.63 Pattern for an articular functional wrist and thumb TM-MP joints neoprene orthosis

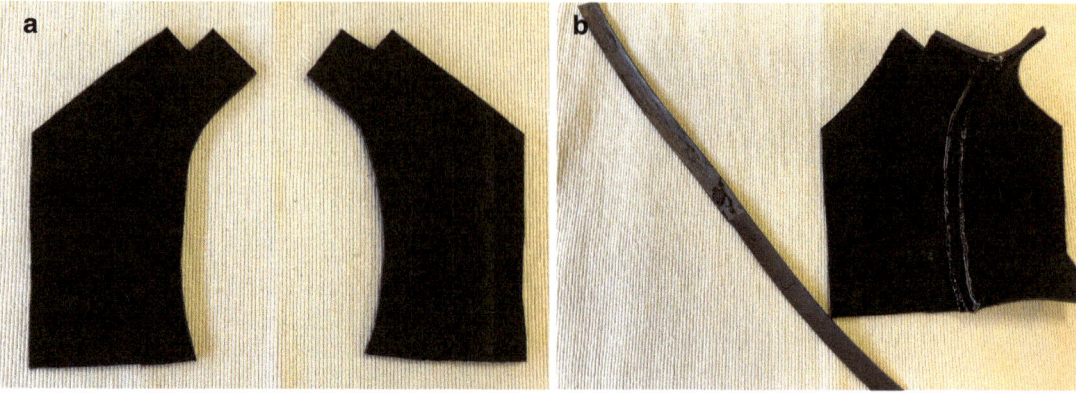

Fig. 11.64 (**a** and **b**) First steps to making an articular functional neoprene orthosis for the wrist and thumb TM-MP joints

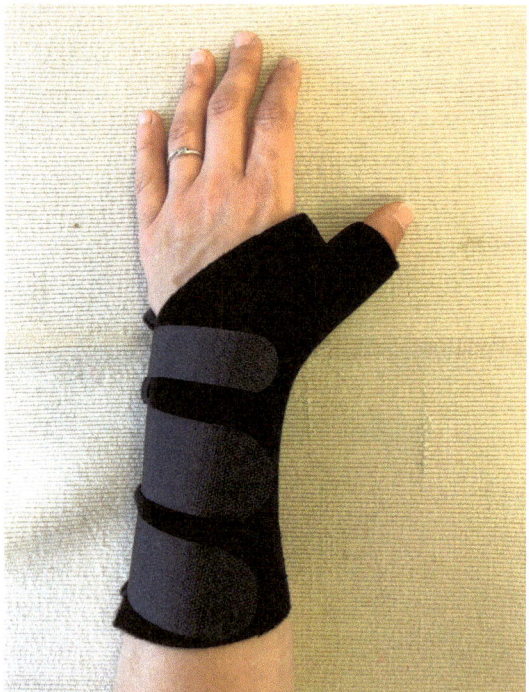

Fig. 11.65 Articular functional neoprene orthosis wrist and thumb TM-MP joints

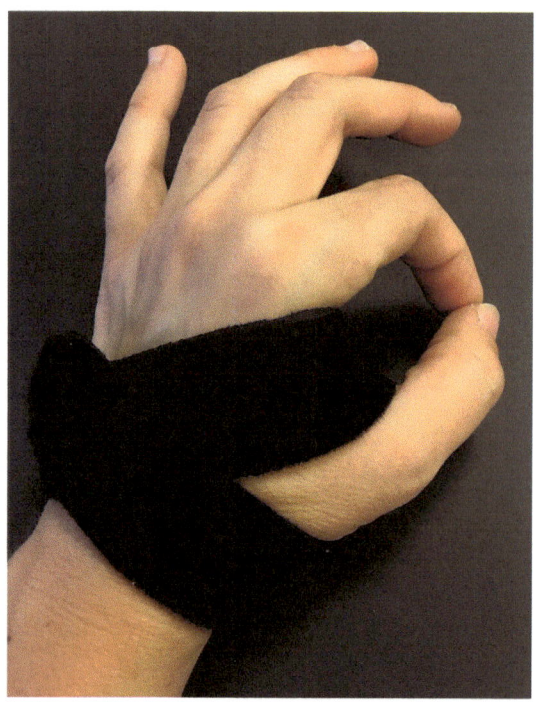

Fig. 11.66 Neoprene strap

velvet side. The strap can be 3–3.5 cm wide and about 36 cm long (which fits most patients).

After measuring the circumference of the patient's hand, a loop is made in the strap and the neoprene is sewn together at that measurement (the loop will go towards the left for the left hand and conversely for the right hand) (Fig. 11.67). A

piece of hook Velcro is sewn on the smooth side of the leftover strap where it shall be fastened on the back of the hand.

11.9.4.2 Made of Thermoplastic

This orthosis is mainly used for patients with rhizarthrosis that are looking for more rigid support than what neoprene orthoses offer for their pro-

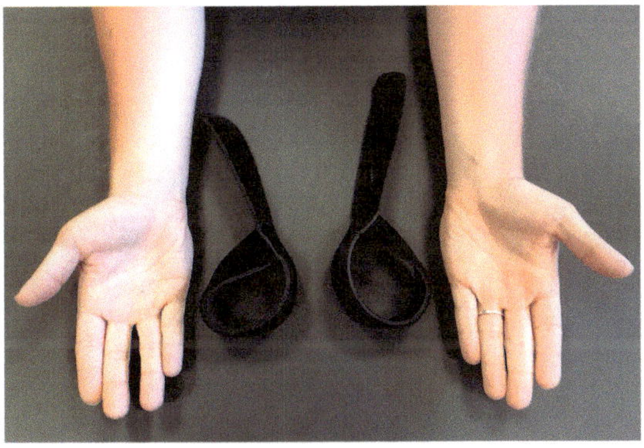

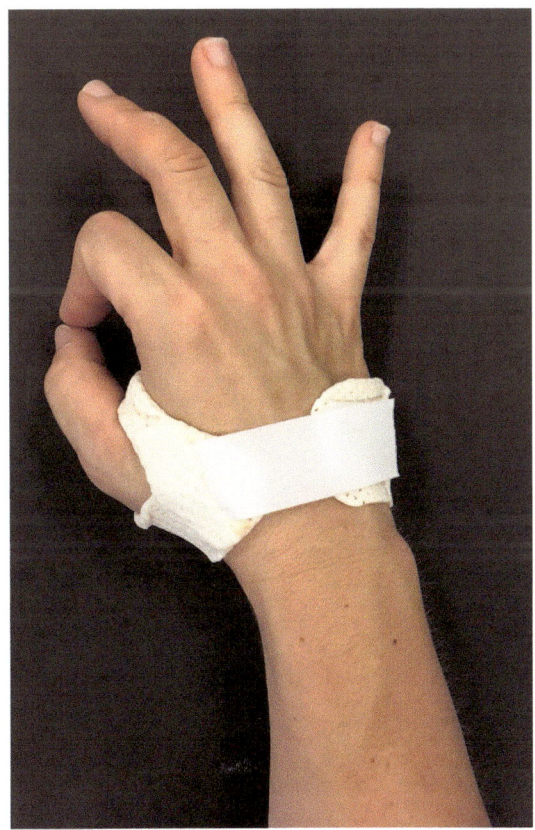

Fig. 11.67 Two symmetrical neoprene straps for the right and left hands (showing the direction of the loop)

fessional and/or leisure activities. This orthosis cannot under any circumstances replace a nocturnal resting orthosis in thermoplastic. It can also be used after surgery (prosthesis or trapeziectomy) or a trapezio-metacarpal joint sprain when patients return to certain activities.

The concept of the carpo-metacarpal (CMC) orthosis is to stabilize the trapezio-metacarpal joint without immobilizing adjacent joints, especially the metacarpophalangeal joint (Fig. 11.68).

The orthosis functions with the idea of creating a "pseudo-hydraulic environment." The orthosis is molded around the thenar eminence while the muscles are relaxed. Thus, during an activity (using a pinch grip, for example), the orthosis will limit muscle expansion when they contract, and the force will be directed internally which will stabilize the bones in the contained space (therefore, the trapezio-metacarpal joint) (Fig. 11.69). Since the orthosis is made completely of thermoplastic, it has the advantage of being extremely sturdy, is suitable for water-based activities, and can be easily cleaned.

The carpo-metacarpal (CMC) orthosis is made of 2.4 mm thick micro-perforated thermoplastic. The pattern is a "Y" shape. The plastic is folded over on the parts that will become the edges of the orthosis, so no fabric protection needs to be used (Fig. 11.70). Molding is completed with the thumb in slight abduction and flexion, while tightly covering the thenar emi-

Fig. 11.68 CMC (carpo-metacarpal) orthosis

nence, making sure that the patient relaxes their muscles. The wrist, the metacarpophalangeal joints, and the interphalangeal joints shall remain free (Fig. 11.71). The orthosis is fastened on the back of the hand with one Velcro strap fused on the ulnar side to help make adjusting easier.

11.9.5 For the Thumb TM-MP Joints

Patients presenting a highly modified trapezio-metacarpal joint can have trouble tolerating neoprene straps because of the material pressing against it. Others do not find the support their looking for in neoprene straps.

In these cases, a more containing orthosis can be proposed, and it can be reinforced with ther-

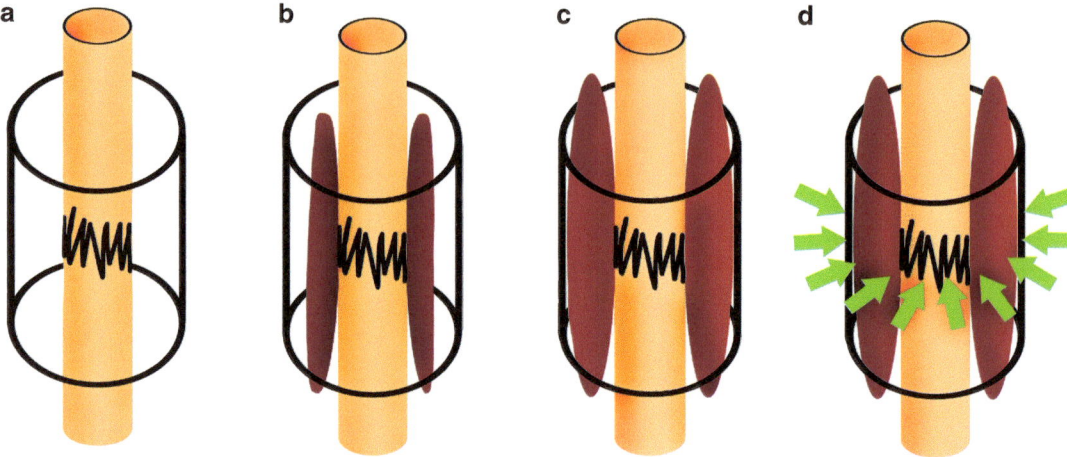

Fig. 11.69 Pseudo-hydraulic environment concept

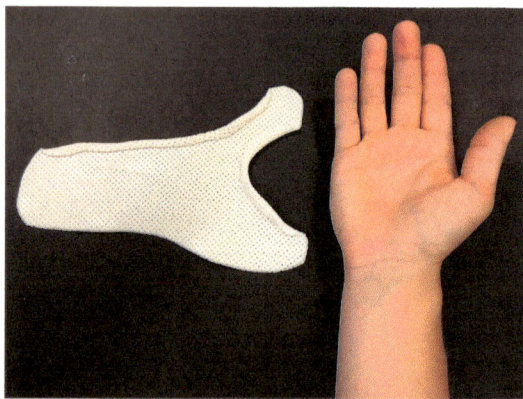

Fig. 11.70 Pattern of a CMC orthosis

moplastic if the patient feels the need. It is made using the same method as the wrist and thumb TM-MP joint orthosis with two symmetrical patterns that are sewed and glued together on the radial side and glued together at the first commissure. It is fastened using one or two Velcro straps.

The painful trapezio-metacarpal joint can be protected with a patch of thermoplastic (on the outside of the orthosis) or with silicone (on the inside of the orthosis) according to the patient's needs. For patients presenting "Z-shaped" thumb deformity during gripping, a U-shaped piece of thermoplastic can be fused to the outside of the neoprene orthosis around the thenar eminence of the first commissure to induce thumb abduction.

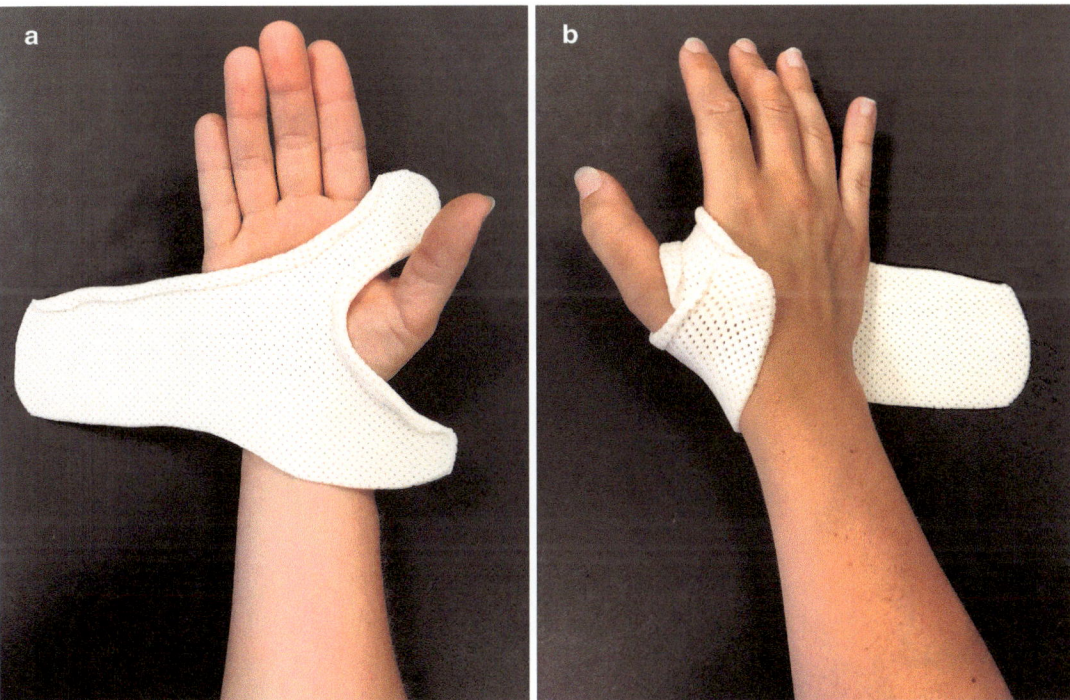

Fig. 11.71 (**a**) Starting point to CMC orthosis molding. (**b**) Molding of a CMC orthosis

References

1. Fess EE. A history of splinting: to understand the present, view the past. J Hand Ther. 2002;15(2):97–132.
2. Fess EE. Hand splinting: principles and methods. St Louis: The C.V. Mosby Company; 1981.
3. Fess EE, et al. Hand and upper extremity splinting: principles and methods. 3rd ed. St. Louis: Mosby Elsevier; 2004.
4. ASHT, Splint Nomenclature Task Force. Splint classification system. Chicago: American Society of Hand Therapists; 1992.
5. Anthonissen M, et al. The effects of conservative treatments on burn scars: a systematic review. Burns. 2016;42(3):508–18.
6. Kapandji IA. Physiologie articulaire tome 1 - Membre supérieur. Paris: Maloine; 2005.
7. Weiss N, et al. Position of the wrist associated with the lowest carpal-tunnel pressure: implications for splint design. J Bone Joint Surg Am. 1995;77(11):1695–9.
8. Cooney W, et al. The kinesiology of the thumb trapeziometacarpal joint. J Bone Joint Surg Am. 1981;63:1371–81.
9. Sun Y, et al. In vivo metacarpophalangeal joint collateral ligament length changes during flexion. J Hand Surg Eur Vol. 2017;42E(6):610–5.
10. Sandhu SS, Dreckmann S, Binhammer PA. Change in the collateral and accessory collateral ligament lengths of the proximal interphalangeal joint using cadaveric model three-dimensional laser scanning. J Hand Surg Eur Vol. 2016;41(4):380–5.
11. Evans RB. Managing the injured tendon: current concepts. J Hand Ther. 2012;25(2):173–189; quiz 190.
12. Rappaport PO, et al. Effect of wrist and interphalangeal thumb movement on zone T2 flexor pollicis longus tendon tension in a human cadaver model. J Hand Ther. 2015;28(4):347–354; quiz 355.
13. Wong AL, et al. The optimal orthosis and motion protocol for extensor tendon injury in zones IV-VIII: a systematic review. J Hand Ther. 2017;30(4):447–56.
14. Howell JW, Merritt WH, Robinson SJ. Immediate controlled active motion following zone 4–7 extensor tendon repair. J Hand Ther. 2005;18(2):182–90.
15. Nguyen T, et al. Effects of cell seeding and cyclic stretch on the fiber remodeling in an extracellular matrix-derived bioscaffold. Tissue Eng Part A. 2009;15(4):957–63.
16. Krotoski J, Breger Stanton DE. The forces of dynamic orthotic positioning: ten questions to ask before applying a dynamic orthosis to the hand. In: Skirven TM, Osterman AL, Fedorczyk J, Amadio PC, editors. Rehabilitation of the hand and upper extremity. 2-volume set: expert consult. St. Louis: Elsevier Health Sciences; 2011.
17. Valdes K, et al. Efficacy of orthotic devices for increased active proximal interphalangeal extension

joint range of motion: a systematic review. J Hand Ther. 2019;32(2):184–93.

18. Flowers KR, LaStayo PC. Effect of total end range time on improving passive range of motion. J Hand Ther. 1994;25(1):48–54; quiz 55.

19. Flowers KR. A proposed decision hierarchy for splinting the stiff joint, with an emphasis on force application parameters. J Hand Ther. 2002;15(2):158–62.

20. Colditz JC. Plaster of Paris: the forgotten hand splinting material. J Hand Ther. 2002;15(2):144–57.

21. Midgley R, Pisano K. Therapist's management of the stiff hand. In: Skirven TM, Osterman AL, Fedorczyk J, Amadio PC, editors. Rehabilitation of the hand and upper extremity. St. Louis: Elsevier Health Sciences; 2021.

22. Midgley R. Case report: the casting motion to mobilize stiffness technique for rehabilitation after a crush and degloving injury of the hand. J Hand Ther. 2016;29(3):323–33.

23. Colditz JC. Active redirection instead of passive motion for joint stiffness. IFSSH Ezine; 2014. p. 41–4.

24. Midgley R. Use of casting motion to mobilize stiffness to regain digital flexion following Dupuytren's fasciectomy. Hand Ther. 2010;15(2):45–51.